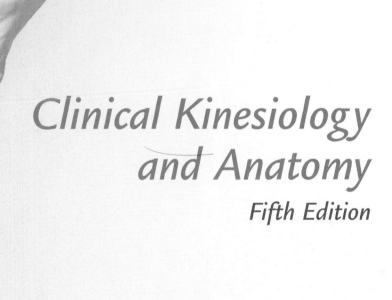

Clinical Kinesiology and Anatomy

Fifth Edition

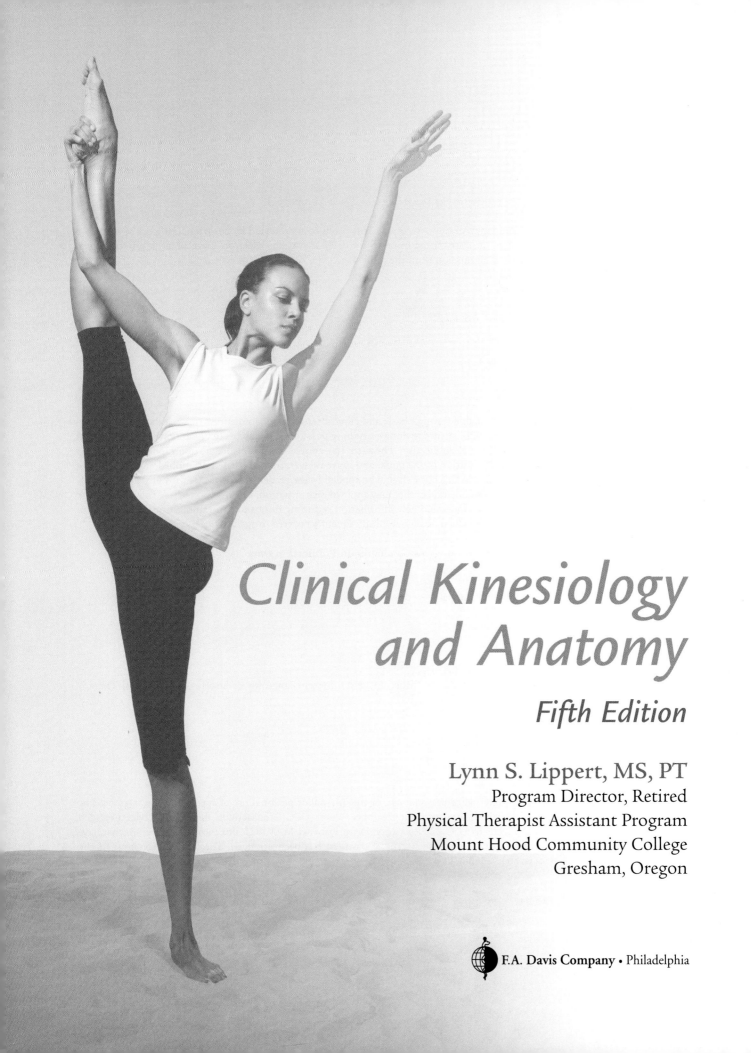

Clinical Kinesiology and Anatomy

Fifth Edition

Lynn S. Lippert, MS, PT
Program Director, Retired
Physical Therapist Assistant Program
Mount Hood Community College
Gresham, Oregon

F.A. Davis Company • Philadelphia

F. A. Davis Company
1915 Arch Street
Philadelphia, PA 19103
www.fadavis.com

Copyright © 2011 by F. A. Davis Company

Printed in the United States of America

Last digit indicates print number: 10 9 8 7 6 5 4 3 2

Acquisitions Editor: Melissa A. Duffield
Manager of Content Development: George W. Lang
Developmental Editor: Karen E. Williams
Art and Design Manager: Carolyn O'Brien

As new scientific information becomes available through basic and clinical research, recommended treatments and drug therapies undergo changes. The author(s) and publisher have done everything possible to make this book accurate, up to date, and in accord with accepted standards at the time of publication. The author(s), editors, and publisher are not responsible for errors or omissions or for consequences from application of the book, and make no warranty, expressed or implied, in regard to the contents of the book. Any practice described in this book should be applied by the reader in accordance with professional standards of care used in regard to the unique circumstances that may apply in each situation. The reader is advised always to check product information (package inserts) for changes and new information regarding dose and contraindications before administering any drug. Caution is especially urged when using new or infrequently ordered drugs.

Library of Congress Cataloging-in-Publication Data

Lippert, Lynn, 1942–
  Clinical kinesiology and anatomy / Lynn S. Lippert. — 5th ed.
    p. ; cm.
  Includes bibliographical references and index.
  ISBN-13: 978-0-8036-2363-7
  ISBN-10: 0-8036-2363-1
  1. Kinesiology. 2. Physical therapy assistants. I. Title.
  [DNLM: 1. Kinesiology, Applied. 2. Movement. 3. Musculoskeletal System—anatomy & histology. 4. Physical Therapy Modalities. WE 103]
  QP303.L53 2011
  612.7'6—dc22

                                                          2010036700

To Sal, who has supported this project from the very beginning. A simple but heartfelt "thank you" seems inadequate. Perhaps dipping it in chocolate first would be more meaningful.

To Hunt, whose creativity has amazed and inspired me throughout my life.

Acknowledgments

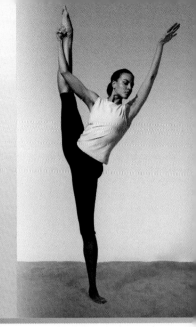

I have some appreciation of what an actor receiving an Academy Award goes through, wanting not to forget anyone who figured importantly in reaching this culminating moment. I feel the same way—I don't want to forget to thank anyone who helped me in creating this Fifth Edition. Like the previous four editions, I need to acknowledge numerous people. Sal Jepson continued to remind me that describing concepts simply is always better than rambling dissertations. Don Davis continued to remind me that physics isn't always as simple as I would like to make it. Authors always dream of an error-proof edition, so Shelby Clayson, MS, PT, applied her eagle-eyes to proofreading. Debbie Van Dover, MEd, PT, and Kristin Kjensrud, MSPT, assisted with proofing the numerous figures. Linda Besant and Damara Bennett of Oregon Ballet Theatre helped me understand human movement through dancers' eyes. I am convinced that we all would have better posture if we took ballet lessons as children. Gwen White, PT, CLT, offered her expertise and knowledge of the lymphatic system and lymphedema, and John Medeiros, PT, PhD, did the same regarding arthrokinematics.

My gratitude goes out to Rob Craven, President, and the many people at F. A. Davis for their commitment to making this textbook one that will continue to make us all proud. Melissa Duffield, Acquisitions Editor, brought new energy and vision. Karen Williams, Developmental Editor, often had a better (i.e., more clearly stated) way of wording a sentence. I have appreciated her calm and honest communication. Margaret Biblis, Publisher, continued to support this project. Carolyn O'Brien, Design Manager, used her expertise in the creation of the book cover and inside art.

Reviewers

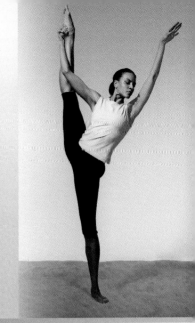

Renee Borromeo, MA, PT
Instructor
Physical Therapist Assistant Program
Penn State Mont Alto
Mont Alto, Pennsylvania

John W. Burns, MS, ATC
Athletic Training Clinical Education Coordinator
Department of Kinesiology
Washburn University
Topeka, Kansas

Steve Hammons, DPT, ACCE
Academic Coordinator of Clinical Education
Physical Therapist Assistant Program
Somerset Community College
Somerset, Kentucky

Kimberly Prevo, OTR/L
Academic Fieldwork Coordinator
Health Science Department
Kirkwood Community College
Cedar Rapids, Iowa

Debbie Van Dover, PT, MEd
Director
Physical Therapist Assistant Program
Mt. Hood Community College
Gresham, Oregon

Peter Zawicki, PT, MS
Director
Physical Therapist Assistant Program
GateWay Community College
Phoenix, Arizona

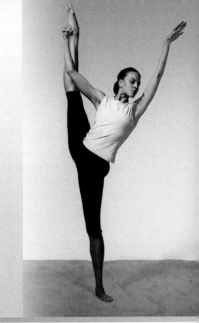

Preface to Fifth Edition

The major addition to the Fifth Edition is the chapter on the circulatory system. The cardiovascular and lymphatic systems are becoming more clinically relevant in the fields of physical and occupational therapy, athletic training, and massage therapy, just as they have in other medical fields. New treatment techniques require basic understanding of these systems.

Individuals wanting a fundamental understanding of kinesiology and anatomy from a clinical perspective will find this text of great value. The anatomical basis of common pathological conditions is briefly described in most chapters to give greater clinical relevance. The functional activities and clinical exercises in the "Review Questions" section of many chapters have been expanded.

The depth and scope of the text remains the same. Emphasis is on basic kinesiology and anatomy. Simple, easy-to-follow descriptions and explanations remain the core of this book. Not all disciplines may need all of the information within this text. For example, some disciplines may not have a need to study arthrokinematics, or the temporomandibular joint, or gait. The book is written so that instructors can omit these and other concepts without putting the student at a disadvantage in terms of understanding other subject matter. The chapters dedicated to the various joints are essentially self-standing, so the order in which they are read can be easily changed. Instead of beginning with joints of the upper extremity, one could begin with the lower extremity or the axial skeleton, and not lose understanding.

Lynn S. Lippert

Preface to the Fourth Edition

Fifteen years ago, this project began as an attempt to provide a basic kinesiology and anatomy text to physical therapist assistant students. Jean-Francois Vilain, publisher at F. A. Davis Company, recognized the need and published this as the first textbook written for the physical therapist assistant. The narrow title *Clinical Kinesiology for Physical Therapist Assistants* was chosen to encourage others to write much-needed books and to encourage publishers to publish them. While many books have been written, there remain content areas that lack appropriate texts that could benefit students if they existed. Our work here is clearly not done.

However, the publisher felt that the time had come to change the title of this text to *Clinical Kinesiology and Anatomy,* opening the market to other disciplines. However, this text remains a basic textbook. Students who want a fundamental understanding of kinesiology and anatomy with a clinical perspective will find this text of great value. Examples, activities, and exercises are not focused solely on physical therapy but have been broadened to be of use to those in occupational therapy, athletic training, massage therapy, and other fields needing this basic level of understanding.

As with previous editions, the emphasis is on basic kinesiology and anatomy. Simple, easy-to-follow descriptions and explanations remain the core of this book. Clinical relevance has been increased by adding the following: (1) brief definitions and descriptions of common pathologies in terms of anatomical location, and (2) questions involving the analysis of functional activities and clinical exercises, in addition to general anatomy review.

Not all disciplines may need all of the information within this text. For example, some disciplines may not place emphasis on the arthrokinematic features. The book is written so that the arthrokinematic chapter can be omitted from study. Examples and questions regarding this subject matter can also be omitted without the student being at a disadvantage in terms of understanding other subject matter. The chapters dedicated to the various joints begin with the upper extremity and proceed to the axial skeleton, and then to the lower extremity. However, because these chapters are essentially self-standing, the order in which they are read can easily be changed. One could begin with the lower extremity or with the axial skeleton and not lose comprehension.

There are several textbooks that give a more in-depth analysis of the subject matter; however, *Clinical Kinesiology and Anatomy* is intended to provide an easy-to-understand basic introduction.

Lynn S. Lippert

Preface to the Third Edition

There are some changes and several new faces in this revision; however, the depth and scope of the text remains the same. It has been satisfying and rewarding to continually hear that one of the main strengths of the book is the simple, easy-to-follow descriptions and explanations.

The muscular system has been expanded to include an explanation of open and closed kinetic chain principles. The gait chapter now includes an explanation of many common pathological gait patterns. Several illustrations have been redrawn for greater clarity.

Five new chapters have been added. A chapter on basic biomechanics provides explanations and examples of the various biomechanical principles commonly used in physical therapy. Chapters describing the temporomandibular joint and the pelvic girdle have been added for those who want a basic description of those joints' structure and function. Normal posture and arthrokinematics, which were included in the *Kinesiology Laboratory Manual for Physical Therapist Assistants,* have been described and expanded upon in this revision.

There is no universal agreement within the physical therapy community regarding the scope of practice of the physical therapist assistant. It is generally felt that joint mobilization is not an entry-level skill. I do not disagree with this. However, physical therapist assistants are exposed to and involved in patient treatments where these skills are utilized. For this reason, they need basic understanding of the terminology and principles, and this text provides them with this information.

This revision of *Clinical Kinesiology for Physical Therapist Assistants* is the result of many suggestions from educators, students, and clinicians. The profession needs good textbooks that cover many additional areas of physical therapist assistant education. I hope that by its fourth edition, this text will have its place on the bookshelf along with those yet-to-be-written texts.

Lynn S. Lippert

Preface to the Second Edition

Most of the people who write and lecture on anatomy agree on what is there and where it is, although they do not always agree on what to call it. Kinesiologists tend to agree that motion occurs, but they certainly do not agree on what muscles cause a motion or on the relative importance of each muscle's action in that motion.

In *Clinical Kinesiology for Physical Therapist Assistants,* the emphasis is on basic kinesiology. In describing joint motion and muscle action, I have focused on describing the commonly agreed-on prime movers, using the terminology most widely accepted within the discipline of physical therapy. Many textbooks exist that describe in greater detail various motions and muscles, in both normal and pathological conditions. For more in-depth analysis, the student should consult these books.

The idea of writing a kinesiology textbook for physical therapist assistant students has been around for several years. Somehow, time constraints and the pressures of other projects always got in the way. When educators gathered to discuss issues regarding physical therapist assistant education, lack of appropriate textbooks was always high on the list of problems. It became evident that if such textbooks were to exist, the physical therapist assistant educators were the ones who needed to write them.

Clinical Kinesiology for Physical Therapist Assistants is the result of those discussions. I hope that it is only the first of many textbooks that emphasize physical therapist assistant education.

Lynn S. Lippert

Contents in Brief

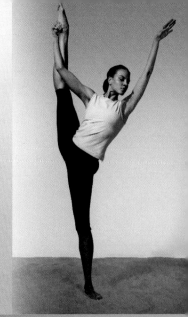

Part I
Basic Clinical Kinesiology and Anatomy

CHAPTER 1	Basic Information	3
CHAPTER 2	Skeletal System	13
CHAPTER 3	Articular System	21
CHAPTER 4	Arthrokinematics	31
CHAPTER 5	Muscular System	39
CHAPTER 6	Nervous System	53
CHAPTER 7	Circulatory System	75
CHAPTER 8	Basic Biomechanics	93

Part II
Clinical Kinesiology and Anatomy of the Upper Extremities

CHAPTER 9	Shoulder Girdle	115
CHAPTER 10	Shoulder Joint	131
CHAPTER 11	Elbow Joint	147
CHAPTER 12	Wrist Joint	161
CHAPTER 13	Hand	171

Part III
Clinical Kinesiology and Anatomy of the Trunk

| CHAPTER 14 | Temporomandibular Joint | 197 |
| CHAPTER 15 | Neck and Trunk | 211 |

| CHAPTER 16 | Respiratory System | 235 |
| CHAPTER 17 | Pelvic Girdle | 247 |

Part IV
Clinical Kinesiology and Anatomy of the Lower Extremities

CHAPTER 18	Hip Joint	261
CHAPTER 19	Knee Joint	283
CHAPTER 20	Ankle Joint and Foot	301

Part V
Clinical Kinesiology and Anatomy of the Body

| CHAPTER 21 | Posture | 329 |
| CHAPTER 22 | Gait | 339 |

Bibliography	*357*
Answers to Review Questions	*361*
Index	*377*

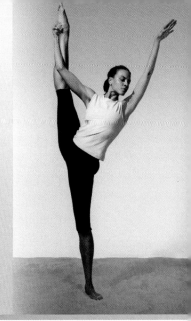

Contents

Part I
Basic Clinical Kinesiology and Anatomy

CHAPTER 1 Basic Information 3
Descriptive Terminology 4
Segments of the Body 5
Types of Motion 6
Joint Movements (Osteokinematics) 7
Review Questions 11

CHAPTER 2 Skeletal System 13
Functions of the Skeleton 13
Types of Skeletons 13
Composition of Bone 13
Structure of Bone 14
Types of Bones 16
Common Skeletal Pathologies 17
Review Questions 19

CHAPTER 3 Articular System 21
Types of Joints 21
Joint Structure 24
Planes and Axes 27
Degrees of Freedom 28
Common Pathological Terms 28
Review Questions 29

CHAPTER 4 Arthrokinematics 31
Osteokinematic Motion 31
End Feel 31
Arthrokinematic Motion 32
Accessory Motion Terminology 32
Joint Surface Shape 32
Types of Arthrokinematic Motion 33
Convex-Concave Rule 34

Joint Surface Positions (Joint Congruency) 35
Accessory Motion Forces 36
Points to Remember 37
Review Questions 37

CHAPTER 5 Muscular System 39
Muscle Attachments 39
Muscle Names 40
Muscle Fiber Arrangement 41
Functional Characteristics of Muscle Tissue 42
Length-Tension Relationship in Muscle Tissue 42
Active and Passive Insufficiency 43
Types of Muscle Contraction 45
Roles of Muscles 48
Angle of Pull 48
Kinetic Chains 49
Points to Remember 50
Review Questions 51

CHAPTER 6 Nervous System 53
Nervous Tissue (Neurons) 54
The Central Nervous System 55
Brain 55
Spinal Cord 58
The Peripheral Nervous System 60
Cranial Nerves 60
Spinal Nerves 60
Functional Significance of Spinal Cord Level 63
Plexus Formation 64

Common Pathologies of the
Central and Peripheral
Nervous Systems   71
  *Common Pathologies
    of the Central Nervous System*   71
  *Common Pathologies
    of the Peripheral Nerves*   71
Review Questions   73

CHAPTER 7 Circulatory System   75
Cardiovascular System   75
  Heart   76
  Blood Vessels   79
Lymphatic System   87
  Functions   87
  Drainage Patterns   89
Common Pathologies   90
Review Questions   91
  Cardiovascular System   91
  Lymphatic System   92

CHAPTER 8 Basic Biomechanics   93
Laws of Motion   94
Force   95
Torque   97
Stability   99
Simple Machines   102
  Levers   102
  Pulleys   108
  Wheel and Axle   109
  Inclined Plane   109
Points to Remember   110
Review Questions   111

Part II
*Clinical Kinesiology and Anatomy
of the Upper Extremities*

CHAPTER 9 Shoulder Girdle   115
Clarification of Terms   115
Bones and Landmarks   116
Joints and Ligaments   117
Joint Motions   119
  *Companion Motions of the Shoulder
    Joint and Shoulder Girdle*   120
  Scapulohumeral Rhythm   120
  Angle of Pull   121

Muscles of the Shoulder Girdle   121
  Muscle Descriptions   121
  Anatomical Relationships   125
  Force Couples   126
  Reversal of Muscle Action   126
  Summary of Muscle Innervation   127
Points to Remember   127
Review Questions   128
  General Anatomy Questions   128
  Functional Activity Questions   128
  Clinical Exercise Questions   128

CHAPTER 10 Shoulder Joint   131
Joint Motions   131
Bones and Landmarks   132
Ligaments and Other Structures   134
Muscles of the Shoulder Joint   135
  Anatomical Relationships   140
  Glenohumeral Movement   141
  Summary of Muscle Action   142
  Summary of Muscle Innervation   142
  Common Shoulder Pathologies   142
Points to Remember   144
Review Questions   144
  General Anatomy Questions   144
  Functional Activity Questions   144
  Clinical Exercise Questions   145

CHAPTER 11 Elbow Joint   147
Joint Structure and Motions   147
Bones and Landmarks   149
Ligaments and Other Structures   151
Muscles of the Elbow and Forearm   152
  Anatomical Relationships   155
  Summary of Muscle Action   156
  Summary of Muscle Innervation   156
  Common Elbow Pathologies   156
Points to Remember   158
Review Questions   159
  General Anatomy Questions   159
  Functional Activity Questions   159
  Clinical Exercise Questions   160

CHAPTER 12 Wrist Joint   161
Joint Structure   161
Joint Motions   162
Bones and Landmarks   162
Ligaments and Other Structures   163

Muscles of the Wrist   163
  Anatomical Relationships   166
  Summary of Muscle Action   167
  Summary of Muscle Innervation   167
Points to Remember   168
Review Questions   169
  General Anatomy Questions   169
  Functional Activity Questions   169
  Clinical Exercise Questions   170

CHAPTER 13 Hand   171
Joints and Motions of the Thumb   171
Joints and Motions of the Fingers   173
Bones and Landmarks   174
Ligaments and Other Structures   174
Muscles of the Thumb and Fingers   176
  Extrinsic Muscles   176
  Intrinsic Muscles   181
  Anatomical Relationships   185
  Common Wrist and Hand Pathologies   186
  Summary of Muscle Actions   187
  Summary of Muscle Innervation   187
Hand Function   189
  Grasps   189
Points to Remember   192
Review Questions   192
  General Anatomy Questions   192
  Functional Activity Questions   193
  Clinical Exercise Questions   193

Part III
Clinical Kinesiology and Anatomy
of the Trunk

CHAPTER 14 Temporomandibular
            Joint   197
Joint Structure and Motions   197
Bones and Landmarks   198
Ligaments and Other Structures   201
Mechanics of Movement   202
Muscles of the TMJ   203
  Anatomical Relationships   207
  Summary of Muscle Action   208
  Summary of Muscle Innervation   208
Points to Remember   208

Review Questions   209
  General Anatomy Questions   209
  Functional Activity Questions   209
  Clinical Exercise Questions   209

CHAPTER 15 Neck and Trunk   211
Vertebral Curves   211
Clarification of Terms   211
Joint Motions   212
Bones and Landmarks   213
Joints and Ligaments   217
Muscles of the Neck and Trunk   219
  Muscles of the Cervical Spine   219
  Muscles of the Trunk   222
  Anatomical Relationships   227
  Summary of Muscle Actions   229
  Summary of Muscle Innervation   229
  Common Vertebral Column
    Pathologies   229
Points to Remember   231
Review Questions   231
  General Anatomy Questions   231
  Functional Activity Questions   231
  Clinical Exercise Questions   232

CHAPTER 16 Respiratory System   235
The Thoracic Cage   235
  Joints and Articulations   236
  Movements of the Thorax   236
Structures of Respiration   237
  Mechanics of Respiration   238
Phases of Respiration   239
Muscles of Respiration   239
  Diaphragm Muscle   239
  Intercostal Muscles   240
  Accessory Inspiratory Muscles   241
  Accessory Expiratory Muscles   242
  Anatomical Relationships   242
  Diaphragmatic Versus
    Chest Breathing   244
  Summary of Innervation of
    the Muscles of Respiration   244
  Valsalva's Maneuver   244
  Common Respiratory
    Conditions or Pathologies   245

Review Questions   245
   General Anatomy Questions   245
   Functional Activity Questions   246
   Clinical Exercise Questions   246

CHAPTER 17 Pelvic Girdle   **247**
Structure and Function   247
False and True Pelvis   248
   Sacroiliac Joint   248
   Pubic Symphysis   252
   Lumbosacral Joint   252
Pelvic Girdle Motions   253
   Muscle Control   256
Review Questions   257
   General Anatomy Questions   257
   Functional Activity Questions   258
   Clinical Exercise Questions   258

Part IV
Clinical Kinesiology and Anatomy
of the Lower Extremities

CHAPTER 18 Hip Joint   **261**
Joint Structure and Motions   262
Bones and Landmarks   262
Ligaments and Other Structures   265
Muscles of the Hip   267
   Anatomical Relationships   274
   Common Hip Pathologies   275
   Summary of Muscle Action   277
   Summary of Muscle Innervation   277
Points to Remember   278
Review Questions   279
   General Anatomy Questions   279
   Functional Activity Questions   280
   Clinical Exercise Questions   281

CHAPTER 19 Knee Joint   **283**
Joint Structure and Motions   283
Bones and Landmarks   286
Ligaments and Other Structures   287
Muscles of the Knee   289
   Anterior Muscles   290
   Posterior Muscles   291
   Anatomical Relationships   293

   Summary of Muscle Action   294
   Summary of Muscle Innervation   294
   Common Knee Pathologies   294
Points to Remember   296
Review Questions   296
   General Anatomy Questions   296
   Functional Activity Questions   297
   Clinical Exercise Questions   298

CHAPTER 20 Ankle Joint and Foot   **301**
Bones and Landmarks   302
   Functional Aspects of the Foot   303
Joints and Motions   304
   Ankle Motions   304
   Ankle Joints   305
   Foot Joints   307
Ligaments and Other Structures   308
   Arches   308
Muscles of the Ankle and Foot   310
   Extrinsic Muscles   310
   Intrinsic Muscles   317
   Anatomical Relationships   317
   Summary of Muscle Innervation   321
   Common Ankle Pathologies   322
Points to Remember   324
Review Questions   324
   General Anatomy Questions   324
   Functional Activity Questions   324
   Clinical Exercise Questions   324

Part V
Clinical Kinesiology and Anatomy
of the Body

CHAPTER 21 Posture   **329**
Vertebral Alignment   329
   Development of Postural Curves   330
Standing Posture   332
   Lateral View   332
   Anterior View   333
   Posterior View   333
Sitting Posture   334
Supine Posture   336
Common Postural Deviations   336

Review Questions   337
    General Anatomy Questions   337
    Functional Activity Questions   337
    Clinical Exercise Questions   337

CHAPTER 22 Gait   **339**
Definitions   339
Analysis of Stance Phase   342
Analysis of Swing Phase   346
Additional Determinants of Gait   347
Age-Related Gait Patterns   348
Abnormal (Atypical) Gait   349
    Muscular Weakness/Paralysis   349
    Joint/Muscle Range-of-Motion
      Limitation   351

    Neurological Involvement   352
    Pain   353
    Leg Length Discrepancy   354
Points to Remember   354
Review Questions   355
    General Anatomy Questions   355
    Functional Activity Questions   355
    Clinical Exercise Questions   355

Bibliography   *357*
Answers to Review Questions   *361*
Index   *377*

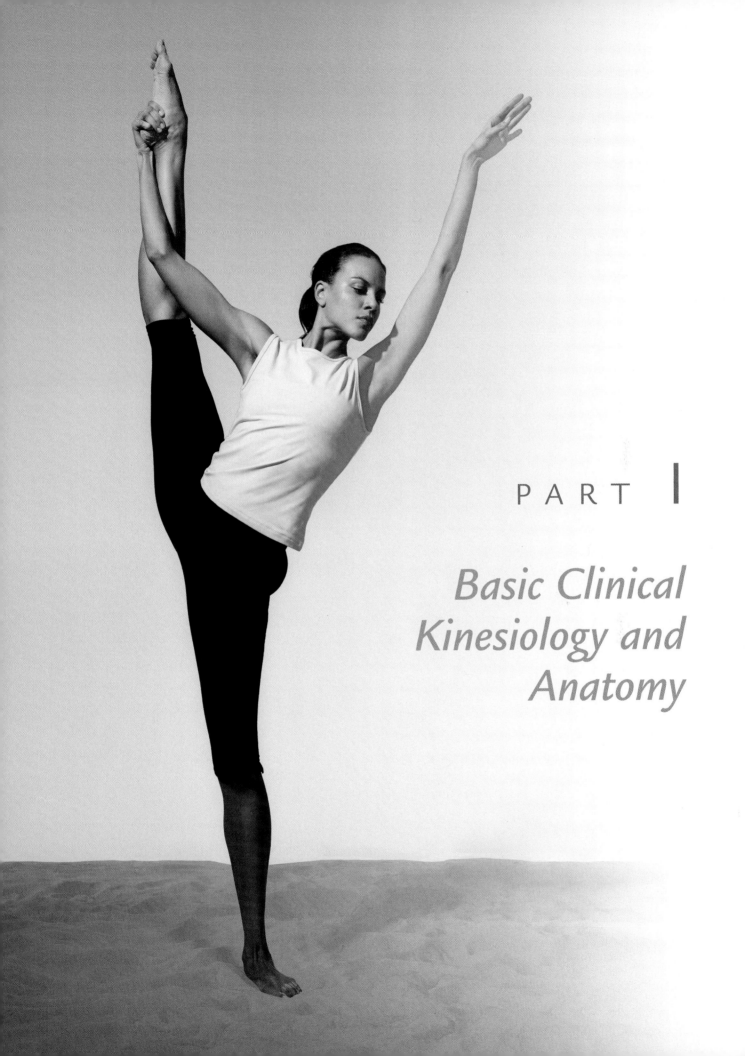

PART I

Basic Clinical
Kinesiology and
Anatomy

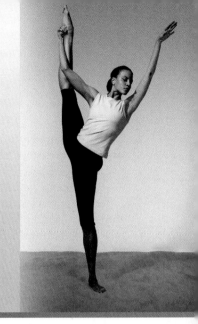

CHAPTER 1
Basic Information

Descriptive Terminology

Segments of the Body

Types of Motion

Joint Movements (Osteokinematics)

Review Questions

By definition, **kinesiology** is the study of movement. However, this definition is too general to be of much use. Kinesiology brings together the fields of anatomy, physiology, physics, and geometry, and relates them to human movement. Thus, kinesiology utilizes principles of mechanics, musculoskeletal anatomy, and neuromuscular physiology.

Mechanical principles that relate directly to the human body are used in the study of **biomechanics.** Because we may use a ball, racket, crutch, prosthesis, or some other implement, we must consider our biomechanical interaction with them as well. This may involve looking at the *static* (nonmoving) and/or *dynamic* (moving) *systems* associated with various activities. Dynamic systems can be divided into kinetics and kinematics. **Kinetics** are those forces causing movement, whereas **kinematics** is the time, space, and mass aspects of a moving system. These and other basic biomechanical concepts will be discussed in Chapter 8.

This text will give most emphasis to the musculoskeletal anatomy components, which are considered the key to understanding and being able to apply the other components. Many students have negative thoughts at the mere mention of the word *kinesiology*. Their eyes glaze over and their brains freeze. Perhaps, based on past experience with anatomy, they feel that their only hope is mass memorization. However, this may prove to be an overwhelming task with no long-term memory gain.

As you proceed through this text, keep in mind a few simple concepts. First, the human body is arranged in a very logical way. Like all aspects of life, there are exceptions. Sometimes the logic of these exceptions is apparent, and sometimes the logic may be apparent only to some higher being. Whichever is the case, you should note the exception and move on. Second, if you have a good grasp of descriptive terminology and can visualize the concept or feature, strict memorization is not necessary. For example, if you know generally where the patella is located and what the structures are around it, you can accurately describe its location using your own words. You do not need to memorize someone else's words to be correct.

By keeping in mind some of the basic principles affecting muscles, understanding individual muscle function need not be so mind-boggling. If you know (1) what motions a particular joint allows, (2) that a muscle must span a particular joint surface to cause a certain motion, and (3) what that muscle's line of pull is, then (4) you will know the particular action(s) of a specific muscle. For example, (1) the elbow allows only flexion and extension; (2) a muscle must span the joint anteriorly to flex and posteriorly to extend; (3) the biceps brachii is a vertical muscle on the anterior surface of the arm; (4) therefore, the bicep flexes the elbow.

Yes, kinesiology *can* be understood by mere mortals. Its study can even be enjoyable. However, a word of caution should be given: Like exercising, it is better to study in small amounts several times a week than to study for a long period in one session before the exam.

Descriptive Terminology

The human body is active and constantly moving; therefore, it is subject to frequent changes in position. The relationship of the various body parts to each other also changes. To be able to describe the organization of the human body, it is necessary to use some arbitrary position as a starting point from which movement or location of structures can be described. This is known as the **anatomical position** (Fig. 1-1A) and is described as the human body standing in an upright position, eyes facing forward, feet parallel and close together, arms at the sides of the body with the palms facing forward. Although the position of the forearm and hands is not a natural one, it does allow for accurate description. The **fundamental position** (Fig. 1-1B) is the same as the anatomical position except that the palms face the sides of the body. This position is often used in discussing rotation of the upper extremity.

Specific terms are used to describe the location of a structure and its position relative to other structures (Fig. 1-2). **Medial** refers to a location or position toward the midline, and **lateral** refers to a location or position farther from the midline. For example, the ulna is on the medial side of the forearm, and the radius is lateral to the ulna.

Anterior refers to the front of the body or to a position closer to the front. **Posterior** refers to the back of the body or to a position more toward the back. For example, the sternum is anterior on the chest wall, and

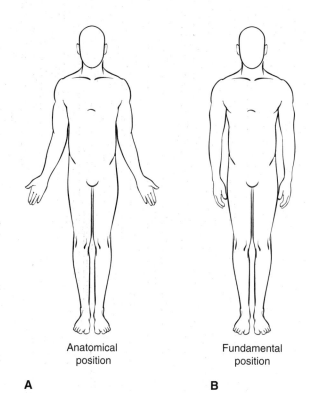

Anatomical position   Fundamental position

A   **B**

Figure 1-1.   Descriptive positions.

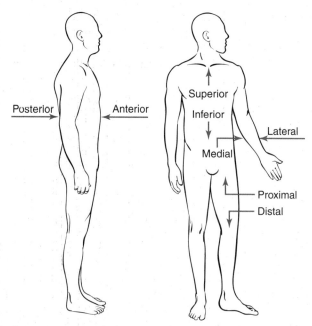

Figure 1-2.   Descriptive terminology.

the scapula is posterior. **Ventral** is a synonym (a word with the same meaning) of *anterior*, and **dorsal** is a synonym of *posterior*; *anterior* and *posterior* are more commonly used in kinesiology. *Front* and *back* also refer to the surfaces of the body, but these are considered lay terms and are not widely used by health-care professionals.

Distal and *proximal* are used to describe locations on the extremities. **Distal** means away from the trunk, and **proximal** means toward the trunk. For example, the humeral head is located on the proximal end of the humerus. The elbow is proximal to the wrist but distal to the shoulder.

Superior is used to indicate the location of a body part that is above another or to refer to the upper surface of an organ or a structure. **Inferior** indicates that a body part is below another or refers to the lower surface of an organ or a structure. For example, the body of the sternum is superior to the xiphoid process but inferior to the manubrium. Sometimes people use **cranial** or *cephalad* (from the word root *cephal*, meaning "head") to refer to a position or structure close to the head. **Caudal** (from the word root *cauda*, meaning "tail") refers to a position or structure closer to the feet. For example, *cauda equina*, which means "horse's tail," is the bundle of spinal nerve roots descending from the inferior end of the spinal cord. Like *dorsal* and *ventral*, cranial and caudal are terms that are best used to describe positions on a quadruped (a four-legged animal). Humans are bipeds, or two-legged animals. You can see that if the dog in Figure 1-3 were to stand on its hind legs, dorsal would become posterior and cranial would become superior, and so on.

A structure may be described as **superficial** or **deep,** depending on its relative depth. For example, in describing the layers of the abdominal muscles, the external oblique is deep to the rectus abdominis but superficial to the internal oblique. Another example is the scalp being described as superficial to the skull.

Supine and *prone* are terms that describe body position while lying flat. When **supine,** a person is lying straight, with the face, or anterior surface, pointed upward. A person in the **prone** position is horizontal, with the face, or anterior surface, pointed downward (the child in Fig. 1-5 is lying prone on the sled).

Bilateral refers to two, or both, sides. For example, bilateral above-knee amputations refer to both right and left legs being amputated above the knee. **Contralateral** refers to the opposite side. For example, a person who has had a stroke affecting the right side of the brain may have contralateral paralysis of the left arm and left leg. On the other hand, **ipsilateral** refers to the same side of the body.

Segments of the Body

The body is divided into segments according to bones (Fig. 1-4). In the upper extremity, the **arm** is the bone (humerus) between the shoulder and the elbow joint. Next, the **forearm** (radius and ulna) is between the elbow and the wrist. The **hand** is distal to the wrist.

The lower extremity is made up of three similar segments. The **thigh** (femur) is between the hip and the knee joint. The **leg** (tibia and fibula) is between the knee and the ankle joint, and the **foot** is distal to the ankle.

The trunk has two segments: the thorax and the abdomen. The **thorax,** or chest, is made up of the ribs,

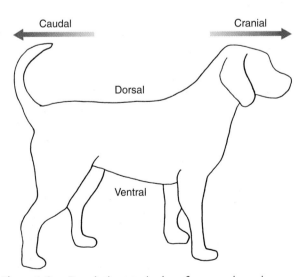

Figure 1-3.   Descriptive terminology for a quadruped.

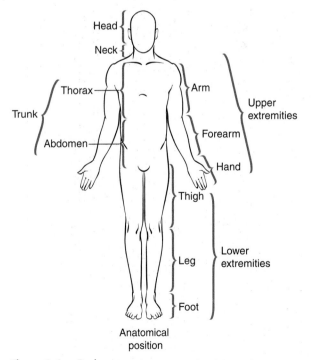

Figure 1-4.   Body segments.

sternum, and mostly thoracic vertebrae. The **abdomen,** or lower trunk, is made up of the pelvis, stomach, and mostly lumbar vertebrae. The **neck** (cervical vertebrae) and **head** (skull) are separate segments.

Arthrokinematic motion (Chapter 4) refers to a joint's surface motion in relation to the body segment's motion. For example, the surface of the proximal end of the humerus moves down, while the body segment (arm) moves up. Body segments are rarely used to describe joint motion. For example, flexion occurs at the shoulder, not the arm. The motion occurs at the joint (shoulder), and the body segment (arm) just goes along for the ride! An exception to this concept is the forearm. It is a body segment but functions as a joint as well. Technically, joint motion occurs at the proximal and distal radioulnar joints; however, common practice refers to this as *forearm pronation* and *supination.*

Types of Motion

Linear motion, also called *translatory motion,* occurs in a more or less straight line from one location to another. All the parts of the object move the same distance, in the same direction, and at the same time. Movement that occurs in a straight line is called **rectilinear motion,** such as the motion of a child sledding down a hill (Fig. 1-5), a sailboarder moving across the water, or a baseball player running from home plate to first base. If movement occurs in a curved path that isn't necessarily circular, it is called **curvilinear motion.** The path a diver takes after leaving the diving board until entering the water is curvilinear motion. Figure 1-6 demonstrates the curvilinear path a skier takes coming down a

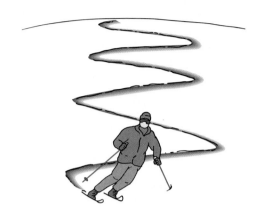

Figure 1-6. Curvilinear motion.

ski slope. Other examples of curvilinear motion are the path of a thrown ball, a javelin thrown across a field, or the Earth's orbit around the sun.

Movement of an object around a fixed point is called **angular motion,** also known as *rotary motion* (Fig. 1-7). All the parts of the object move through the same angle, in the same direction, and at the same time, but they do not move the same distance. When a person flexes his or her knee, the foot travels farther through space than does the ankle or leg.

It is not uncommon to see both types of movement occurring at the same time—the entire object moving in a linear fashion and the individual parts moving in an angular fashion. In Figure 1-8, the skateboarder's whole body moves down the street (linear motion), while individual joints on the "pushing" leg (i.e., the hip, knee, and ankle) rotate about their axes (angular motion). Another example of combined motions is walking. The whole body exhibits linear motion walking from point A to point B, while the hips, knees, and ankles exhibit

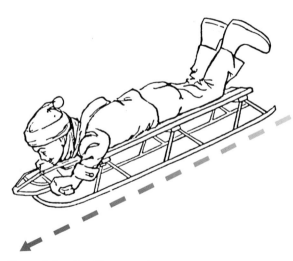

Figure 1-5. Rectilinear motion.

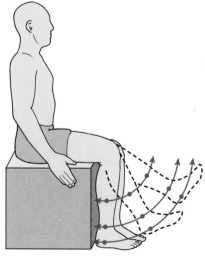

Figure 1-7. Angular motion.

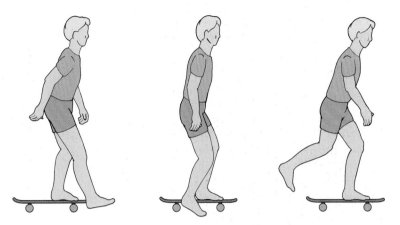

Figure 1-8. Combination of linear and angular motion.

angular motion. A person throwing a ball uses the upper extremity joints in an angular direction. The ball travels in a curvilinear path.

Generally speaking, most movement within the body is angular; movement outside the body tends to be linear. Exceptions to this statement can be found. For example, the movement of the scapula in elevation/depression and protraction/retraction is essentially linear. However, the movement of the clavicle, which is attached to the scapula, is angular and gets its angular motion from the sternoclavicular joint.

Joint Movements (Osteokinematics)

Joints move in many different directions. As will be discussed, movement occurs around joint axes and through joint planes. The following terms are used to describe the various joint movements that occur at synovial joints (Fig. 1-9). Synovial joints are freely movable joints where most joint motion occurs. These joints are discussed in more detail in Chapter 3. This type of joint

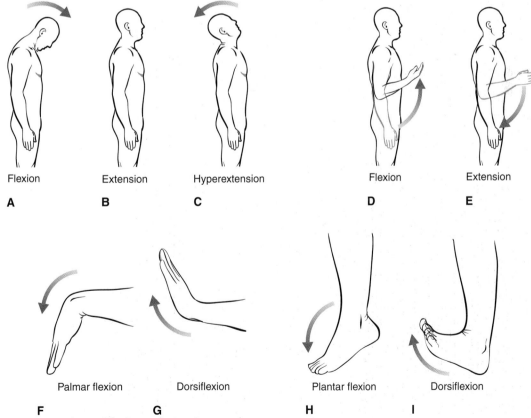

Figure 1-9. Joint motions of flexion and extension.

motion is also called **osteokinematics,** which deals with the relationship of the *movement of bones around a joint axis* (e.g., humerus moving on scapula), as opposed to **arthrokinematics,** which deals with the relationship of *joint surface movement* (humeral head's movement within glenoid fossa of scapula). This will be discussed in more detail in Chapter 4.

Flexion is the bending movement of one bone on another, bringing the two segments together and causing an increase in the joint angle. Usually this occurs between anterior surfaces of articulating bones, and surfaces move toward each other. In the case of the neck, flexion is a "bowing down" motion (Fig. 1-9A) in which the head moves toward the anterior chest. With elbow flexion, the forearm and arm move toward each other. With the knee, however, the posterior surfaces (thigh and leg) move toward each other, causing flexion. With hip flexion, the thigh moves toward the trunk when the lower extremity is the moving part. When the lower extremities are fixed and the trunk becomes the moving part, the trunk flexes. Actually, whether flexion represents an increase or decrease in joint angle will depend on your point of reference. When performing a goniometric measurement of elbow flexion, you would begin in the anatomical position (full extension), which is considered zero. The amount of flexion increases toward 180 degrees. In this case, flexion would represent an increase in the joint angle (Fig. 1-9D). In other references, flexion begins at 180 degrees (full extension) and moves toward 0 degrees; thus, it is a decrease in the joint angle.

Conversely, **extension** is the straightening movement of one bone away from another, causing an increase of the joint angle. This motion usually returns the body part to the anatomical position after it has been flexed (Fig. 1-9B, E). The joint surfaces tend to move away from each other. Extension occurs when the head moves up and away from the chest, and the thigh moves away from the trunk and returns to anatomical position. **Hyperextension** is the continuation of extension beyond the anatomical position (Fig. 1-9C). The shoulder, hip, neck, and trunk can hyperextend. Flexion at the wrist may be called **palmar flexion** (Fig. 1-9F), and flexion at the ankle may be called **plantar flexion** (Fig. 1-9H). Extension at the wrist and ankle joints may be called **dorsiflexion** (Fig. 1-9G, I).

Abduction is movement away from the midline of the body (Fig. 1-10A), and **adduction** (Fig. 1-10B) is movement toward the midline. The shoulder and hip can abduct *and* adduct. Exceptions to this midline definition are the fingers and toes. The reference point for the fingers is the middle finger. Movement away from the middle finger is abduction (see Fig. 13-5). It should be noted that the middle finger abducts (to the right

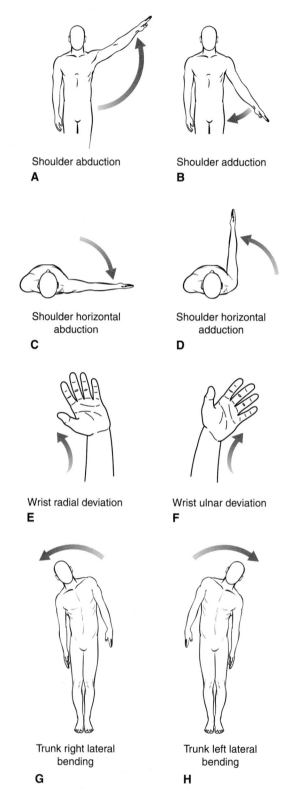

Shoulder abduction
A

Shoulder adduction
B

Shoulder horizontal abduction
C

Shoulder horizontal adduction
D

Wrist radial deviation
E

Wrist ulnar deviation
F

Trunk right lateral bending
G

Trunk left lateral bending
H

Figure 1-10.   Joint motions of abduction and adduction.

and to the left) but adducts only as a return movement from abduction to the midline. The point of reference for the toes is the second toe (see Fig. 20-13). Similar to the middle finger, the second toe abducts to the right and the left but does not adduct except as a return movement from abduction.

Horizontal abduction and adduction are motions which cannot occur from anatomical position. They must be preceded by either flexion or abduction of the shoulder joint so that the arm is at shoulder level. From this position, shoulder movement backward is **horizontal abduction** (Fig. 1-10C) and movement forward is **horizontal adduction** (Fig. 1-10D). There are similar movements at the hip, but the ranges of motion are not usually as great.

Radial deviation and *ulnar deviation* are terms more commonly used to refer to wrist abduction and adduction. When the hand moves laterally, or toward the thumb side, it is **radial deviation** (Fig. 1-10E). When the hand moves medially from the anatomical position toward the little finger side at the wrist, it is **ulnar deviation** (Fig. 1-10F).

When the trunk moves sideways, the term **lateral bending** is used. The trunk can laterally bend to the right or to the left (Fig. 1-10G, H). If the right side of the trunk bends, moving the shoulder toward the right hip, it is called *right lateral bending*. The neck also laterally bends in the same way. The term *lateral flexion* is sometimes used to describe this sideward motion. However, because this term is easily confused with *flexion,* it will not be used in this book.

Circumduction is motion that describes a circular, cone-shaped pattern. It involves a combination of four joint motions: (1) flexion, (2) abduction, (3) extension, and (4) adduction. For example, if the shoulder moves in a circle, the hand would move in a much larger circle. The entire arm would move in a cone-shaped sequential pattern of flexion to abduction to extension to adduction, bringing the arm back to its starting position (Fig. 1-11).

Rotation is movement of a bone or part around its longitudinal axis. If the anterior surface rolls inward toward the midline, it is called **medial rotation** (Fig. 1-12A). This is sometimes referred to as *internal rotation.* Conversely, if the anterior surface rolls outward, away from the midline, it is called **lateral rotation** (Fig. 1-12B), or *external rotation.* The neck and trunk rotate to either the right or left side (Fig. 1-12C, D). Visualize the neck rotating as you look over your right shoulder. This would be "right neck rotation."

Rotation of the forearm is referred to as *supination* and *pronation.* In anatomical position, the forearm is in

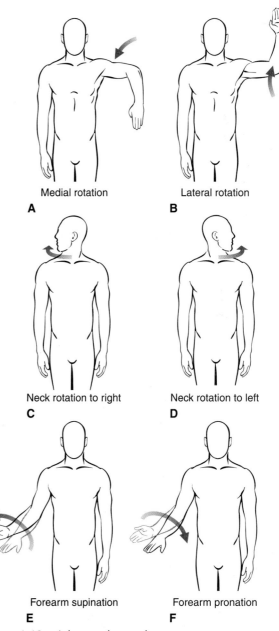

Medial rotation   Lateral rotation

A   B

Neck rotation to right   Neck rotation to left

C   D

Forearm supination   Forearm pronation

E   F

Figure 1-12. Joint rotation motions.

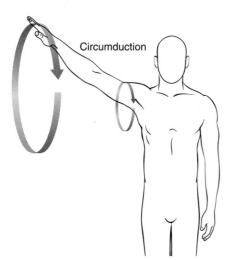

Circumduction

Figure 1-11. Circumduction motion.

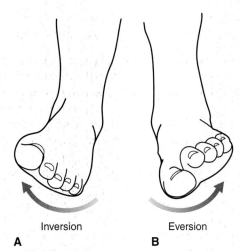

Inversion   Eversion
A   **B**

Figure 1-13.   Inversion and eversion of left foot.

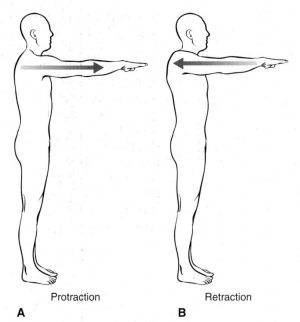

Protraction   Retraction
A   **B**

Figure 1-14.   Protraction and retraction.

supination (Fig. 1-12E). This faces the palm of the hand forward, or anteriorly. In **pronation** (Fig. 1-12F), the palm is facing backward, or posteriorly. When the elbow is flexed, the "palm up" position refers to supination and "palm down" refers to pronation.

The following are terms used to describe motions specific to certain joints. **Inversion** is moving the sole of the foot inward at the ankle (Fig. 1-13A), and **eversion** is the outward movement (Fig. 1-13B). **Protraction** is mostly a linear movement along a plane parallel to the ground and away from the midline (Fig. 1-14A), and

retraction is mostly a linear movement in the same plane but toward the midline (Fig. 1-14B). Protraction of the shoulder girdle moves the scapula away from the midline, as does protraction of the jaw, whereas retraction in both of these cases returns the body part toward the midline, or back to anatomical position.

Review Questions

1. Using descriptive terminology, complete the following:
   a. The sternum is _____ to the vertebral column.
   b. The calcaneus is on the _____ portion of the foot.
   c. The hip is _____ to the chest.
   d. The femur is _____ to the tibia.
   e. The radius is on the _____ side of the forearm.

2. When a football is kicked through the goalposts, what type of motion is being demonstrated by the football? By the kicker?

3. Looking at a spot on the ceiling directly over your head involves what joint motion?

4. Putting your hand in your back pocket involves what shoulder joint rotation?

5. Picking up a pencil on the floor beside your chair involves what trunk joint motion?

6. Putting your right ankle on your left knee involves what type of hip rotation?

7. What is the only difference between *anatomical* position and *fundamental* position?

8. If you place your hand on the back of a dog, that is referred to as what surface? If you place your hand on the back of a person, that is referred to as what surface?

9. A person wheeling across a room in a wheelchair uses both linear and angular motion. Describe when each type of motion is being used.

10. A person lying on a bed staring at the ceiling is in what position?

11. When touching the left shoulder with the left hand, is a person using the contralateral or ipsilateral hand?

Refer to Figure 1-15 below.

12. Identify the three main positions of the left hip.

13. What is the position of the left knee?

14. What is the position of the right forearm?

15. Identify the two main positions of the neck (not the head).

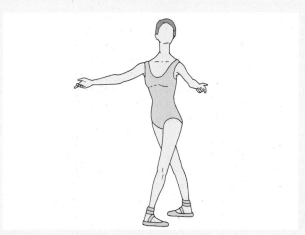

Figure 1-15. Ballet position.

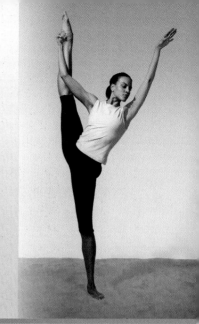

CHAPTER 2
Skeletal System

Functions of the Skeleton

Types of Skeletons

Composition of Bone

Structure of Bone

Types of Bones

Common Skeletal Pathologies

Review Questions

Functions of the Skeleton

The skeletal system, which is made up of numerous bones, is the rigid framework of the human body. It gives support and shape to the body. It protects vital organs such as the brain, spinal cord, and heart. It assists in movement by providing a rigid structure for muscle attachment and leverage. The skeletal system also manufactures blood cells in various locations. The main sites of blood formation are the ilium, vertebra, sternum, and ribs. This formation occurs mostly in flat bones. Calcium and other mineral salts are stored throughout all osseous tissue of the skeletal system.

Types of Skeletons

The bones of the body are grouped into two main categories: axial and appendicular (Fig. 2-1 on page 15). The **axial skeleton** forms the upright part of the body. It consists of approximately 80 bones of the head, thorax, and trunk. The **appendicular skeleton** attaches to the axial skeleton and contains the 126 bones of the extremities. There are 206 bones in the body. Individuals may have additional sesamoid bones, such as in the flexor tendons of the great toe and the thumb.

Table 2-1 lists the bones of the adult human body. The sacrum, coccyx, and hip bones are each made up of several bones fused together. In the hip bone, these fused bones are known as the *ilium, ischium,* and *pubis.*

Composition of Bone

Bones can be considered organs, because they are made up of several different types of tissue (fibrous, cartilaginous, osseous, nervous, and vascular), and they function as integral parts of the skeletal system.

Table 2-1	Bones of the Human Body		
	Single	**Paired**	**Multiple**
Axial Skeleton			
Cranium (8)	Frontal Sphenoid Ethmoid Occipital	Parietal Temporal	None
Face (14)	Mandible Vomer	Maxilla Zygomatic Lacrimal Inferior concha Palatine Nasal	None
Other (7)	Hyoid	Ear ossicles (3)	None
Vertebral column (26)	Sacrum (5)* Coccyx (3)*	None	Cervical (7) Thoracic (12) Lumbar (5)

Thorax (25)	Sternum	Ribs (12 Pairs)
		  True: 7
		  False: 3
		  Floating: 2
			None

Appendicular Skeleton			
Upper extremity (64)	None	Scapula Clavicle Humerus Ulna Radius	Carpals (8) Metacarpals (5) Phalanges (14)
Lower extremity (62)	None	Hip (3)* Femur Tibia Fibula Patella	Tarsals (7) Metatarsals (5) Phalanges (14)

*Denotes bones that are fused together.

Bone is made up of one-third *organic* (living) material and two-thirds *inorganic* (nonliving) material. The organic material gives the bone elasticity, whereas the inorganic material provides hardness and strength, which makes bone opaque on an x-ray. Just how hard is bone? It has been estimated that if you took a human skull and slowly loaded weight onto it, the skull could support three tons before it broke!

Compact bone makes up a hard, dense outer shell. It always completely covers bone and tends to be thick along the shaft and thin at the ends of long bones. It is also thick in the plates of the flat bones of the skull.

Cancellous bone is the porous and spongy inside portion called the *trabeculae*, which means "little beams" in Latin. They are arranged in a pattern that resists local stresses and strains (Fig. 2-2A). Trabeculae tend to be filled with marrow and make the bone lighter. Cancellous bone makes up most of the articular ends of bones.

Structure of Bone

The **epiphysis** is the area at each end of a long bone. This area tends to be wider than the shaft (Fig. 2-3). In adult bone, the epiphysis is osseous; in growing bone, the epiphysis is cartilaginous material called the **epiphyseal plate.** Longitudinal growth occurs here through the manufacturing of new bone.

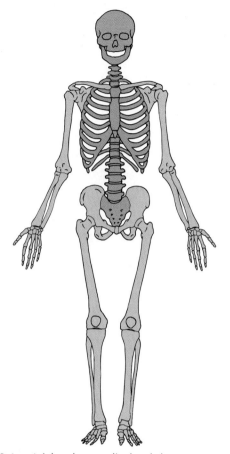

Figure 2-1.   Axial and appendicular skeleton.

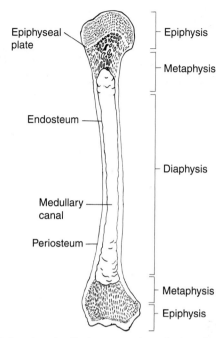

Figure 2-3.   Longitudinal cross section of a long bone.

The **diaphysis** is the main shaft of bone. It is made up mostly of compact bone, which gives it great strength. Its center, the **medullary canal,** is hollow, which, among other features, decreases the weight of the bone. This canal contains marrow and provides passage for nutrient arteries. The **endosteum** is a membrane that lines the medullary canal. It contains **osteoclasts,** which are mainly responsible for bone resorption.

In long bones, the flared part at each end of the diaphysis is called the **metaphysis.** It is made up mostly of cancellous bone and functions to support the epiphysis.

Periosteum is the thin fibrous membrane covering all of the bone except the articular surfaces that are covered with hyaline cartilage. The periosteum contains nerve and blood vessels that are important in providing nourishment, promoting growth in diameter of immature bone, and repairing the bone. It also serves as an attachment point for tendons and ligaments.

On an x-ray, a growing bone will show a distinct line between the epiphyseal plate and the rest of the bone (Fig. 2-4A). Because this line does not exist in the normal adult bone, its absence indicates that bone growth has stopped (Fig. 2-4B).

There are two types of epiphyses found in children whose bones are still growing (Fig. 2-5). A **pressure epiphysis** is located at the ends of long bones, where they receive pressure from the opposing bone making up that joint. This is where growth of long bones occurs. Because

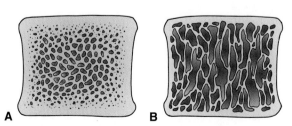

Figure 2-2.   Normal **(A)** and osteoporotic **(B)** bone composition.

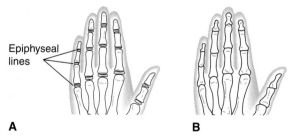

Figure 2-4.   Epiphyseal lines in the hand bones of a child **(A)** and an adult **(B)**.

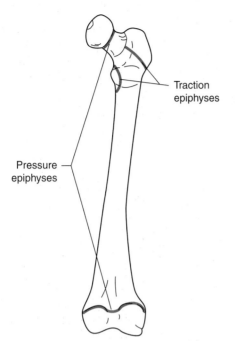

Figure 2-5.   Types of epiphyses found in an immature bone.

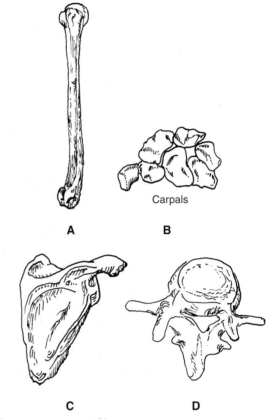

Figure 2-6.   Types of bones.

the epiphysis of a growing bone is not firmly attached to the diaphysis, it can slip or become misshapen. A **traction epiphysis** is located where tendons attach to bones and are subjected to a pulling, or traction, force. Examples would be the greater and lesser trochanters of the femur and tibial tuberosity.

Types of Bones

Long bones are so named because their length is greater than their width (Fig. 2-6A). They are the largest bones in the body and make up most of the appendicular skeleton. Long bones are basically tube-shaped with a shaft (diaphysis) and two bulbous ends (epiphysis). The wide part of the shaft nearest the epiphysis is called the *metaphysis* (see Fig. 2-3). The diaphysis consists of compact bone surrounding the marrow cavity. The metaphysis and epiphysis consist of cancellous bone covered by a thin layer of compact bone. Over the articular surfaces of the epiphysis is a thin layer of hyaline cartilage. Bone growth occurs at the epiphysis.

Short bones tend to have more equal dimensions of height, length, and width, giving them a cube shape (Fig. 2-6B). They have a great deal of articular surface and, unlike long bones, usually articulate with more than one bone. Their composition is similar to long bones: a thin layer of compact bone covering cancellous bone, which has a marrow cavity in the middle.

Examples of short bones include the bones of the wrist (carpals) and ankle (tarsals).

Flat bones have a very broad surface but are not very thick. They tend to have a curved surface rather than a flat one (Fig. 2-6C). These bones are made up of two layers of compact bone with cancellous bone and marrow in between. The ilium and scapula are good examples of flat bones.

Irregular bones have a variety of mixed shapes, as their name implies (Fig. 2-6D). Examples of irregular bones include the vertebrae and sacrum, which do not fit into the other categories. They are also composed of cancellous bone and marrow encased in a thin layer of compact bone.

Sesamoid bones, which resemble the shape of sesame seeds, are small bones located where tendons cross the ends of long bones in the extremities. They develop within the tendon and protect it from excessive wear. For example, the tendon of the flexor hallucis longus spans the bottom (plantar surface) of the foot and attaches on the great toe. If this tendon were not protected in some way at the ball of the foot, it would constantly be stepped on. Mother Nature is too clever to allow this to happen. Sesamoid bones are located on either side of the tendon near the head of the first metatarsal, providing a protective "groove" for the tendon to pass through this weight-bearing area.

Sesamoid bones also change the angle of a tendon's attachment. The patella can be considered a sesamoid bone because it is encased in the quadriceps tendon and improves the mechanical advantage of the quadriceps muscle. As previously mentioned, sesamoid bones are also found in the flexor tendons that pass posteriorly into the foot on either side of the ankle. In the upper extremity, they are found in the flexor tendons of the thumb, near the metacarpophalangeal and interphalangeal joints. Occasionally, a sesamoid bone is located near the metacarpophalangeal joint of the index and little fingers.

Table 2-2 summarizes the types of bones of the axial and appendicular skeletons. It should be noted that there are no long or short bones in the axial skeleton, and there are no irregular bones in the appendicular skeleton. Sesamoid bones are not included in Table 2-2 because they are considered accessory bones, and their shape and number vary greatly.

When looking at various bones, you will see holes, depressions, ridges, bumps, grooves, and various other kinds of markings. Each of these markings serves different purposes. Table 2-3 describes the different kinds of bone markings and their purposes.

Common Skeletal Pathologies

Fracture, *broken bone,* or *cracked bone* are all synonymous. It is a break in the continuity of the bony cortex caused by direct force, indirect force, or pathology. Fractures in children tend to be incomplete ("greenstick") or at the epiphysis. Fractures in the elderly mostly happen in the hip (proximal femur), resulting from a fall, or they happen in the upper extremity, resulting from a fall on the outstretched hand. Fractures are often described by type (e.g., closed), direction of fracture line (e.g., transverse), or position of bone parts (e.g., overriding).

Osteoporosis is a condition characterized by loss of normal bone density, or bone mass (see Fig. 2-2B). This condition can weaken a bone to the point it will fracture. The vertebra of an elderly person is a common site for osteoporosis. **Osteomyelitis** is an infection of the bone usually caused by bacteria. A fracture that breaks through the skin (open fracture) poses a greater risk of developing osteomyelitis than a fracture that does not break the skin (closed fracture).

Because the epiphysis of a growing bone is not firmly attached to the diaphysis, it can slip or become misshapen. The proximal head of the femur is a common site for problems at the pressure epiphysis, such as **Legg-Calvé-Perthes disease** and **slipped femoral capital epiphysis.** Overuse can cause irritation and

Table 2-2	Types of Bones		
Type	**Appendicular Skeleton**		**Axial Skeleton**
	Upper Extremity	Lower Extremity	
Long bones	Clavicle Humerus Radius Ulna Metacarpals Phalanges	Femur Fibula Tibia Metatarsals Phalanges	None
Short bones	Carpals	Tarsals	None
Flat bones	Scapula	Hip Patella	Cranial bones (frontal, parietal) Ribs Sternum
Irregular bones	None	None	Vertebrae Cranial bones (sphenoid, ethmoid) Sacrum Coccyx Mandible, facial bones

Table 2-3	Bone Markings	

Depressions and Openings

Marking	Description	Examples
1. Foramen	Hole through which blood vessels, nerves, and ligaments pass	Vertebral foramen of cervical vertebra
2. Fossa	Hollow or depression	Glenoid fossa of scapula
3. Groove	Ditchlike groove containing a tendon or blood vessel	Bicipital (intercondylar) groove of humerus
4. Meatus	Canal or tubelike opening in a bone	External auditory meatus
5. Sinus	Air-filled cavity within a bone	Frontal sinus in frontal bone

Projections or Processes That Fit Into Joints

Marking	Description	Examples
1. Condyle	Rounded knucklelike projection	Medial condyle of femur
2. Eminence	Projecting, prominent part of bone	Intercondylar eminence of tibia
3. Facet	Flat or shallow articular surface	Articular facet of rib
4. Head	Rounded articular projection beyond a narrow, necklike portion of bone	Femoral head

Projections/Processes That Attach Tendons, Ligaments, and Other Connective Tissue

Marking	Description	Examples
1. Crest	Sharp ridge or border	Iliac crest of hip
2. Epicondyle	Prominence above or on a condyle	Medial epicondyle of humerus
3. Line	Less prominent ridge	Linea aspera of femur
4. Spine	Long, thin projection (spinous process)	Scapular spine
5. Tubercle	Small, rounded projection	Greater tubercle of humerus
6. Tuberosity	Large, rounded projection	Ischial tuberosity
7. Trochanter	Very large prominence for muscle attachment	Greater trochanter of femur

inflammation of any traction epiphysis where tendons attach to bone. A common condition at the traction epiphysis of the tibial tuberosity in children whose bones are still growing is called **Osgood-Schlatter disease.** Problems at these pressure and traction epiphyses usually exist only during the bone-growing years and not after the epiphyses have fused and bone growth stops.

Review Questions

1. What are the differences between the axial and appendicular skeletons?

2. Give one example of compact bone and one of cancellous bone.

3. Which is heavier, compact bone or cancellous bone? Why?

4. What type of bone is mainly involved in an individual's growth in height? In what portion of the bone does this growth occur?

5. What is the purpose of sesamoid bone?

6. Name the bone markings that can be classified as
   a. depressions and openings;
   b. projections or processes that fit into joints;
   c. projections or processes that attach connective tissue.

In Questions 7–9, classify the bone markings.

7. Bicipital groove

8. Humeral head

9. Acetabulum

10. What is the name of the membrane that lines the medullary canal?

11. The main shaft of bone is called what?

12. In children, does long bone growth occur at a traction epiphysis or at a pressure epiphysis?

13. Is the humerus part of the axial or appendicular skeleton?

14. Is the clavicle part of the axial or appendicular skeleton?

15. Is the sternum part of the axial or appendicular skeleton?

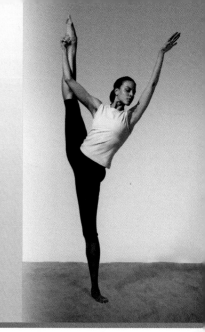

CHAPTER 3

Articular System

Types of Joints

Joint Structure

Planes and Axes

Degrees of Freedom

Common Pathological Terms

Review Questions

A joint is a connection between two bones. Although joints have several functions, perhaps the most important is to allow motion. Joints also help to bear the body's weight and to provide stability. This stability may be mostly due to the shape of the bones making up the joint, as with the hip joint, or may be due to soft tissue features, as seen in the shoulder and knee. Joints also contain synovial fluid, which lubricates the joint and nourishes the cartilage.

Types of Joints

A joint may allow a great deal of motion, as in the shoulder, or very little motion, as in the sternoclavicular joint. As with all differences, there are trade-offs. A joint that allows a great deal of motion will provide very little stability. Conversely, a joint that is quite stable tends to have little motion. There is often more than one term that can be used to describe the same joint. These terms tend to describe either the structure or the amount of motion allowed.

A **fibrous joint** has a thin layer of fibrous periosteum between the two bones, as in the sutures of the skull. There are three types of fibrous joints: synarthrosis, syndesmosis, and gomphosis. A **synarthrosis,** or suture joint, has a thin layer of fibrous periosteum between the two bones, as in the sutures of the skull. The ends of the bones are shaped to allow them to interlock (Fig. 3-1A). With this type of joint, there is essentially no motion between the bones; its purpose is to provide shape and strength. Another type of fibrous joint is a **syndesmosis,** or ligamentous joint. There is a great deal of fibrous tissue, such as ligaments and interosseous membranes, holding the joint together (Fig. 3-1B). A small amount of twisting or stretching movement can occur in this type of joint. The distal tibiofibular joint at the ankle and the distal radioulnar joint are examples. The third type of fibrous joint is called a **gomphosis,** which is Greek for

A. Synarthrosis (suture type)

B. Syndesmosis (ligamentous type)

C. Gomphosis (peg-in-socket)

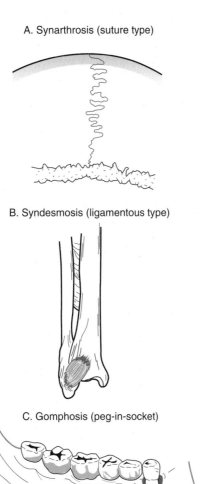

Figure 3-1.   Fibrous joints.

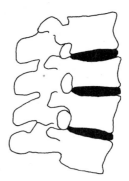

Figure 3-2.   Cartilaginous joint.

capsule. The outer layer of the capsule is made up of a strong fibrous tissue that holds the joint together. The inner layer is lined with a synovial membrane that secretes the synovial fluid. The articular surface is very smooth and covered with cartilage called *hyaline* or *articular cartilage.* The synovial joint is also called a **diarthrodial joint** because it allows free motion. It is not as stable as the other types of joints but does allow a great deal more motion. Table 3-1 provides a summary of the joint types. The number of axes, the shape of the joint, and the type of motion allowed by the joint could further classify synovial, or diarthrodial, joints (Table 3-2).

In a **nonaxial joint,** movement tends to be linear instead of angular (Fig. 3-4). The joint surfaces are relatively flat and glide over one another instead of one moving around the other and can be described as a **plane joint.** The motion that occurs between the carpal bones is an example of this type of motion. Unlike most other types of diarthrodial joint motion, nonaxial motion occurs secondarily to other motion. For example, you can flex and extend your elbow without moving other joints; however, you cannot move your carpal bones by themselves. Motion of the carpals occurs when

"bolting together." This joint occurs between a tooth and the wall of its dental socket in the mandible and maxilla (Fig. 3-1C). It's structure is referred to as *peg-in-socket.*

A **cartilaginous joint** (Fig. 3-2) has either hyaline cartilage or fibrocartilage between the two bones. The vertebral joints are examples of joints in which disks of fibrocartilage are directly connecting the bones. The first sternocostal joint is an example of the direct connection made by hyaline cartilage. Cartilaginous joints are also called **amphiarthrodial joints,** because they allow a small amount of motion, such as bending or twisting, and some compression. At the same time, these joints provide a great deal of stability.

A **synovial joint** (Fig. 3-3) has no direct union between the bone ends. Instead, there is a cavity filled with synovial fluid contained within a sleevelike

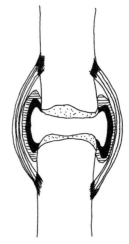

Figure 3-3.   Synovial joint.

Table 3-1	Joint Classification		
Type	**Motion**	**Structure**	**Example**
Synarthrosis	None	Fibrous—suture	Bones in the skull
Syndesmosis	Slight	Fibrous—ligamentous	Distal tibiofibular
Gomphosis	None	Fibrous—peg-in-socket	Teeth in mandible and maxilla
Amphiarthrosis	Little	Cartilaginous	Symphysis pubis, intervertebral disks
Diarthrosis	Free	Synovial	Hip, elbow, knee

Table 3-2	Classification of Diarthrodial Joints		
Number of Axes	**Shape of Joint**	**Joint Motion**	**Example**
Nonaxial	Plane (Irregular)	Gliding	Intercarpals
Uniaxial	Hinge	Flexion/extension	Elbow and knee
	Pivot	Rotation	Atlas/axis, radius/ulna
Biaxial	Condyloid (Ellipsoidal)	Flexion/extension, abduction/adduction	Wrist, MPs
	Saddle	Flexion/extension, abduction/adduction, rotation (accessory)	Thumb CMC
Triaxial (multiaxial)	Ball and socket	Flexion/extension, abduction/adduction, rotation	Shoulder, hip

the wrist joint moves in either flexion and extension or abduction and adduction.

A **uniaxial joint** has angular motion occurring in one plane around one axis, much like a hinge. The elbow, or humeroulnar joint, is a good example of a **hinge joint** with the convex shape of the humerus fitting into the concave-shaped ulna (Fig. 3-5). The only motions possible are flexion and extension, which occur in the sagittal plane around the frontal axis. No other motions are possible at this joint. The interphalangeal joints of the hand and foot also have this hinge motion. The knee is a hinge joint, but this example must be clarified. During the last few degrees of extension, the femur rotates medially on the tibia. This rotation is not an active motion but rather the result of certain mechanical features present. Therefore, the knee is best classified as a uniaxial joint, because it has *active* motion around only one axis.

Also at the elbow is the radioulnar joint, which as a **pivot joint,** demonstrates another type of uniaxial motion. The head of the radius pivots on the stationary ulna during pronation and supination of the forearm (Fig. 3-6). This pivot motion is in the transverse plane around the longitudinal axis. The motion of the atlantoaxial joint of C1 and C2 is also pivotal. The first cervical vertebra *(atlas),* on which the head rests, rotates

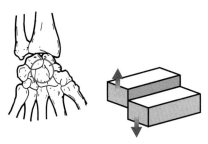

Figure 3-4.   Plane joint.

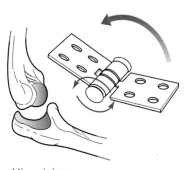

Figure 3-5.   Hinge joint.

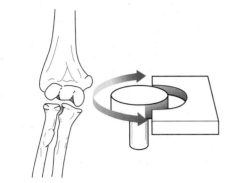

Figure 3-6.   Pivot joint.

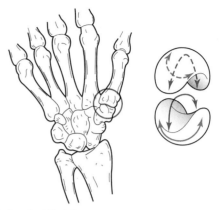

Figure 3-8.   Saddle joint.

around the odontoid process of the second cervical vertebra *(axis)*. This allows the head to rotate.

Biaxial joint motion, such as that found at the wrist, occurs in two different directions (Fig. 3-7). Flexion and extension occur around the frontal axis, and radial and ulnar deviation occur around the sagittal axis. This bidirectional motion also occurs at the metacarpophalangeal (MCP) joints, which are referred to as **condyloid joints,** or *ellipsoidal joints,* because of their shape.

The carpometacarpal (CMC) joint of the thumb is biaxial but differs somewhat from the condyloid joint. In this joint, the articular surface of each bone is concave in one direction and convex in the other. The bones fit together like a horseback rider in a saddle, which is why this joint is also descriptively called a **saddle joint** (Fig. 3-8).

Unlike the condyloid joint, the CMC joint allows a slight amount of rotation. Like the motion within the carpal bones, this rotation cannot occur by itself. If you try to rotate your thumb without also flexing and abducting, you find that you cannot do it. Yet, rotation does occur. Look at the direction to which the pad of your thumb is pointing when it is adducted. Abduct and flex your thumb and notice that the direction to which the pad is pointing has changed by approximately 90 degrees. This rotation has not occurred actively; rotation has

occurred because of the joint's shape. Therefore, although the CMC joint of the thumb is not a true biaxial joint due to the rotation allowed, it fits best into this category because the *active* motion allowed is around two axes.

With a **triaxial joint,** sometimes referred to as a *multiaxial joint,* motion occurs actively in all three axes (Fig. 3-9). This joint allows more motion than any other type of joint. The hip and shoulder allow motion around the frontal axis (flexion and extension), around the sagittal axis (abduction and adduction), and around the vertical axis (rotation). The triaxial joint is also referred to as a **ball-and-socket joint** because in the hip, for example, the ball-shaped femoral head fits into the concave socket of the acetabulum.

Joint Structure

There are many other structures associated with synovial joints (Fig. 3-10). First, there are **bones,** usually two, that

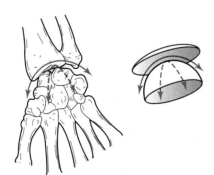

Figure 3-7.   Condyloid joint.

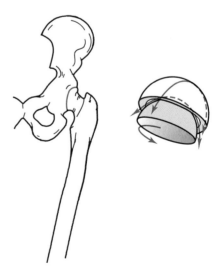

Figure 3-9.   Ball-and-socket joint.

articulate with each other. The amount and direction of motion allowed at each joint are dictated by the shape of the bone ends and by the articular surface of each bone. For example, the shoulder joint has a smooth articular surface over most of the humeral head and over the glenoid fossa (shoulder socket). As a result, there is a great deal of shoulder motion, and that motion occurs in all directions. The knee, on the other hand, has a great deal of motion but in a specific direction. In examining the distal end of the femur, you will note that there are two ridges much like the rocker surfaces of a rocking chair. The proximal end of the tibia has two articular surfaces with a high area (intercondylar eminence) in between them. These articular surfaces allow a great deal of motion but, like the rocking chair, in only one direction.

The two bones of a joint are held together and supported by **ligaments,** which are bands of fibrous connective tissue. Ligaments also provide attachment for cartilage, fascia, or, in some cases, muscle. Ligaments are flexible but not elastic. This flexibility is needed to allow joint motion, but the nonelasticity is needed to keep the bones in close approximation to each other and to provide some protection to the joint. In other words, ligaments prevent excessive joint movement. When ligaments surround a joint, they are called *capsular ligaments.*

Every synovial joint has a **capsule** that surrounds and encases the joint and protects the articular surfaces of the bones (Fig. 3-11). In the shoulder joint, the capsule completely encases the joint, forming a partial vacuum that helps hold the head of the humerus against the glenoid fossa. In other joints, the capsule may not be as complete.

The joint capsule has two layers: an outer layer and an inner layer. The outer layer consists of fibrous tissue and supports and protects the joint. This layer is usually reinforced by ligaments. The inner layer is lined with a **synovial membrane,** a thick, vascular connective tissue that secretes synovial fluid. **Synovial fluid** is a thick, clear fluid (similar to an egg white) that lubricates the articular cartilage; this reduces friction and helps the joint move freely. This fluid provides some shock absorption and is the major source of nutrition for articular cartilage.

Cartilage is a dense, fibrous connective tissue that can withstand great amounts of pressure and tension. The body has three basic types of cartilage: hyaline, fibrocartilage, and elastic. **Hyaline cartilage,** also called **articular cartilage,** covers the ends of opposing bones. With the help of synovial fluid, it provides a smooth articulating surface in all synovial joints. Because hyaline cartilage lacks its own blood or nerve supply and must get its nutrition from the synovial fluid, it cannot repair itself if it is damaged.

Fibrocartilage acts as a shock absorber. This is especially important in weight-bearing joints such as the knee and vertebrae. At the knee, the semilunar-shaped cartilage called **menisci** builds up the sides of the relatively flat articular surface of the tibia. Intervertebral **disks** (see Fig. 3-2) lie between the vertebral bones. Because of their very dense structure, these disks are capable of absorbing an amazing amount of shock that is transmitted upward from weight-bearing forces.

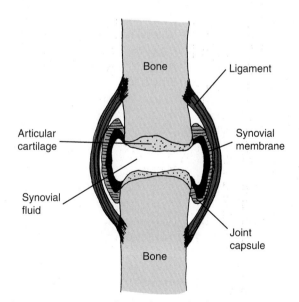

Figure 3-10.   Synovial joint, longitudinal cross section.

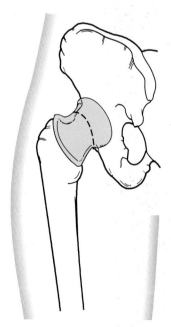

Figure 3-11.   Joint capsule.

In the upper extremity, a fibrocartilaginous disk located between the clavicle and sternum is important for absorbing the shock transmitted along the clavicle to the sternum should you fall on your outstretched hand. This disk helps prevent dislocation of the sternoclavicular joint. It is also important in allowing motion. The disk, which is attached to the sternum at one end and the clavicle at the other, is much like a swinging door hinge that allows motion in both directions. This double-hung hinge allows the clavicle to move on the sternum as the acromial end is elevated and depressed. In effect, the fibrocartilage divides the joint into two cavities, allowing two sets of motion.

There are other functions of fibrocartilage in joints. The shoulder fibrocartilage, called **labrum,** deepens the shallow glenoid fossa, making it more of a socket to hold the humeral head (Fig. 3-12). Fibrocartilage also fills the gap between two bones. If you examine the wrist, you will notice that the ulna does not extend all the way to the carpal bones, as does the radius. A small triangular disk located in this gap acts as a space filler and allows force to be exerted on the ulna and carpals without causing damage.

The third type of cartilage, **elastic cartilage,** is designed to help maintain a structure's shape. It is found in the external ear and eustachian (auditory) tube. It is also found in the larynx, where its motion is important to speech.

Muscles provide the contractile force that causes joints to move. Therefore, they must span the joint to have an effect on that joint. Muscles are soft and cannot attach directly to the bone. A **tendon** must connect them to bone. The tendon may be a cylindrical cord, like the long head of the biceps tendon, or a flattened band, like the rotator cuff. In certain locations, tendons are encased in **tendon sheaths.** These fibrous sleeves surround the tendon when it is subject to pressure or friction, such as when it passes between muscles and bones or through a tunnel between bones. The tendons passing over the wrist all have tendon sheaths. These sheaths are lubricated by fluid secreted from their lining.

An **aponeurosis** is a broad, flat tendinous sheet. Aponeuroses are found in several places where muscles attach to bones. The large, powerful latissimus dorsi muscle is attached at one end over a large area to several bones by means of an aponeurosis. In the anterior abdominal wall, aponeuroses provide a base of muscular attachment where no bone is present but where great strength is needed. As the abdominal muscles approach the midline from both sides, they attach to an aponeurosis called the **linea alba.**

Bursae are small, padlike sacs found around most joints. They are located in areas of excessive friction, such as under tendons and over bony prominences (Fig. 3-13). Lined with synovial membrane and filled with a clear fluid, bursae reduce friction between moving parts. For example, in the shoulder, the deltoid muscle passes directly over the acromion process. Repeated motion would cause excessive wearing of the muscle tissue. However, the subdeltoid bursa that is located between the muscle and acromion process prevents excessive friction and reduces the likelihood of damage. The same arrangement occurs in the elbow, where the triceps tendon attaches to the olecranon process. Some joints, such as the knee, have many bursae. There are two types of bursae: natural bursae (which has just been described) and acquired bursae. A bursa can appear in an area that normally does not have excessive friction if such friction occurs in that area. These *acquired bursae* tend to occur in places other than joints. For example, a person may develop a bursa on the lateral side of the third finger of the writing hand. This is often called the "student's bursa," because students often do a lot of writing and note taking. These bursae disappear when the activity is stopped or greatly reduced.

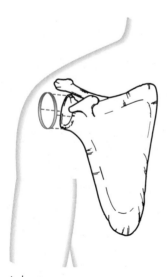

Figure 3-12.   Labrum.

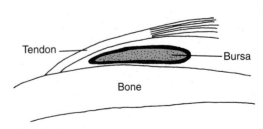

Figure 3-13.   Bursa.

Planes and Axes

Planes of action are fixed lines of reference along which the body is divided. There are three planes, and each plane is at right angles, or perpendicular, to the other two planes (Fig. 3-14).

The **sagittal plane** passes through the body from front to back and divides the body into right and left parts. Think of it as a vertical wall that the extremity moves along. Motions occurring in this plane are flexion and extension.

The **frontal plane** passes through the body from side to side and divides the body into front and back parts. It is also called the *coronal plane*. Motions occurring in this plane are abduction and adduction.

The **transverse plane** passes through the body horizontally and divides the body into top and bottom parts. It is also called the *horizontal plane*. Rotation occurs in this plane.

Whenever a plane passes through the midline of a part, whether it is the sagittal, frontal, or transverse plane, it is referred to as a *cardinal plane,* because it divides the body into equal parts. The point where the three cardinal planes intersect each other is the **center of gravity.** In the human body, that point is in the midline at about the level of, though slightly anterior to, the second sacral vertebra (Fig. 3-15).

Axes are points that run through the center of a joint around which a part rotates (Fig. 3-16). The **sagittal axis** is a point that runs through a joint from front to back. The **frontal axis** runs through a joint from side to side. The **vertical axis,** also called the *longitudinal axis,* runs through a joint from top to bottom.

Joint movement occurs around an axis that is always perpendicular to its plane. Another way of stating this is that joint movement occurs *in a plane* and *around an axis.* A particular motion will always occur in the same plane and around the same axis. For example, flexion/extension will always occur in the sagittal plane around the frontal axis. Abduction/adduction will always occur in the frontal plane around the sagittal axis. Similar motions, such as radial and ulnar deviation of the wrist, will also

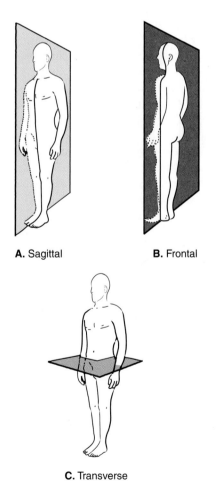

A. Sagittal

B. Frontal

C. Transverse

Figure 3-14. The planes of the body. **(A)** Sagittal plane. **(B)** Frontal plane. **(C)** Transverse plane.

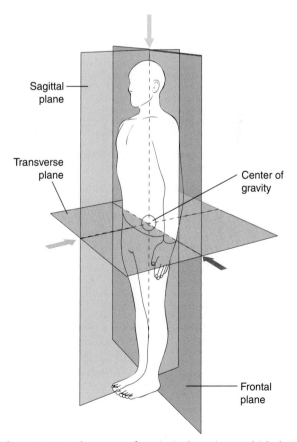

Sagittal plane

Transverse plane

Center of gravity

Frontal plane

Figure 3-15. The center of gravity is the point at which the three cardinal planes intersect.

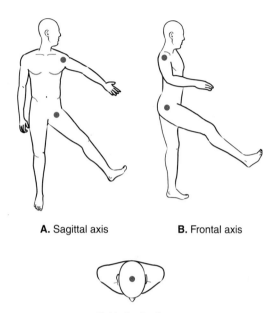

A. Sagittal axis   **B.** Frontal axis

C. Vertical axis

Figure 3-16.   The axes of the body. **(A)** Sagittal axis.
(B) Frontal axis. **(C)** Vertical axis.

occur in the frontal plane around the sagittal axis. The
thumb is the exception, because flexion/extension and
abduction/adduction do not occur in these traditional
planes. (These thumb motions, and their planes and axes,
will be described in Chapter 13.) Table 3-3 summarizes
joint motion in relation to planes and axes.

Degrees of Freedom

Joints can also be described by the degrees of freedom,
or number of planes, in which they can move. For example, a uniaxial joint has motion around one axis and in
one plane. Therefore, it has one degree of freedom. A
biaxial joint would have two degrees of freedom, and a

Table 3-3	Joint Motions	
Plane	**Axis**	**Joint Motion**
Sagittal	Frontal	Flexion/extension
Frontal	Sagittal	Abduction/adduction
		Radial/ulnar deviation
		Eversion/inversion
Transverse	Vertical	Medial/lateral rotation
		Supination/pronation
		Right/left rotation
		Horizontal abduction/
		adduction

triaxial joint would have three, the maximum number
of degrees of freedom that an individual joint can have.

This concept becomes significant when dealing with
one or more distal joints. For example, the shoulder has
three degrees of freedom, the elbow and radioulnar
joints each have one, and together they have five degrees
of freedom. The entire limb from the finger to the
shoulder would have 11 degrees of freedom.

Common Pathological Terms

Dislocation refers to the complete separation of the two
articular surfaces of a joint. A portion of the joint capsule
surrounding the joint will be torn. **Subluxation,** a partial dislocation of a joint, usually occurs over a period of
time. A common example is a shoulder subluxation that
develops after a person has had a stroke. Muscle paralysis
and the weight of the arm slowly subluxes the shoulder
joint.

Osteoarthritis is a type of arthritis that is caused by
the breakdown and eventual loss of the cartilage of one
or more joints. Also known as *degenerative arthritis,* it
occurs more frequently as we age and commonly affects
the hands, feet, spine, and large weight-bearing joints,
such as the hips and knees.

Sprains are a partial or complete tearing of ligament
fibers. A *mild* sprain involves the tearing of a few fibers
with no loss of function. With a *moderate* sprain, there is
partial tearing of the ligament with some loss of function. In a *severe* sprain, the ligament is completely torn
(ruptured) and no longer functions. **Strain** refers to the
overstretching of muscle fibers. As with sprains, strains
are graded depending on severity.

Tendonitis is an inflammation of a tendon.
Synovitis is an inflammation of the synovial membrane. **Tenosynovitis** is an inflammation of the tendon sheath and is often caused by repetitive use. The
tendon of the long head of the biceps and the flexor
tendons of the hand are common sites. **Bursitis** is an
inflammation of the bursa. **Capsulitis** is an inflammation of the joint capsule.

Review Questions

1. What are the three types of joints that allow little or no motion?

2. What are the two terms for a joint that allows a great deal of motion?

3. What are the three features that describe diarthrodial joints?

4. What type of joint structure connects bone to muscle?

5. What type of joint structure pads and protects areas of great friction?

6. How does hyaline cartilage differ from fibrocartilage? Give an example of each type of cartilage.

7. When the anterior surface of the forearm moves toward the anterior surface of the humerus, what joint motion is involved? In what plane is the motion occurring? Around what axis?

8. What joint motions are involved in turning the palm of the hand? In what plane and around what axis does that joint motion occur?

9. What joint motion is involved in returning the fingers to anatomical position from the fully spread position? In what plane and around what axis does the joint motion occur?

10. Identify the 11 degrees of freedom of the upper extremity.

11. Give an example of a synarthrodial joint in the axial skeleton.

12. *Diarthrodial, synovial, triaxial,* and *ball-and-socket* are all terms that could be used to describe which joint of the upper extremity? Could these same terms apply to a joint in the lower extremity? If so, what joint is it?

13. *Diarthrodial, synovial, biaxial,* and *saddle* are all terms that could be used to describe which joint?

14. What are two joint terms that could be used to describe the symphysis pubis?

15. What joint structure surrounds and encases the joint and protects the articular surfaces?

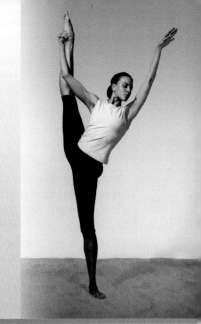

CHAPTER 4
Arthrokinematics

Osteokinematic Motion

   End Feel

Arthrokinematic Motion

   Accessory Motion Terminology

   Joint Surface Shape

   Types of Arthrokinematic Motion

   Convex-Concave Rule

   Joint Surface Positions (Joint Congruency)

   Accessory Motion Forces

Points to Remember

Review Questions

Osteokinematic Motion

Joint movement is commonly thought of as one bone moving on another, causing such motions as flexion, extension, abduction, adduction, or rotation. These movements, which are done under voluntary control, are often referred to as **classical, physiological,** or **osteokinematic motion.** This type of motion can be done in the form of isometric, isotonic, or even isokinetic exercises. When performed actively, muscles move joints through ranges of motion (ROMs). As we move our joints throughout the day, we are actively performing osteokinematic movements. These movements were described in Chapter 1. When a person moves a joint passively through its range of motion, it is usually done to assist in maintaining full motion or to determine the nature of the resistance at the end of the range. The latter is called the *end feel* of a joint.

End Feel

End feel is a subjective assessment of the *quality* of the feel when slight pressure is applied at the end of the joint's passive range of motion. It was first described by Cyriax (1983), who stressed the importance of the tactile sensation end feel that the examiner senses during passive motion.

An end feel may be either normal or abnormal. A normal end feel exists when there is full passive ROM at a joint, and the normal anatomical structures (e.g., bone, capsule, muscle, or muscle length) stop the movement. Abnormal end feel may be present when pain, muscle guarding, swelling, or abnormal anatomy stops the joint movement.

The three types of normal end feel are bony, soft tissue stretch, and soft tissue approximation. *Bony* is sometimes used to describe normal or abnormal end feel. Normal **bony end feel** is characterized by a hard and abrupt limit to passive joint motion. This occurs when bone contacts bone at the end of the ROM, and sometimes it is called *hard end feel*. An example would be normal terminal elbow extension as the bony olecranon process contacts the bony olecranon fossa. Normal **soft tissue stretch** is characterized by a firm sensation that has slight give when the joint is taken to the end-range of motion. This *firm end feel*, as it is sometimes called, results from tension in the surrounding ligaments, capsule, and muscles. This is the most common end feel. Examples would be shoulder medial and lateral rotation, hip and knee extension, and ankle dorsiflexion. **Soft tissue approximation** occurs when muscle bulk is compressed, giving a *soft end feel*, as it is sometimes called. For example, elbow flexion is stopped by the approximation of the forearm and arm. This is particularly evident on a person with well-developed muscles or who is extremely obese.

Abnormal end feel can be described as bony, boggy, muscle spasm, empty, and springy block. These terms can be used to quantify the limitation of joint motion. An **abnormal bony end feel** is the sudden hard stop usually felt well before the end of normal ROM, when abnormal bony structures such as an osteophyte (bone spur) block the joint's motion. **Boggy end feel** is often found in acute conditions in which soft tissue edema is present, such as immediately after a severe sprained ankle or with synovitis. It has a soft, "wet sponge" feel. **Muscle spasm** is a reflexive muscle guarding during motion. It is a protective response seen with acute injury. Palpation of the muscle will reveal the muscle in spasm. The ability to palpate normal end feel and to distinguish changes from normal end feel is important in protecting joints during ROM exercises. **Empty end feel** occurs when movement produces considerable pain. There is no mechanical limitation at the end of the range, because the individual will not let you move the part through further ROM. With **springy block**, a rebound movement is felt at the end of the ROM. It usually occurs with internal derangement of a joint, such as torn cartilage.

Arthrokinematic Motion

Another way of viewing joint movement is to look at what is taking place within the joint at the joint surfaces. Called **arthrokinematic motion,** it is defined as the manner in which adjoining joint surfaces move on each other during osteokinematic joint movement. Therefore, osteokinematic motion is referred to as *joint motion,* and arthrokinematic motion is referred to as *joint surface motion.*

Accessory Motion Terminology

Terminology can be somewhat confusing, because various experts use terminology somewhat differently. That said, there are two types of accessory motion that must be described. **Component movements** are motions that accompany active motion but are not under voluntary control. For example, the shoulder girdle must rotate upward for the shoulder joint to flex. The femur rotates on the tibia during the last few degrees of knee extension. Rotation occurs at the thumb during opposition. None of these motions can be done independently, but they must occur for normal joint motion to occur. **Joint play** movements are passive movements between joint surfaces done by passively applying external force. These movements are also not under voluntary control. This includes such motions as glide, spin, and roll, which will be defined later.

Regardless of how these accessory movements are defined, it is generally agreed that they are necessary for joint mobilization. **Joint mobilization** is generally described as a passive oscillatory motion or sustained stretch that is applied at a slow enough speed by an external force that the individual can stop the motion. It is used to improve joint mobility or to decrease pain originating in joint structures. Further discussion of joint mobilization is beyond the scope of this book. These terms and related concepts are introduced to provide a basic understanding of joint movement. Another term, **manipulation,** is defined as a passive movement applied within a short range and with a very forceful thrust that cannot be stopped. It is applied under anesthesia. This maneuver, too, is well beyond the scope of this text.

Joint Surface Shape

To understand arthrokinematics, one must recognize that the type of motion occurring at a joint depends on the shape of the articulating surfaces of the bones. Most joints have one concave bone end and one convex bone end (Fig. 4-1). A convex surface is rounded outward, much like a mound. A concave surface is "caved" in, much like a cave.

All joint surfaces are either ovoid or sellar. An **ovoid joint** has two bones forming a convex-concave relationship. For example, in the metacarpophalangeal joint, one surface is concave (proximal phalanx) and the other is convex (metacarpal; see Fig. 4-1). Most synovial joints are ovoid. In an ovoid joint, one bone end is usually larger than its adjacent bone end. This permits a greater ROM on a less articular surface, which reduces the size of the joint.

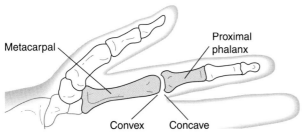

Figure 4-1. Shape of bone surfaces of an ovoid joint—MCP joint of finger.

In a **sellar,** or **saddle-shaped, joint,** each joint surface is concave in one direction and convex in another. The carpometacarpal (CMP) joint of the thumb is perhaps the best example of a sellar joint (Fig. 4-2). If you look at the carpal bone (trapezium), it is concave in a front-to-back direction and convex in a side-to-side direction. The first metacarpal bone that articulates with the carpal bone has just the opposite shape. It is convex in a front-to-back direction and concave in a side-to-side direction.

Types of Arthrokinematic Motion

The types of arthrokinematic motion are roll, glide, and spin. Most joint movement involves a combination of all three of these motions. **Roll** is the rolling of one joint surface on another. New points on each surface come into contact throughout the motion (Fig. 4-3). Examples include the surface of your shoe on the floor during walking, or a ball rolling across the ground. **Glide,** or

slide, is linear movement of a joint surface parallel to the plane of the adjoining joint surface (Fig. 4-4). In other words, one point on a joint surface contacts new points on the adjacent surface. An ice-skater's blade (one point) sliding across the ice surface (many points) demonstrates the glide motion. **Spin** is the rotation of the movable joint surface on the fixed adjacent surface (Fig. 4-5). Essentially the same point on each surface remains in contact with each other. An example of this type of movement would be a top spinning on a table. If the top remains perfectly upright, it spins in one place. Examples in the body would be any pure (relatively speaking) rotational movement, such as the humerus rotating medially and laterally in the glenoid fossa, or the head of the radius spinning on the capitulum of the humerus.

As we will discuss in Chapter 19, the knee joint motion clearly demonstrates that all three types of arthrokinematic motion are necessary to obtain full knee flexion and extension. In this motion during weight-bearing, the femoral condyles roll on the tibial condyles. Because of the large range of flexion and extension permitted at the knee, the femur would roll

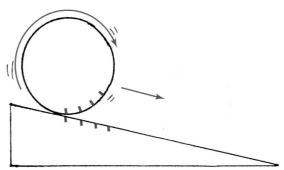

Figure 4-3. Roll—movement of one joint surface on another. New points on each surface make contact.

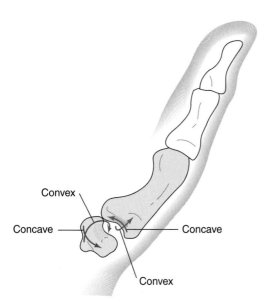

Figure 4-2. Shape of bone surfaces of a sellar joint—CMP joint of thumb.

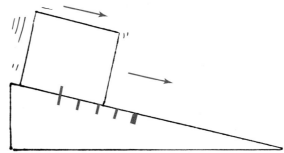

Figure 4-4. Glide—linear movement of one joint surface parallel to the other joint surface. One point on one surface contacts new points on other surface.

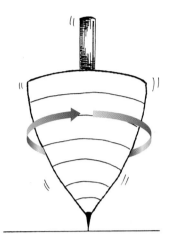

Figure 4-5. Spin—rotation of one joint surface on another. Same point on each surface remains in contact.

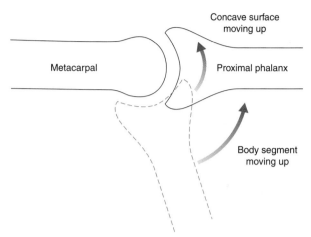

Figure 4-6. The concave surface moves in the same direction as the body segment.

off the tibia if the femoral condyles did not also glide posteriorly on the tibia. Because the medial and lateral femoral condyles are different sizes, and the medial and lateral aspects of the knee joint move at different speeds, there must be spin (medial rotation) of the femur on the tibia during the last 15 degrees of knee extension. In a non-weight-bearing activity, the same motions are occurring except that the tibia is moving on the femur, and the spin motion is lateral rotation of the tibia on the femur (see Fig. 19-3B).

Convex-Concave Rule

Knowing that a joint surface is concave or convex is important, because shape determines motion. The **concave-convex rule** describes how the differences in shapes of bone ends require joint surfaces to move in a specific way during joint movement.

The rule is described as follows: A concave joint surface will move on a fixed convex surface in the same direction the body segment is moving. For example, the proximal portion of the proximal phalanx is concave, and the distal portion of the metacarpal is convex (Fig. 4-6). During finger extension (from finger flexion), the proximal phalanx moves in the same direction as the phalanx itself while moving on the convex metacarpal joint surface. To summarize, the **concave joint surface** moves in the **same direction** as the body segment's motion. On the other hand, a convex joint surface will move on a fixed concave surface in the opposite direction as the moving body segment. For example, the head of the humerus is convex, whereas the glenoid fossa of the scapula, in which it articulates, is concave (Fig. 4-7). During shoulder flexion, the convex surface of the humeral head moves in the opposite direction (downward) from the rest of the humerus,

which is moving upward. Thus, the **convex joint surface** moves in the **opposite direction** of the body segment's movement.

There is an easy visual way to remember this rule. To represent a joint, make a fist with your left hand and place it inside your cupped right hand. Your left fist represents a convex joint surface of one bone. The left forearm represents the bone. Your cupped right hand represents a concave surface of the other bone. Keeping your hands at the same level, your wrist straight, and your left fist rotating inside the cupped hand, raise your left

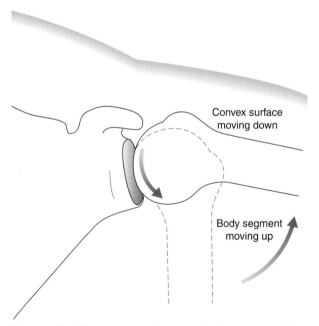

Figure 4-7. The convex surface moves in the opposite direction from the body segment.

elbow. Notice that as your forearm (body segment) moves up, your fist (joint surface) rotates down. In other words, the convex surface moves in the opposite direction as the body segment's motion. Repeat the action, with the cupped hand moving on the fist. Raise your right elbow and notice that your cupped right hand is moving up and over the left fist. The concave surface (cupped hand) is moving in the same direction as the body segment's (right forearm) motion.

Joint Surface Positions (Joint Congruency)

How well joint surfaces match or fit is called *joint congruency*. The surfaces of a joint are congruent in one position and incongruent in all other positions. When a joint is **congruent,** the joint surfaces have maximum contact with each other, are tightly compressed and are difficult to distract (separate). The ligaments and capsule holding the joint together are taut. This is known

as the **close-packed,** or **closed-pack, position.** It usually occurs at one extreme of the ROM. For example, if you place your knee in the fully extended position, you can manually move the patella slightly from side to side and up and down. However, if you flex your knee, such patellar movement is *not* possible. Therefore, the close-packed position of the patellofemoral joint is knee flexion. Other close-packed positions are ankle dorsiflexion; metacarpophalangeal flexion; and extension of the elbow, wrist, hip, knee, and interphalanges. Table 4-1 gives a more detailed listing of the close-packed positions of joints.

When ligaments and capsular structures are tested for stability and integrity, the joint is usually placed in the close-packed position. By the nature of the characteristics of a close-packed position, a joint is often in this position when injured. For example, a knee joint that sustains a lateral force when it is extended (closed-packed position) is much more likely to be injured than when it is in a flexed or semiflexed position (loose-packed position). Also,

Table 4-1	Comparison of Close-Packed and Loose-Packed Position of Joints	
Joint(s)	**Close-Packed Position**	**Loose Packed Position**
Facet (spine)	Extension	Midway between flexion and extension
Temporomandibular	Clenched teeth	Mouth slightly open (freeway space)
Glenohumeral	Abduction and lateral rotation	55° abduction, 30° horizontal adduction
Acromioclavicular	Arm abducted to 30°	Arm resting by side in normal physiological position
Ulnohumeral (elbow)	Extension	70° flexion, 10° supination
Radiohumeral	Elbow flexed 90°, forearm supinated 5°	Full extension and supination
Proximal radioulnar	5° supination	70° flexion, 35° supination
Radiocarpal (wrist)	Extension with ulnar deviation	Neutral with slight ulnar deviation
Carpometacarpal	N/A	Midway between abduction/adduction and flexion/extension
Metacarpophalangeal (fingers)	Full flexion	Slight flexion
Metacarpophalangeal (thumb)	Full opposition	Slight flexion
Interphalangeal	Full extension	Slight flexion
Hip	Full extension and medial rotation*	30° flexion, 30° abduction and slight lateral rotation
Knee	Full extension and lateral rotation of tibia	25° flexion
Talocrural (ankle)	Maximum dorsiflexion	10° plantar flexion, midway between maximum inversion and eversion
Metatarsophalangeal	Full extension	Neutral
Interphalangeal	Full extension	Slight flexion

*Some authors include abduction.
Adapted from Magee, DJ: Orthopedic Physical Assessment, ed 4. WB Saunders, Philadelphia, 2002, p 50, with permission.

when a joint is swollen, it cannot be moved into the close-packed position.

In all other positions, the joint surfaces are incongruent. The position of maximum incongruence is called the **open-packed** or **loose-packed position.** It is also referred to as the **resting position.** Parts of the capsule and supporting ligaments are lax. There is minimal congruency between the articular surfaces. Further passive separation of the joint surfaces can occur in this position. Because the ligaments and capsular structures tend to be more relaxed, joint mobilization techniques are best applied in the open-packed position. It is these open-packed positions that allow for the roll, spin, and glide that are necessary for normal joint motion. Table 4-1 gives a more detailed listing of the loose-packed positions of joints and compares these positions with those of the close-packed positions.

Also, a certain amount of **accessory motions,** or **joint play,** can be demonstrated in these open-packed positions. This is the passive movement of one articular surface over another. Because joint play is not a voluntary movement, it requires relaxed muscles and the external force of a trained practitioner to correctly demonstrate it.

Accessory Motion Forces

When applying joint mobilization, three main types of forces are used: traction, compression, and shearing. Bending and torsional forces are the result of a combination of forces.

Traction, also called **distraction** or **tension,** occurs when external force is exerted on a joint, causing the joint surfaces to pull apart (Fig. 4-8). Carrying a heavy suitcase or hanging from an overhead bar causes traction to the shoulder, elbow, and wrist joints. You can demonstrate this on another person by grasping their index finger at the proximal end of the middle phalanx with one thumb and index finger. Next, grasp the distal end of the proximal phalanx with your other thumb and index finger. Move the proximal interphalangeal (PIP) joint into a slightly flexed position (loose-packed position), and pull gently in opposite directions. This

description, and others to follow, is meant to illustrate the various forces and is not a description of therapeutic technique. *Extreme care must be exercised when performing these motions.*

Approximation, also called **compression,** occurs when an external force is exerted on a joint, causing the joint surfaces to be pushed closer together (Fig. 4-9). Doing a chair or floor push-up causes the joint surfaces of the shoulder, elbow, and wrist to be approximated. As a general rule, traction can assist a joint's mobility and approximation can assist a joint's stability.

Shear forces occur parallel to the surface (Fig. 4-10). Shear force results in a glide motion at the joint. Using the positions described with distraction, grasp another person's index finger at the proximal end of the middle phalanx with one thumb and index finger. Next, grasp the distal end of the proximal phalanx with your other thumb and index finger. With the PIP joint slightly flexed, gently move your two hands in an opposite up-and-down motion. This motion describes anterior/posterior glide of the PIP joint (a shearing force).

Bending and torsional forces are actually a combination of forces. **Bending** occurs when an other-than-vertical force is applied, resulting in compression on the concave side and distraction on the convex side (Fig. 4-11). Rotary or torsional forces involve a twisting motion. One force is trying to turn one end or part about a longitudinal axis while the other force is fixed or turning in the opposite direction (Fig. 4-12).

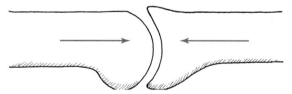

Figure 4-9.   Compression force causes bone ends to move toward each other.

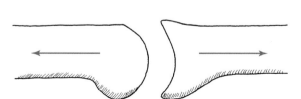

Figure 4-8.   Traction force causes bone ends to move apart from each other.

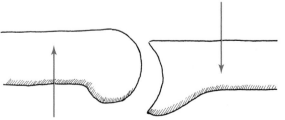

Figure 4-10.   Shear force causes bone ends to move parallel to and in opposite direction from each other.

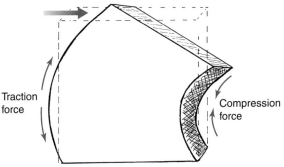

Figure 4-11.   Bending force causes compression on one side and traction on the other side.

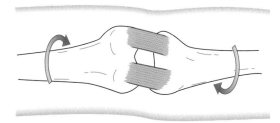

Figure 4-12.   Rotary or torsional force is a twisting motion.

Points to Remember

- Normal end feel can be described as bony, soft tissue stretch, or soft tissue approximation.
- Abnormal end feel can be described as bony, boggy, empty, springy block, or muscle spasm.
- Joint surface shape can be ovoid or sellar.
- Types of arthrokinematic motion are roll, glide, or spin.

- According to the concave-convex rule, concave joint surfaces move in the same direction as the joint or body segment's motion, while convex surfaces move in the opposite direction as the joint motion.
- When a joint is congruent, it is in the close-packed position. When the joint is incongruent, it is in the open-packed position.
- When mobilizing a joint, traction, compression, shear, bending, or torsional forces may be used.

Review Questions

1. a. Is shoulder flexion and extension an arthrokinematic or osteokinematic type of motion?
   b. Is shoulder distraction an arthrokinematic or osteokinematic type of motion?
2. You would feel what type of end feel at the end of the knee flexion range?
3. Flex the shoulder from an extended position.
   a. Is the humerus moving on the scapula, or is the scapula moving on the humerus?
   b. Is the proximal end of the humerus a concave or convex joint surface?
   c. Does the glenoid fossa of the scapula have a concave or convex joint surface?
   d. Is the concave surface moving on a fixed convex surface, or is a convex surface moving on a fixed concave surface?
   e. Is the joint surface moving in the same or opposite direction as the joint motion?
4. Identify the accessory motion force(s) occurring in the following activities:
   a. Leaning on a table with your elbows extended
   b. Transferring from a wheelchair to the car using a sliding board
   c. Picking up one end of a table
   d. Opening a jar
   e. Swinging a child around by her arms
5. Is the temporomandibular joint (TMJ) (jaw) in the close-packed position when the teeth are clenched or when the mouth is slightly open?
6. In terms of joint congruency, describe how a stack of Pringles potato chips fits together (see Fig. 13-2). Place a stack of two chips in front of you with the long end pointing toward you in an anterior-posterior position. Consider the joint surfaces of each chip in contact with the other:
   a. Is the anterior/posterior shape of the bottom surface of the top chip concave or convex?
   b. Is the anterior/posterior shape of the top surface of the bottom chip concave or convex?
   c. Is the medial/lateral shape of the bottom surface of the top chip concave or convex?
   d. Is the medial/lateral shape of the top surface of the bottom chip concave or convex?
   e. If these chips represented a joint, would the shape of the joint be ovoid or sellar?

(continued on next page)

Review Questions—cont'd

7. Rotating a quarter on its edge across the table demonstrates what type of arthrokinematics motion?

8. Lay the quarter flat on the table and hit it with your finger, sending it across the table. This would be what type of arthrokinematics motion?

9. In comparing the size of a quarter and a nickel, note that the quarter is larger. Place a pencil mark on the quarter at the 6 and 12 o'clock positions. Lay a nickel flat on the table. Roll the quarter across the flat surface of the nickel, starting with the quarter at the 6 o'clock position at the edge of the nickel.
   a. Will the quarter reach the edge of the nickel before reaching the 12 o'clock position?
   b. Which arthrokinematic motion will you have to use on the quarter, in addition to roll, so that the 12 o'clock mark can reach the opposite side of the nickel?

10. Hold a pencil vertically with the lead end on the table. Holding the eraser end between your thumb and index finger, roll the pencil between your fingers, keeping the lead end in contact with the table. This is demonstrating which type of arthrokinematic motion?

11. Assuming muscles are of normal length and taking a person's ankle into dorsiflexion, you would expect what type of end feel?

12. A person bends down to touch the floor in the sagittal plane.
    a. What type of force is applied to the anterior part of the vertebra?
    b. What type of force is applied to the posterior part of the vertebra?

13. Sitting in a chair, a man turns around to look behind him. What type of force is being applied to the vertebral column?

14. The surfaces of the thumb metacarpophalangeal (MCP) joint are what shape?

15. Is the rotational motion at the thumb carpometacarpal (CMC) joint considered a classical movement or an accessory movement? Why?

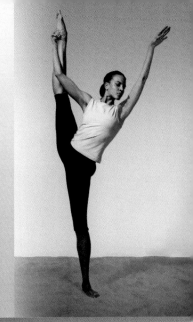

CHAPTER 5
Muscular System

Muscle Attachments

Muscle Names

Muscle Fiber Arrangement

Functional Characteristics
of Muscle Tissue

Length-Tension Relationship
in Muscle Tissue

Active and Passive Insufficiency

Types of Muscle Contraction

Roles of Muscles

Angle of Pull

Kinetic Chains

Points to Remember

Review Questions

Muscle Attachments

When a muscle contracts, it knows no direction—it simply shortens. If a muscle were unattached at both ends and stimulated, the two ends would move toward the middle. However, muscles are attached to bones and cross at least one joint, so when a muscle contracts, one end of the joint moves toward the other. The more movable bone, often referred to as the **insertion,** moves toward the more stable bone, called the **origin.** For example, when the biceps brachii muscle contracts, the forearm moves toward the humerus, as when bringing a glass toward your mouth (Fig. 5-1A). The humerus is more stable because it is attached to the axial skeleton at the shoulder joint. The forearm is more movable because it is attached to the hand, which is quite movable. Therefore, the insertion is moving toward the

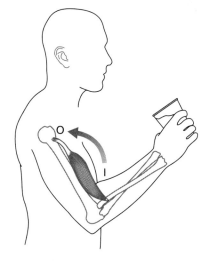

Insertion moves toward origin

A

Figure 5-1. **(A)** Direction of movement of biceps muscle attachments.

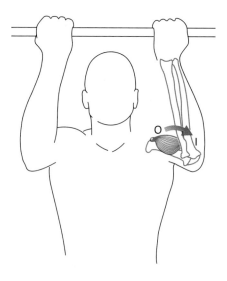

Origin moves toward insertion

B

Figure 5-1. **(B)** Direction of movement of biceps muscle attachments in reversal of muscle actions.

origin; explained another way, the more movable end is traveling toward the more stable end. Another point that can be made about muscle attachments is that origins tend to be closer to the trunk, and insertions tend to be closer to the distal end.

This arrangement can be reversed if the more movable end becomes less movable. For example, what happens when the hand is holding on to a chin-up bar when the biceps contract? The biceps still flex the elbow, but now the humerus moves toward the forearm. In other words, the origin moves toward the insertion (Fig. 5-1B). Some sources refer to this as **reversal of muscle action.** However, you should realize that the same joint motion is occurring (in this case, elbow flexion). What has changed is that instead of the insertion moving toward the origin, the origin is now moving toward the insertion. The proximal bone, which is usually more stable, has become more movable.

Consider another example in a very simplistic form. Lying on your back, bring your knees up toward your chest. Using your hip flexors to flex your hip, you are moving the femur (more movable) toward your chest (more stable), or moving the insertion toward the origin. If someone holds your feet down, your femur would become the more stable end and your trunk would become the more movable end. When your hip flexors contract, the origin moves toward the insertion. Closed kinetic chain exercises are based on the distal

segment being fixed and the proximal end being moved. This is another way of applying reversal of muscle action. Open and closed kinetic chains will be discussed later in this chapter.

Muscle Names

The name of a muscle can often tell you a great deal about that muscle. Muscle names tend to fall into one or more of the following categories:

1. Location
2. Shape
3. Action
4. Number of heads or divisions
5. Attachments = origin/insertion
6. Direction of the fibers
7. Size of the muscle

The tibialis anterior, as its name indicates, is located on the anterior surface of the tibia. The rectus (meaning "straight" in Latin) abdominis muscle is a vertical muscle located on the abdomen. The trapezius muscle has a trapezoid shape, and the serratus anterior muscle (Fig. 5-2) has a serrated or jagged-shaped attachment anteriorly. The name of the extensor carpi ulnaris muscle tells you that its action is to extend the wrist (carpi) on the ulnar side. The triceps brachii muscle is a three-headed muscle on the arm, and the biceps femoris muscle is a two-headed muscle on the thigh. The sternocleidomastoid muscle (Fig. 5-3) attaches on the sternum, clavicle, and mastoid bones. The names of the external and internal oblique muscles describe the

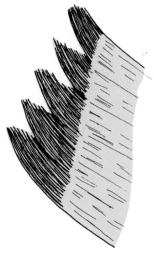

Figure 5-2. The serratus anterior muscle has a saw-toothed shape.

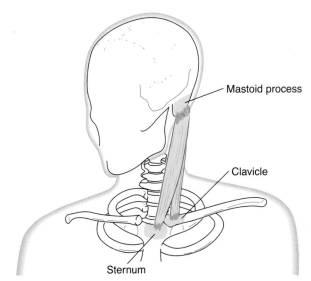

Figure 5-3. The sternocleidomastoid muscle is named for its attachments on the sternum, clavicle, and mastoid bone.

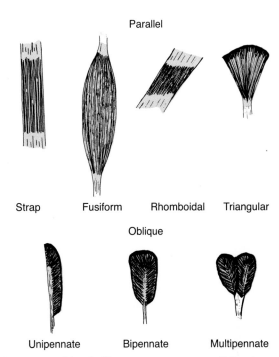

Figure 5-4. Muscle fiber arrangements, parallel and oblique.

direction of the fibers and their location to one another. In the same way, the names *pectoralis major* and *pectoralis minor* indicate that although both of these muscles are in the same area, one is larger than the other.

Muscle Fiber Arrangement

Muscle fibers are arranged within the muscle in a direction that is either parallel or oblique to the muscle's long axis (Fig. 5-4). **Parallel muscle** fibers tend to be longer and thus have a greater range of motion potential. **Oblique muscle** fibers tend to be shorter but are more numerous per given area than parallel fibers, which means that oblique-fibered muscles tend to have a greater strength potential but a smaller range-of-motion potential than parallel-fibered muscles. There are many types of each muscle fiber arrangement in the body.

Parallel-fibered muscles can be strap, fusiform, rhomboidal (rectangular), or triangular in shape. **Strap muscles** are those that are long and thin with fibers running the entire length of the muscle. The sartorius muscle in the lower extremity, the rectus abdominis in the trunk, and the sternocleidomastoid in the neck are examples of strap muscles.

A **fusiform muscle** has a shape similar to that of a spindle. It is wider in the middle and tapers at both ends where it attaches to tendons. Most, but not all, fibers run the length of the muscle. The muscle may be any length or size, from long to short or large to small. Examples of fusiform muscles can be found in the elbow flexors; that is, the biceps, brachialis, and brachioradialis muscles.

A **rhomboidal muscle** is four-sided, usually flat, with broad attachments at each end. Examples of this muscle shape are the pronator quadratus in the forearm, the rhomboids in the shoulder girdle, and the gluteus maximus in the hip region.

Triangular muscles are flat and fan-shaped, with fibers radiating from a narrow attachment at one end to a broad attachment at the other. An example of this type of muscle is the pectoralis major in the chest.

Oblique-fibered muscles have a feather arrangement in which a muscle attaches at an oblique angle to its tendon, much like feather tendrils attach to the quill. The different types of oblique-fibered muscles are unipennate, bipennate, and multipennate.

Unipennate muscles look like one side of a feather. There are a series of short fibers attaching diagonally along the length of a central tendon. Examples are the tibialis posterior muscle of the ankle, the semimembranosus of the hip and knee, and the flexor pollicis longus muscle of the hand.

The **bipennate muscle** pattern looks like that of a common feather. Its fibers are obliquely attached to both sides of a central tendon. The rectus femoris muscle of the hip and the interossei muscles of the hand are examples of this pattern.

Multipennate muscles have many tendons with oblique fibers in between. The deltoid and subscapularis muscles at the shoulder demonstrate this pattern.

Functional Characteristics of Muscle Tissue

Muscle tissue has the properties of irritability, contractility, extensibility, and elasticity. No other tissue in the body has all of these characteristics. To better understand these properties, you might find it helpful to know that muscles have a **normal resting length.** This is defined as the length of a muscle when it is unstimulated—that is, when there are no forces or stresses placed upon it. **Irritability** is the ability to respond to a stimulus. A muscle contracts when stimulated. This can be a natural stimulus from a motor nerve or an artificial stimulus such as from an electrical current. **Contractility** is the muscle's ability to shorten or contract when it receives adequate stimulation. This may result in the muscle shortening, staying the same, or lengthening. **Extensibility** is the muscle's ability to stretch or lengthen when a force is applied. **Elasticity** is the muscle's ability to recoil or return to normal resting length when the stretching or shortening force is removed. Saltwater taffy has extensibility but not elasticity. You can stretch it, but once the force is removed, the taffy will remain stretched. A wire spring has both extensibility and elasticity. Stretch the spring, and it will lengthen. Remove the stretch, and the spring will return to its original length. The same can be said of a muscle. However, unlike the taffy or the wire spring, a muscle is able to shorten beyond its normal resting length.

The properties of a muscle are summarized as follows: Stretch a muscle, and it will lengthen (extensibility). Remove the stretch, and it will return to its normal resting position (elasticity). Stimulate a muscle, and it will respond (irritability) by shortening (contractility); then remove the stimulus and it will return to its normal resting position (elasticity).

Length-Tension Relationship in Muscle Tissue

Tension refers to the force built up within a muscle. Stretching a muscle builds up *passive tension,* much like stretching a rubber band. It involves the noncontractile units of a muscle. *Active tension* comes from the contractile units and can be compared to releasing one end of a stretched rubber band. The total tension of a muscle is a combination of passive and active tension. **Tone** is the

slight tension that is present in a muscle at all times, even when the muscle is resting. It is a state of readiness that allows the muscle to act more easily and quickly when needed.

Although there is variation between muscles, it can generally be said that a muscle is capable of being shortened to approximately one-half of its normal resting length. For example, a muscle that is approximately 6 inches long can shorten to approximately 3 inches. Also, a muscle can be stretched about twice as far as it can be shortened. Therefore, this same muscle can be stretched 3 inches beyond its resting length to an overall length of 9 inches. The **excursion** of a muscle is that distance from maximum elongation to maximum shortening. In this example, the excursion would be 6 inches (Fig. 5-5).

Usually a muscle has sufficient excursion to allow the joint to move through its entire range. This is certainly true of muscles that span only one joint. However, a muscle spanning two or more joints may not have sufficient excursion to allow the joint to move through the combined range of all the joints it crosses.

One of the factors determining the amount of tension in a muscle is its length. It has been demonstrated that a muscle is strongest if put on a stretch prior to contracting. There are many examples of this concept. For instance, think of what you do when kicking a ball. First you hyperextend your hip and then forcefully flex it. In other words, you put the hip flexors on a stretch before contracting them. This is similar to pulling back on a rubber band before snapping it.

There is an optimum range of a muscle within which it contracts most effectively. As with a rubber band, a muscle contraction is strongest when it is on a stretch and it loses power quickly as it shortens. Therefore, two-joint muscles have the advantage over one-joint muscles in that they maintain greater contractile force through a

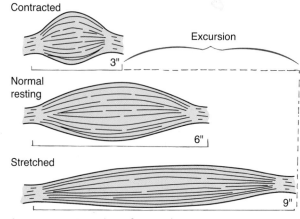

Figure 5-5.   Excursion of a muscle.

wider range. They do so by contracting over one joint while being elongated over another. Consider your hamstring muscles when climbing stairs. Hamstring function is to extend the hip and flex the knee. When you go up stairs, you start by flexing the hip and knee (Fig. 5-6A). This elongates the hamstrings over the hip and shortens them over the knee. Next, your hip goes into extension (shortening the muscle), while your knee also goes into extension (elongating the muscle; Fig. 5-6B). In other words, the hamstring muscles are being shortened over the hip while they are being elongated over the knee. Therefore, they are able to maintain an optimal length-tension relationship throughout the range.

Active and Passive Insufficiency

In a one-joint muscle, the excursion of the muscle will be greater than the range of motion allowed by the joint. However, with a two-joint or multijoint muscle, the muscle's excursion is less than the combined range allowed by the joints. The tension within the muscle becomes insufficient at both extremes. It can neither be elongated nor shortened any farther. Brunnstrom uses the terms *active* and *passive insufficiency* to describe these conditions.

The point at which a muscle cannot shorten any farther is called **active insufficiency.** Active insufficiency occurs to the agonist (the muscle that is contracting). Consider the hamstrings as an example. The hamstring muscles are two-joint muscles located on the posterior thigh. They extend the hip and flex the knee. There is sufficient tension to perform either hip extension or knee flexion, but not both simultaneously. Notice that if you flex your knee while your hip is extended, you cannot complete the full knee range. The muscles have "insufficient power" to contract (shorten) over both joints at the same time (Fig. 5-7A). They have become actively insufficient. To see that more range of motion exists, grab your ankle and pull the knee into more flexion (Fig. 5-7B). Be careful when trying this exercise that you do not get a muscle cramp. In other words, in this two-joint muscle that is contracting over both joints at the same time, the muscle (hamstring) will run out of the contractility before the joints (hip and knee) run out of range of motion.

Passive insufficiency occurs when a muscle cannot be elongated any farther without damage to its fibers. Passive insufficiency occurs to the antagonist (the muscle that is relaxed and on the opposite side of the joint from the agonist). *Agonist* and *antagonist* are terms described in more detail later in this chapter.

Consider the hamstring muscle as an example of passive insufficiency. The hamstring is long enough to be stretched over each joint individually (hip flexion or knee extension), but not both. If you flex your hip with

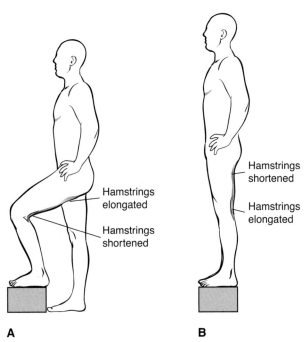

A   **B**

Figure 5-6. Optimal length-tension relationship of hamstrings when going up stairs. **(A)** When the foot is placed on the step, the hamstrings are being stretched over the hip while shortened over the knee. **(B)** Stepping up requires the hip to extend (hamstrings are contracting = shortening) and the knee to extend (hamstrings are being stretched).

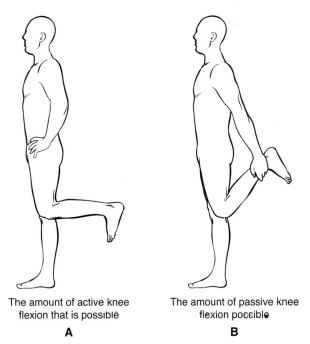

The amount of active knee flexion that is possible
A

The amount of passive knee flexion possible
B

Figure 5-7. Active insufficiency of the hamstring muscle.

your knee flexed, you can complete the range. As you can see in Figure 5-8A, the individual can touch the toes by flexing the hip and the knee. The hamstrings are being stretched over only one joint (the hip). You can also extend your knee fully when the hip is extended (see Fig. 5-6B), because the hamstrings are being stretched over only the knee. However, if you try to flex your hips to touch your toes with your knee extended (Fig. 5-8B), you will experience pain in the posterior thigh well before you reach full hip flexion. Your hamstring muscles are telling you to stop. They are being stretched over both joints at the same time and have become passively insufficient. They cannot be stretched any farther.

Stretching

Generally speaking, an agonist usually becomes actively insufficient (cannot contract any farther) before the antagonist becomes passively insufficient (cannot be stretched farther). We can use this concept to good advantage when we purposely stretch a muscle to either maintain or regain its normal resting length. Some activities require a great deal of flexibility, so stretching is done to lengthen the resting length of a muscle. In all of these situations, stretching should be performed on relaxed muscles. A person is put in a position that will stretch a muscle, usually a two-joint muscle, over all joints simultaneously within the pain limits of that muscle. If you want to stretch your hamstring muscles, put the knee in extension and slowly flex the hip to the point where you feel discomfort but not to the point of extreme pain. To stretch a one-joint muscle, it is necessary to put any two-joint muscles on a slack over the joint not crossed by the one joint-muscle. For example, to stretch the soleus muscle (which crosses the ankle only), the gastrocnemius muscle (which crosses the ankle and knee) must be put on a slack over the knee. This can be accomplished by flexing the knee while dorsiflexing the ankle. Otherwise, if you attempt to dorsiflex the ankle when the knee is extended, you may be stretching the gastrocnemius more than the soleus.

There are various methods of stretching used for different situations and sometimes for different results. These different methods are important but are beyond the scope of this discussion.

Tendon Action of a Muscle (Tenodesis)

Some degree of opening and closing the hand can be accomplished by using the principle of passive insufficiency. The finger flexors and extensors are multijoint muscles. They cross the wrist, the metacarpophalangeal (MCP) joints, the proximal interphalangeal joints (PIP), and sometimes the distal interphalangeal joints (DIP). We have already noticed that a two-joint or multijoint muscle does not have sufficient length to be stretched over all joints simultaneously. Something has to give. If you rest your flexed elbow on the table in a pronated position, relax, and let your wrist drop into flexion, you will notice that your fingers have a tendency to extend passively (Fig. 5-9A). Conversely, if you supinate your forearm and relax your wrist into extension, your fingers will have a tendency to close (Fig. 5-9B). If these tendons were a little tight, this opening and closing would be more pronounced. This is called **tenodesis** or **tendon action of a muscle.** A person who is quadriplegic and has no voluntary ability to open and close the fingers can use this principle to grasp and release light objects. By supinating the forearm, the weight of the hand and gravity causes the wrist to fall into hyperextension. This closes the fingers, creating a slight grasp. Pronating the forearm causes the wrist to fall into flexion, thus opening the fingers and releasing an object.

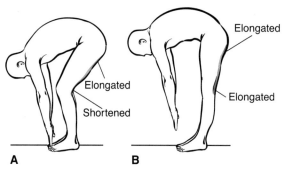

A **B**

Figure 5-8. Passive insufficiency of the hamstring muscle. **(A)** The hamstring being stretched (elongated) over only one joint allows more joint range of motion. **(B)** Stretching the muscle over both joints (the hip and knee) allows less individual joint range of motion.

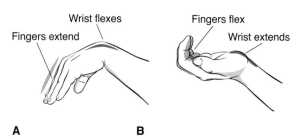

A **B**

Figure 5-9. Tenodesis, the functional use of passive insufficiency, demonstrated on the finger flexor and extensor muscles. Each group cannot be stretched over the wrist, MP, PIP, and DIP joints at the same time. **(A)** Passive insufficiency of the finger extensors occurs when the wrist is flexed, causing the fingers to extend. **(B)** Passive insufficiency of the finger flexors occurs when the wrist is extended, causing the fingers to flex.

Types of Muscle Contraction

There are three basic types of muscle contraction: isometric, isotonic, and isokinetic. An **isometric contraction** occurs when a muscle contracts, producing force without changing the length of muscle (Fig. 5-10A). The term *isometric* originates from the Greek word meaning "same length." To demonstrate this action, get in a sitting position and place your right hand under your thigh and place your left hand on your right biceps muscle. Now, pull up with your right hand—in other words, attempt to flex your right elbow. Note that there was no real motion at the elbow joint, but you did feel the muscle contract. This is an isometric contraction of your right biceps muscle. The muscle contracted, but no joint motion occurred.

Next, hold a weight in your hand while flexing your elbow to bring the weight up toward your shoulder (Fig. 5-10B). You will feel the biceps muscle contract, but this time there is joint motion. This is an **isotonic contraction,** which occurs when a muscle contracts and the muscle length and joint angle changes.

Occasionally you will read a text that describes an isometric contraction as a *static,* or *tonic, contraction* and an isotonic contraction as *phasic.* Although these terms mean essentially the same thing, they have fallen into disuse, and specific differences between these terms no longer seem relevant.

The term *isotonic* originates from the Greek word meaning "same tone or tension." Use of this term is not without its critics, because it is felt that tension created within a muscle does not remain constant throughout its range. Therefore, this term is not as significant as its two types. An isotonic contraction can be subdivided into concentric and eccentric contractions. A **concentric contraction** occurs when there is joint movement, the muscles shorten, and the muscle attachments (O and I) move toward each other (Fig. 5-10B). It is sometimes referred to as a *shortening contraction.* Picking up the weight, as described earlier, is an example of a concentric contraction of the biceps muscle.

If you continue to palpate the biceps muscle while setting the weight back down on the table, you will feel that the biceps muscle (not the triceps muscle) continues to contract, even though the joint motion is elbow extension. What is occurring is an eccentric contraction of the biceps muscle. An **eccentric contraction** occurs when there is joint motion but the muscle appears to lengthen; that is, the muscle attachments separate (Fig. 5-10C). After bringing the weight up to shoulder level, realize that if you relaxed your biceps muscle, the pull of gravity on your hand, forearm, and the weight would cause them to drop to the table. If you used your triceps muscle to extend the elbow (concentrically), your hand and weight would crash onto the tabletop with great force and speed. However, what you did by slowly returning the weight to the tabletop was to slow down (decelerate) the pull of gravity. You did this by eccentrically contracting the biceps (elbow flexor).

Eccentric contractions are sometimes referred to as *lengthening contractions.* This is somewhat misleading, because although the muscle is lengthening at a gross level, it is shortening microscopically. What the muscle is actually doing is returning to its normal resting

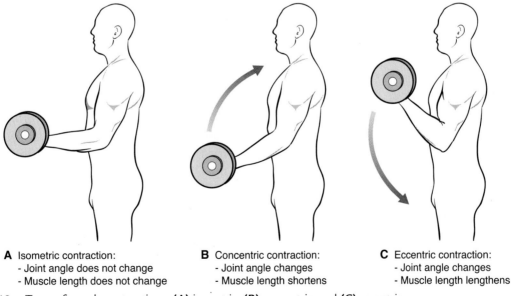

A Isometric contraction:
 - Joint angle does not change
 - Muscle length does not change

B Concentric contraction:
 - Joint angle changes
 - Muscle length shortens

C Eccentric contraction:
 - Joint angle changes
 - Muscle length lengthens

Figure 5-10.   Types of muscle contractions: **(A)** isometric, **(B)** concentric, and **(C)** eccentric.

position from a shortened position. An eccentric contraction can produce much greater forces than can a concentric contraction.

Frequently, different types of muscle contractions are used in various exercises. Quadriceps "setting" exercises are isometric contractions of the quadriceps muscle. Flexing and extending the knee are isotonic contractions. Sitting on a chair and extending the knee is a concentric contraction of the quadriceps muscle (Fig. 5-11), whereas flexing the knee and returning it to the starting position is an eccentric contraction of the quadriceps muscle. If you lie on the floor in a prone position and flex your knee to 90 degrees, you are doing a concentric contraction of the hamstring muscles. Straightening your knee is an eccentric contraction of the same muscles. What is happening? Straightening the knee while sitting and bending the knee while prone involves moving the lower leg *against gravity*. Muscles need to accelerate to move against gravity. Bending the knee while sitting and straightening the knee while prone involve moving the part *with gravity* and actually slowing down gravity. Generally speaking, eccentric contractions are used in deceleration activities, and concentric contractions are used in acceleration activities.

Therefore, it can be summarized that the two types of isotonic contractions have the following features.

Concentric Contractions
1. Muscle attachments move closer together.
2. Movement is usually occurring against gravity (a "raising" motion).
3. It is an acceleration activity.

Eccentric Contractions
1. Muscle attachments move farther apart.
2. Movement usually occurs with gravity (a "lowering" motion).
3. The contraction is used with a deceleration activity.

Table 5-1 shows many examples to emphasize the difference between concentric and eccentric contractions and how they change depending on the action performed. You could say the same thing about any two opposing muscle actions (e.g., supinators and pronators).

However, not all concentric and eccentric contractions work against or with gravity. Of course, there are exceptions. Here is an example. In the sitting position, have someone give resistance while you flex your knee. What type of contraction is this, and what muscle group is contracting? The answer is a concentric contraction of the hamstring muscles (knee flexors). In this case, your lower leg is moving down (with gravity), but gravity is not being slowed down. This is because a force (the other person's resistance) greater than the pull of gravity is being overcome. So, the knee flexors are contracting against an external resistance greater than gravity.

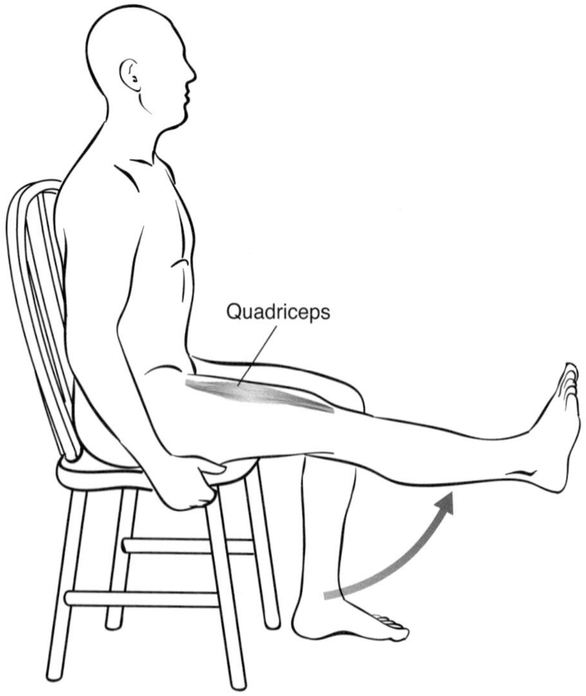

Figure 5-11. Concentric contraction of quadriceps muscle.

Table 5-1	Comparison of Concentric and Eccentric Contractions	
Type of Contraction	Active Muscle Group (Contacting)	Joint Motion
Concentric	Flexors	Flexion
Concentric	Extensors	Extension
Concentric	Abductors	Abduction
Concentric	Adductors	Adduction
Concentric	Medial rotators	Medial rotation
Concentric	Lateral rotators	Lateral rotation
Type of Contraction	Muscle Group Active (Contacting)	Joint Motion Occurring
Eccentric	Flexors	Extension
Eccentric	Extensors	Flexion
Eccentric	Abductors	Adduction
Eccentric	Adductors	Abduction
Eccentric	Medial rotators	Lateral rotation
Eccentric	Lateral rotators	Medial rotation

Consider another example. Normally, you use your shoulder flexors to lower your arm into extension in an eccentric contraction, because you are slowing down gravity. However, if you hold on to the handle of an overhead pulley and pull down into shoulder extension, you are doing a concentric contraction of the shoulder extensors. While your arm is moving in the same direction as gravity, you are overcoming a force greater than gravity (i.e., the overhead pulley weight). To prove this, keep holding the pulley handle but relax your shoulder muscles. Notice that your arm does not fall toward the ground. Why? The pulley weight is greater than the gravity weight (force of gravity).

Next, if you slowly, and under control, return the pulley handle to the starting position (shoulder flexion), you are doing an eccentric contraction of the shoulder extensors. Why? You are moving against gravity (a "raising" motion). However, in this case, you are decelerating the external force (the pulley weights).

Elastic tubing is a common method of providing resistance while exercising. While it can be used effectively with concentric contractions, it has greater limitations with eccentric contractions. If you attached elastic tubing over the top of a door and pulled down, you would be duplicating the action of the overhead pulley. Pulling down would be a concentric contraction of the shoulder extensors. However, returning to the starting position using elastic tubing is not as effective as an eccentric contraction with the pulleys. The initial motion is a strong eccentric contraction, but the elasticity quickly loses its tension. Therefore, using tubing for eccentric contraction must be done only in the early part of the motion and must not be considered effective throughout the entire range. It is possible to have effective eccentric contraction through smaller ranges using elastic tubing, such as forearm pronation and supination, but not with wide ranges, such as elbow flexion and extension.

When you put a person in a position to minimize the effects of gravity, muscle contractions are concentric. If you lie in a supine position and flex and extend your shoulder, the contractions of the flexors and extensors are concentric. If a muscle is too weak to move against gravity, the therapist might put the person in a **gravity-eliminated** position to exercise. For flexion and extension, the gravity-eliminated position is side-lying. The muscle may have enough strength to move but not to overcome or slow down gravity. Sit or kneel next to a table and rest your arm at shoulder level on the table. An example of a gravity-eliminated motion is moving your arm forward and backward in horizontal adduction and abduction with the weight of your arm being supported by the table.

Another, though less common, type of muscle contraction is an **isokinetic contraction.** This can be done only with special equipment. The Cybex Orthotron was the first machine to produce such contractions. With an isokinetic contraction, resistance to the part varies, but the velocity, or speed, stays the same. This differs from an isotonic contraction, in which the resistance remains constant but the velocity varies.

Consider the example of a person with a 5-pound weight attached to the leg. While the person straightens and flexes the knee (isotonic contraction), the amount of resistance stays the same. That 5-pound weight remained 5 pounds throughout the range. Because of other factors, such as the angle of pull, it is easier to move the leg in the middle and at the end of the range than at the beginning. In other words, the speed at which the person is able to move the leg varies throughout the range.

In an isokinetic contraction, the speed is preset and will stay the same no matter how hard a person pushes. However, the resistance will vary. If the person pushes harder, the machine will give more resistance, and if the person does not push as hard, there will be less resistance.

Why are isokinetic muscle contractions significant? A complete discussion of the merits of isokinetic exercise in comparison with other forms of exercise is best covered in a more detailed discussion of therapeutic exercise, which is beyond the scope of this book. However, there are two significant advantages. Isokinetic exercises can alter or adjust the amount of resistance given through the range of motion, whereas an isotonic exercise cannot. This is important because a muscle is not as strong at the beginning or end of its range as it is in the middle. Because the muscle is strongest in the midrange, more resistance should be given there and less resistance should be given at the beginning and end. An isotonic exercise cannot do this; therefore, there may be too much resistance in the weaker parts of the range and not enough resistance in the stronger parts.

Accommodating resistance is also important because of the pain factor. If pain suddenly develops during the exercise, the person's response is to stop exercising or not to work as hard. With an isotonic contraction, this response cannot happen quickly or even safely. With an isokinetic exercise, if the person stops working, the machine also stops. If the person does not contract as hard, the machine does not give as much resistance.

Hopefully this will give you some idea of the value of isokinetic exercise. However, there are some drawbacks. For example, isokinetic exercise requires special

Table 5-2	Types of Muscle Contraction		
Type	Speed	Resistance	Joint Motion
Isometric	Fixed	Fixed (0 degrees/sec)	No
Isotonic	Variable	Fixed	Yes
Isokinetic	Fixed	Variable (accommodating)	Yes

equipment, and that equipment is expensive. There is a time and place for all of these types of muscle contractions. It is important that you recognize the differences among them. Table 5-2 summarizes the major differences among these three types of muscle contractions.

Roles of Muscles

Muscles assume different roles during joint motion, depending on such variables as the motion being performed, the direction of the motion, and the amount of resistance the muscle must overcome. If any of these variables change, the muscle's role may also change. The roles a muscle can assume are those of an agonist, antagonist, stabilizer, or neutralizer. An **agonist** is a muscle or muscle group that causes the motion. It is sometimes referred to as the **prime mover.** A muscle that is not as effective but does assist in providing that motion is called an **assisting mover.** Factors that determine whether a muscle is a prime mover or an assisting mover include size, angle of pull, leverage, and contractile potential. During elbow flexion, the biceps muscle is an agonist, and because of its size and angle of pull, the pronator teres muscle is an assisting mover.

An **antagonist** is a muscle that performs the opposite motion of the agonist. In the case of elbow flexion, the antagonist is the triceps muscle. Keep in mind that the role of a muscle is specific to a particular joint action. In the case of elbow extension, the triceps muscle is the agonist and the biceps muscle is the antagonist. However, in elbow flexion, the biceps muscle is the agonist and the triceps muscle is the antagonist.

The antagonist has the potential to oppose the agonist, but it is usually relaxed while the agonist is working. When the antagonist contracts at the same time as the agonist, a **cocontraction** results. A cocontraction occurs when there is a need for accuracy. Some experts feel that cocontractions are common when a person learns a task, especially a difficult one; thus, as the task is learned, cocontraction activity tends to disappear.

A **stabilizer** is a muscle or muscle group that supports, or makes firm, a part and allows the agonist to work more efficiently. For example, when you do a push-up, the agonists are the elbow extensor muscles. The abdominal muscles (trunk flexor muscles) act as stabilizers to keep the trunk straight, while the arms move the trunk up and down. A stabilizer is sometimes referred to as a *fixator.*

Remember, a muscle knows no direction when it contracts. If a muscle can do two (or more) actions but only one is wanted, a **neutralizer** contracts to prevent the unwanted motion. For example, the biceps muscle can flex the elbow and supinate the forearm. If only elbow flexion is wanted, the supination component must be ruled out. Therefore, the pronator teres muscle, which pronates the forearm, contracts to counteract the supination component of the biceps muscle, and only elbow flexion occurs. A neutralizer may also allow a muscle to perform more than one role. Wrist ulnar deviation is such an example. The flexor carpi ulnaris muscle causes flexion and ulnar deviation of the wrist. The extensor carpi ulnaris muscle causes extension and ulnar deviation. In ulnar deviation, these muscles contract and accomplish two things: They neutralize each other's flexion/extension component while acting as agonists in wrist ulnar deviation.

A **synergist** is a muscle that works with one or more other muscles to enhance a particular motion. Some authors use this term to encompass the role of agonists, assisting movers, stabilizers, and neutralizers. The disadvantage of this term is that although it indicates that the muscle is working, it does not indicate how.

Angle of Pull

Several factors determine the role that a muscle will play in a particular joint motion. Determining whether a muscle has a major role (prime mover), a minor role (assisting mover), or no role at all will depend on such factors as its size, angle of pull, the joint motions possible, and the location of the muscle in relation to the joint axis. Visualizing the muscle, particularly in relation to other muscles performing the same action, will give you an idea about size as a factor. For example, compare the size of the triceps with that of the anconeus (see Figs. 11-17 and 11-18). It is easy to see that the anconeus will have little effect on joint motion compared to the triceps. Next, you know the motions that a particular joint allows. In the case of the elbow, the motions possible are flexion and extension. The triceps and anconeus cross the joint posterior to the joint axis. Because the triceps is much larger than the anconeus, it crosses the elbow posteriorly, and because extensors must cross the elbow posteriorly, it is logical that the triceps is a prime mover in elbow extension.

Not all muscles are so obvious in their action. Angle of pull is usually a major factor. Most muscles pull at a diagonal. As will be discussed in Chapter 8 regarding torque, most muscles have a diagonal line of pull. That diagonal line of pull is the resultant force of a vertical force and a horizontal force. In the case of the shoulder girdle, muscles with a greater vertical angle of pull will be effective in pulling the scapula up or down (elevating or depressing the scapula). Muscles with a greater horizontal pull will be more effective in pulling the scapula in or out (protracting or retracting). Muscles with a more equal horizontal and vertical pull will have a role in both motions. Figure 5-12 gives an example of each. The levator scapula has a stronger vertical component, the middle trapezius has a stronger horizontal component, and the rhomboids have a more equal pull in both directions. As you will see when these muscles are described later in Chapter 9, the levator scapula is a prime mover in scapular elevation and the middle trapezius is a prime mover in retraction, whereas the rhomboids are prime movers in both elevation and retraction.

Kinetic Chains

The concept of open versus closed kinetic chain exercises has evolved into movement and exercise. In engineering terms, a kinetic chain consists of a series of rigid links connected in such a way as to allow motion. Because these links are connected, movement of one link causes motion at other links in a predictable way. Applying this to the human body, a **closed kinetic chain** requires that the distal segment is fixed (closed) and the proximal segment(s) moves (Fig. 5-13). For example, when you rise from a sitting position, your knees extend, causing your hips and ankles to move as well. With your foot fixed on the ground, there is no way you can move your knee without causing movement at the hip and knee.

However, if you were to remain seated and extend your knee, your hip and ankle would not move. This is an **open kinetic chain** activity. The distal segment is free to move while the proximal segment(s) can remain stationary (Fig. 5-14). With open-chain activities, the limb segments are free to move in many directions. For example, if you are lying on a bed with your arm in the air, you can move your shoulder, elbow, wrist, and hand in many directions, either together or individually. This is open-chain activity. The distal segment is not fixed but is free to move.

However, if you grab an overhead trapeze, your hand, the distal segment, is fixed, or closed. As you flex your elbow, your shoulder has to go into some extension. As your elbow extends, your shoulder must go into some flexion. With closed-chain activities, the limb segments

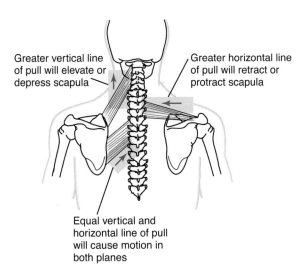

Figure 5-12.   Angle of pull as a determinant of muscle action.

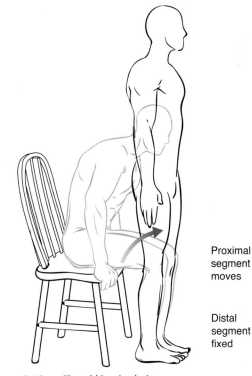

Figure 5-13.   Closed kinetic chain.

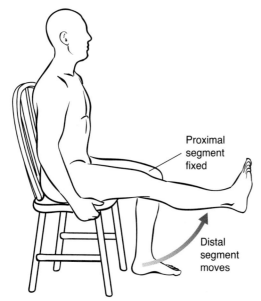

Proximal segment fixed

Distal segment moves

Figure 5-14.   Open kinetic chain.

Table 5-3	Exercise Terminology
Concentric	**Eccentric**
Usually open chain	Can be open or closed chain
Usually non-weight-bearing	Can be weight-bearing or non-weight-bearing
Open Chain	**Closed Chain**
Can be concentric or eccentric	Can be concentric or eccentric
Usually non-weight-bearing	Usually weight-bearing
Non-Weight-Bearing	**Weight-Bearing**
Can be concentric or eccentric	Usually eccentric
Usually open chain	Usually closed chain

move in limited and predictable directions. Other examples of upper-extremity closed-chain activities occur during crutch walking and pushing a wheelchair. The crutch tip (distal segment) is fixed on the ground and the body (proximal segment) moves. The hands on the wheelchair rims are the distal segments, and joints proximal to the hands move in a connected fashion (i.e., the elbows extend and the shoulders flex).

Closed-chain exercise equipment includes such things as the bench press, rowing machine, stationary bicycle, and stair stepper. Examples of open-chain exercise equipment include the Cybex and free weights. Manual muscle testing is all open-chain movement. The treadmill is a combination of open- and closed-chain exercise. The weight-bearing portion is the closed-chain movement, and the non-weight-bearing portion is the open-chain movement.

Table 5-3 illustrates the interrelationships of the concepts discussed in this chapter. Keep in mind that these are general statements and are not absolute.

Points to Remember
- The two ends of a muscle are referred to as the origin or insertion.
- Usually the insertion moves toward the origin.
- When the origin moves toward the insertion, it is referred to as reversal of muscle action.
- Active insufficiency is when a muscle cannot contract any farther.
- Passive insufficiency is when a muscle cannot be elongated any farther.
- Muscle tissue has the properties of irritability, contractility, extensibility, and elasticity.
- Muscle fibers are arranged in either a parallel or an oblique pattern, which favors range or power, respectively.
- Muscle contractions are of three basic types: isometric, concentric, or eccentric.
- A muscle can assume the role of agonist, antagonist, stabilizer, or neutralizer, depending on a particular situation.
- Kinetic chain movement depends on whether the distal segment is fixed (closed) or free to move (open).

Review Questions

1. Usually when a muscle contracts, the distal attachment moves toward the proximal attachment.
   a. What is another name to describe the distal attachment?
   b. What is another name for the proximal attachment?

2. What is the term for describing a muscle contraction in which the proximal end moves toward the distal end?

3. The flexor carpi radialis performs wrist flexion and radial deviation. The flexor carpi ulnaris performs wrist flexion and ulnar deviation.
   a. In what wrist action do the two muscles act as agonists?
   b. In what wrist action do they act as antagonists?

4. The following chart identifies the hip motions of three muscles. Hip extension is the desired motion.

Muscle	Extension	Lateral Rotation	Medial Rotation
Gluteus maximus	X	X	
Hamstrings	X		
Gluteus minimus			X

   a. Which of these muscles are acting as agonists in hip extension?
   b. What motion must be neutralized so the agonists can do only hip extension?
   c. What muscle must act as a neutralizer to rule out the undesired motion?

5. What is the term for the situation in which a muscle contracts until it can contract no farther even though more joint range of motion is possible?

6. Is walking downhill a concentric or an eccentric contraction of your quadriceps muscle?

7. Sitting with a weight in your hand, forearm pronated, elbow extended, and shoulder medially rotated, slowly move your hand out to the side and raise it.
   a. What is the joint motion at the shoulder?
   b. Is an isometric, concentric, or eccentric muscle contraction occurring at the shoulder?
   c. What muscle group is contracting at the shoulder?
   d. What type of muscle contraction is occurring at the elbow?
   e. What muscle group is contracting at the elbow?

8. While lying supine with your arm at your side and with a weight in your hand, raise the weight up and over your shoulder. (*Hint:* Think about gravity's effect throughout the range.)
   a. What is the joint motion at the shoulder?
   b. Is the muscle action during the first 90 degrees of the motion concentric or eccentric?
   c. Are the shoulder flexors or extensors responsible for this action?
   d. Is the muscle action during the second 90 degrees of the motion concentric or eccentric?
   e. Are the shoulder flexors or extensors responsible for this action?

9. Identify the following in terms of open or closed kinetic chain activities:
   a. Wheelchair push-ups
   b. Exercises with weight cuffs
   c. Overhead wall pulleys

10. What position would a person have to be in to perform shoulder abduction and adduction in a gravity-eliminated position?

11. For a muscle to have an effective angle of pull to be a shoulder flexor and not a shoulder abductor, it would have to span the shoulder on what surface?

12. The rectus femoris flexes the hip and extends the knee. The vastus medialis extends only the knee. In what position must the hip and knee be placed to be able to stretch the vastus medialis?

13. If you wanted a muscle to lift a very strong load, what muscle fiber arrangement would you want?

14. If you wanted a muscle to contract through a very great range, what muscle fiber arrangement would you want?

15. In terms of muscle tissue characteristics:
    a. What can a muscle do that a rubber band cannot?
    b. What characteristic does a rubber band have that chewing gum does not?

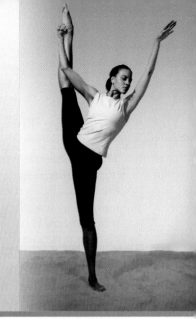

CHAPTER 6
Nervous System

Nervous Tissue (Neurons)

The Central Nervous System

Brain

Spinal Cord

The Peripheral Nervous System

Cranial Nerves

Spinal Nerves

Functional Significance of Spinal Cord Level

Plexus Formation

Common Pathologies of the Central and Peripheral Nervous Systems

Common Pathologies of the Central Nervous System

Common Pathologies of the Peripheral Nerves

Review Questions

The nervous system is the highly complex mechanism in our bodies that controls, stimulates, and coordinates all other body systems. As outlined in Figure 6-1, it can be divided anatomically into the central nervous system (CNS), which includes the brain and spinal cord; the peripheral nervous system (PNS), which includes nerves outside the spinal cord; and the autonomic nervous system (ANS), which controls mostly visceral structures. The subdivisions of the ANS are the sympathetic and the parasympathetic nervous systems. These operate as a check-and-balance system for each other. The sympathetic system deals with stress and stimulation and the parasympathetic system deals with conserving energy.

A specific description of the various parts of each system and their functions is beyond the scope of this text. However, we will provide a fairly brief anatomical and functional description of the CNS and PNS as they affect muscle movement. This description will be focused at the gross, not the cellular, level.

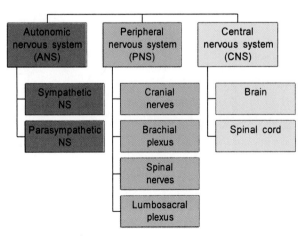

Figure 6-1. The nervous system.

Nervous Tissue (Neurons)

The fundamental unit of nervous tissue is the neuron (Fig. 6-2). Each neuron contains a **cell body** from which extends a single process, called an *axon,* and a variable number of branching processes, called *dendrites.* The term *nerve cell* is synonymous with *neuron* and includes all of its processes (dendrites and axons).

Dendrites are fiber branches that receive impulses from other parts of the nervous system and bring those impulses toward the cell body. **Axons** transmit impulses away from the cell body. They are located on the side opposite the dendrites and usually consist of a single branch. The inner part of the axon is often surrounded by a fatty sheath called **myelin.** The myelin is interrupted approximately every half millimeter. This break in the myelin is referred to as the **node of Ranvier.**

Myelin is a white, fatty substance found in the CNS and PNS. One of its functions is to increase the speed of impulse conduction in the myelinated fiber. Myelin does not cover cell bodies or certain nerve fibers. Areas that contain mostly unmyelinated fibers are referred to as **gray matter,** and areas that contain mostly myelinated fibers are called **white matter** (Fig. 6-3). Areas of gray matter include the cerebral cortex and the central portion of the spinal cord. White matter includes the major tracts within the spinal cord and fiber systems, such as the internal capsule within the brain.

A **nerve fiber** is the conductor of impulses from the neuron. Transmission of impulses from one neuron to another occurs at a **synapse,** which is a small gap between neurons involving very complex physiological actions.

A **tract** is a group of myelinated nerve fibers within the CNS that carries a specific type of information from one area to another. Depending on its location within the CNS, the group of fibers may be referred to as a *fasciculus, peduncle, brachium, column,* or *lemniscus.* A group of fibers within the PNS may be called a *spinal nerve, nerve root, plexus,* or *peripheral nerve,* depending on its location. (An example of the pathway of a tract can be seen in Fig. 6-15.)

Motor and sensory neurons are the two major types of nerve fibers in peripheral nerves. A **motor (efferent) neuron** has a large cell body with multibranched dendrites and a long axon (see Fig. 6-2A). This cell body and dendrites are located within the anterior horn of the spinal cord (see Fig. 6-3). Depending on an author's use of terms, *anterior* and *ventral* are synonymous, as are *posterior* and *dorsal.* The axon leaves the anterior horn through the white matter and is organized with other similar axons in the **anterior root,** which is located just outside the spinal cord in the area of the intervertebral foramen. The axon continues down the peripheral nerve to its termination in a **motor endplate (axon terminal)** of a muscle fiber. A motor neuron conducts **efferent** impulses from the spinal cord to the periphery (see Figs. 6-3 and 6-4).

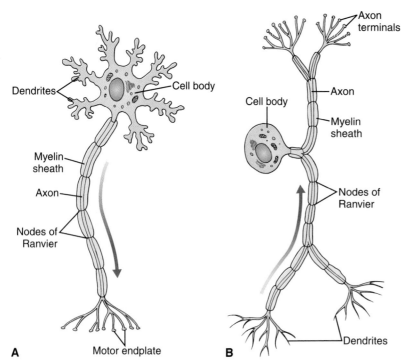

Figure 6-2. Typical **(A)** motor and **(B)** sensory neurons. Arrows indicate the direction that impulses travel.

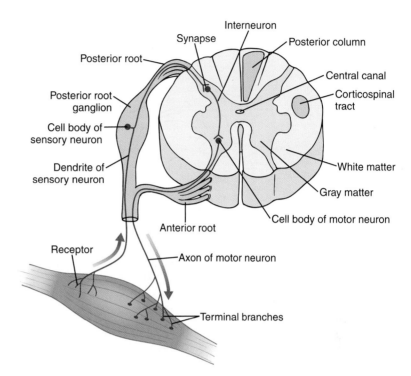

Figure 6-3. Cross section of spinal cord. Note the sensory neuron going into the cord, the motor neuron coming out, and the interneuron connecting the two neurons.

The **sensory (afferent) neuron** has a dendrite, which arises in the skin and runs all the way to its cell body in the posterior root ganglion (Figs. 6-2B and 6-3), located in the intervertebral foramen. The axon travels through the posterior (dorsal) root of the spinal nerve and into the spinal cord through the posterior horn. The axon may end at this point, or it may enter the white matter and ascend to a different level of the spinal cord or to the brainstem. A sensory neuron sends **afferent** impulses from the periphery to the spinal cord (see Figs. 6-3 and 6-4).

Both sensory and motor impulses travel along nerve fibers located outside the spinal cord but within peripheral nerves. As described earlier, motor impulses travel from the CNS to the periphery. Sensory impulses travel from the periphery to the CNS (see Fig. 6-4).

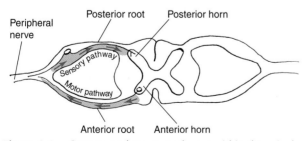

Figure 6-4. Sensory and motor pathways within the spinal cord.

A third type of neuron is an **interneuron** (see Fig. 6-3). It is found within the CNS. Its function is to transmit or integrate signals from one or more sensory neurons and relay impulses to motor neurons.

The Central Nervous System

The main components of the CNS are the brain and the spinal cord. The brain is made up of the cerebrum, brainstem, and cerebellum. (Trivia fans will note that the brain weighs about 3 pounds.)

Brain

Cerebrum

The **cerebrum** is the largest and main portion of the brain (Fig. 6-5), and it is responsible for the highest mental functions. It occupies the anterior and superior area of the cranium above the brainstem and cerebellum. The cerebrum is made up of right and left **cerebral hemispheres** joined in the center by the **corpus callosum.**

Each cerebral hemisphere has a **cortex,** or outer coating, that is many cell layers deep, and each hemisphere is divided into four **lobes** (Fig. 6-6). Each lobe has many known functions. Specific locations of some functions

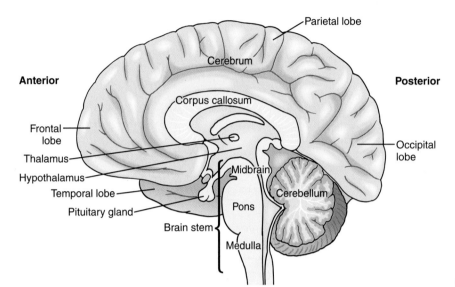

Figure 6-5.   Mid-sagittal section of the brain.

remain undetermined. The **frontal lobe** occupies the anterior portion of the skull. The area of brain activity that controls personality is located here. The frontal lobe also controls motor movement and expressive speech. The **occipital lobe** takes up the posterior portion of the skull. It is responsible for vision and recognition of size, shape, and color. The **parietal lobe** lies between the frontal and occipital lobes. This area controls gross sensation, such as touch and pressure. It also controls fine sensation, such as the determination of texture, weight, size, and shape. Brain activity associated with reading skills is also located in the parietal lobe. The **temporal lobe** lies under the frontal and parietal lobes just above the ear. This is the center for behavior, hearing, language reception, and understanding. These four lobes can also be seen in Figure 6-6.

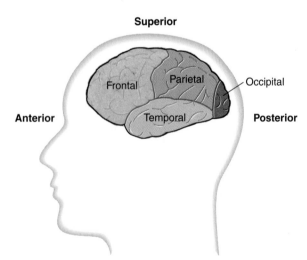

Figure 6-6.   The four lobes of the cerebral hemisphere.

Deep within the cerebral hemispheres, beneath the cortex, is the **thalamus** (see Fig. 6-5). This mass of nerve cells serves as a relay station for body sensations; it is here where pain is perceived. Deep inside the brain is the **hypothalamus,** which is important for hormone function and behavior. Also in this area is the **basal ganglia** (not shown in figure), which is important in coordination of motor movement.

Brainstem

Lying below the cerebrum is the brainstem, which can be divided into three parts: the midbrain, the pons, and the medulla (see Fig. 6-5). The upper portion of the brainstem is the midbrain, located somewhat below the cerebrum. The **midbrain** is the center for visual reflexes. Pons is Latin for "bridge" and is located between the midbrain and the medulla. The **medulla oblongata** is the most caudal, or inferior, portion of the brainstem. It is usually referred to simply as the *medulla*. The medulla is continuous with the spinal cord, with the transition being at the base of the skull, where it passes through the foramen magnum. The medulla is the center for automatic control of respiration and heart rate.

Most of the cranial nerves come from the brainstem area, and all fiber tracts from the spinal cord and peripheral nerves to and from higher centers of the brain go through this area.

Cerebellum

In Latin, **cerebellum** means "little brain." It is located in the posterior portion of the cranium behind the pons and medulla (see Fig. 6-5). It is covered superiorly by the posterior portion of the cerebrum. The main functions of the cerebellum are control of muscle coordination, tone, and posture.

Brain Protection

The brain has three basic levels of protection: bony, membranous, and fluid. Surrounding the brain is the **skull,** which is made up of several bones with joints fused together for greater strength (Fig. 6-7).

Within the skull are three layers of membrane called *meninges* (Fig. 6-8). These cover the brain and provide support and protection. The thickest, most fibrous, tough outer layer is called the **dura mater,** which means "hard mother" in Latin. The middle, thinner layer is called **arachnoid** or, less commonly, *arachnoid mater.* (*Arachnoid,* from Greek for *spider,* means "spider-like.") The inner, delicate layer is called the **pia mater** (Latin for "tender mother"), which carries blood vessels to the brain. These cranial meninges are continuous

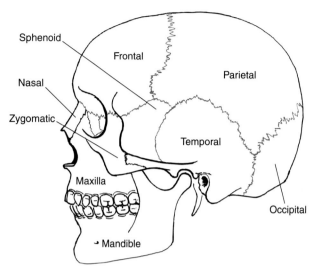

Figure 6-7.   The bones of the skull. The fibrous, immovable joints between these bones offer maximum protection.

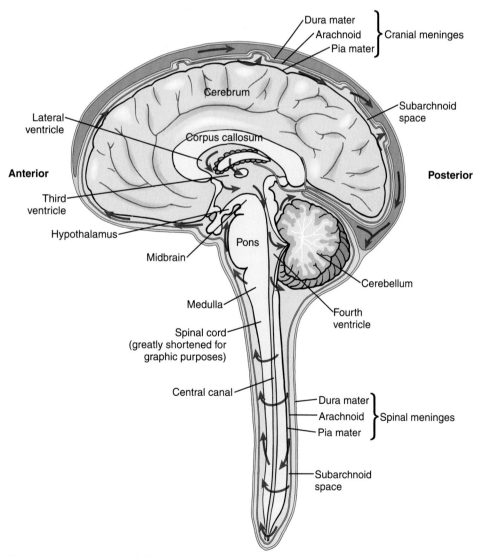

Figure 6-8.   Circulation of cerebrospinal fluid. The arrows indicate direction of flow.

with the spinal meninges that surround the spinal cord, which will be described later in the chapter.

Between the layers of the arachnoid and pia mater is the **subarachnoid space** through which circulates **cerebrospinal fluid** (see Fig. 6-8). This fluid surrounds the brain and fills the four **ventricles** within the brain. The ventricles are four small cavities containing a capillary network that produces cerebrospinal fluid. There are two lateral ventricles, a third ventricle, and a fourth ventricle. The main function of the cerebrospinal fluid is shock absorption.

Spinal Cord

A continuation of the medulla, the spinal cord runs within the vertebral canal from the foramen magnum to the cone-shaped **conus medullaris** at approximately the level of the second lumbar vertebra in an adult (Fig. 6-9). Below this level is a collection of nerve roots running down from the spinal cord; they look much like a horse's tail, hence the name **cauda equina.** The cauda equina is made up of the nerve roots for L2 through S5. The **filum terminale** is a threadlike, nonneural filament that runs from the conus medullaris and attaches to the coccyx.

The spinal cord is approximately 17 inches in length. It is enclosed in the same three protective layers as the brain: the outer dura mater, the arachnoid membrane, and the inner pia mater (Fig. 6-10). As with the brain, cerebrospinal fluid flows in the space between the arachnoid layer and the pia mater (see Fig. 6-8).

The **vertebral foramen,** the passageway for the spinal cord, is surrounded and protected by the bony structures of each individual vertebra (Fig. 6-11). Each vertebra is made up of the **body,** which is the anterior weight-bearing portion, and the posterior **neural arch,** which consists of pedicles, transverse processes, lamina, and a spinous process (Fig. 6-12). The opening formed between these two parts is the vertebral foramen. This opening is not to be confused with the **intervertebral foramen,** located on the sides of the vertebral column. The intervertebral foramen is the opening formed by the superior vertebral notch of the vertebra below and the inferior vertebral notch of the vertebra above (Fig. 6-13). Through this opening, the spinal nerve root exits the vertebral canal.

A cross-sectional view of the spinal cord reveals peripheral white matter and central gray matter (Fig. 6-14). The **gray matter** is in the middle of the cord in an **H** or "butterfly" shape. It contains neuronal cell bodies and synapses. The top portion of the **H** is the **posterior horn,** which transmits sensory impulses. The lower portion, the **anterior horn,** transmits motor impulses.

The **posterior columns,** also called the *dorsal columns,* are located in the posterior medial portions of the spinal cord. These columns transmit the sensations of proprioception, pressure, and vibration (see Fig. 6-14).

White matter contains ascending (sensory) and descending (motor) fiber pathways. Each pathway carries a particular type of impulse, such as touch, from and to a specific area. These various pathways cross over from one side of the body to the other at different levels. It is this crossover phenomenon that results in a

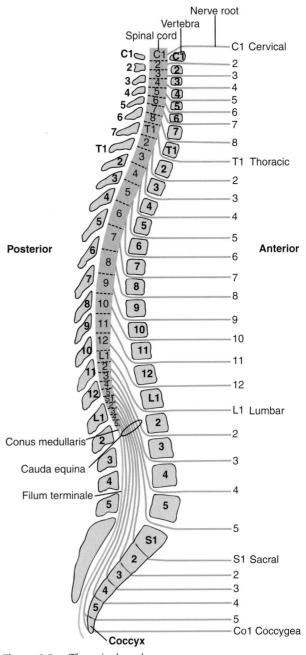

Figure 6-9.   The spinal cord.

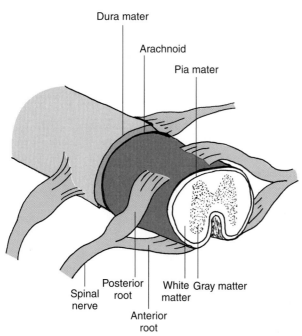

Figure 6-10. The three layers of the meninges surround the spinal cord and the brain.

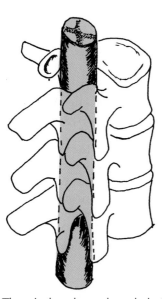

Figure 6-11. The spinal cord runs through the bony vertebral foramen.

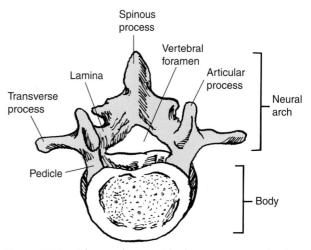

Figure 6-12. The vertebra provides bony protection for the spinal cord.

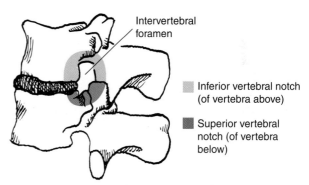

Inferior vertebral notch (of vertebra above)

Superior vertebral notch (of vertebra below)

Figure 6-13. Two vertebrae combine to form an opening (intervertebral foramen) on each side through which passes a spinal nerve root.

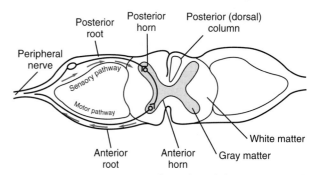

Figure 6-14. Cross section of spinal cord showing gray and white matter.

stroke on the left side of the brain affecting the right side of the body.

The pathway of particular significance to muscle control is the lateral **corticospinal tract** (Fig. 6-15). It is located lateral to the posterior column and posterior horn. As its name implies, it runs from the motor area of the cerebral cortex to the spinal cord, crossing over at about the level of the lower part of the brainstem. Corticospinal pathways synapse in the anterior horn just prior to leaving the spinal cord.

Motor neurons that synapse above this level are called **upper motor neurons.** Those that synapse at

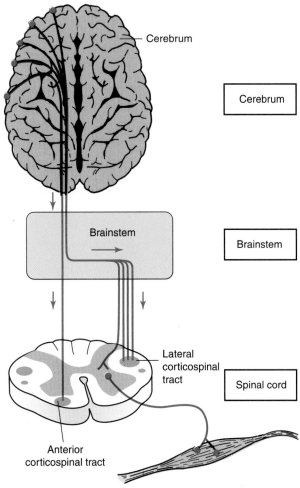

Cerebrum

Cerebrum

Brainstem

Brainstem

Lateral
corticospinal
tract

Spinal cord

Anterior
corticospinal tract

Figure 6-15. Pathway of corticospinal tract from the brain's motor cortex to the spinal cord.

or below the anterior horn are called **lower motor neurons.** Injury to these two types of neurons results in quite different clinical signs. In other words, if a lesion occurs proximal to the anterior horn, it is considered an upper motor neuron lesion. If the lesion occurs to the cell bodies or axons of lower motor neurons, it is considered a lower motor neuron lesion. Paralysis will usually result in either case; however, clinical signs differ greatly (these are contrasted in Table 6-1).

Examples of diagnoses involving upper motor neuron lesions include spinal cord injuries, multiple sclerosis, parkinsonism, cerebral vascular accident, and various types of head injuries. Examples of diagnoses involving lower motor neuron lesions are muscular dystrophy, poliomyelitis, myasthenia gravis, and peripheral nerve injuries.

To summarize, motor impulses travel from the brain, down the spinal cord, through the anterior horn,

and out to the periphery via peripheral nerves. Sensory impulses from the periphery travel up the peripheral nerves, into the spinal cord via the posterior (or dorsal) horn, then up the spinal cord to the brain.

The Peripheral Nervous System

The PNS is, for the most part, made up of all the nervous tissue outside the vertebral canal. It actually begins at the anterior horn of the spinal cord, sending motor impulses out to the muscles and receiving sensory impulses from the skin.

Cranial Nerves

There are 12 pairs of cranial nerves, which are numbered and named (Fig. 6-16). They are sensory nerves, motor nerves, or mixed nerves (a combination of both). Their functions are summarized in Table 6-2.

Of the 12 cranial nerves, the trigeminal (V), facial (VII), and spinal accessory (XI)—often shortened to *accessory*—nerves are the most significant in terms of their control over certain muscles. The chapters in Parts 2, 3, and 4 will identify innervation of muscles, along with a summary description of each muscle.

Spinal Nerves

There are 31 pairs of spinal nerves, including 8 cervical nerves, 12 thoracic nerves, 5 lumbar nerves, 5 sacral nerves, and 1 coccygeal nerve (see Fig. 6-9). The first seven cervical nerves (C1 to C7) exit the vertebral column *above* the corresponding vertebra. For example, the C3 nerve exits above the C3 vertebra. Because there is one more cervical nerve than cervical vertebra, this arrangement changes with the eighth cervical nerve. The C8 nerve exits *under* the C7 vertebra and *over* the T1 vertebra. The T1 nerve exits *under* the T1 vertebra, and so on down the vertebral column (Fig. 6-17).

Branches of Spinal Nerves

Once outside the spinal cord, the anterior (motor) and posterior (sensory) roots join together to form the spinal nerve (Fig. 6-18), which passes through the bony intervertebral foramen. Almost immediately, the nerve sends a branch called the **posterior (dorsal) ramus.** As a rule, this branch tends to be smaller than the anterior ramus. It innervates the muscles and skin of the posterior trunk. The spinal nerve continues as the **anterior (ventral) ramus.** These rami (plural of *ramus*)

Table 6-1	Clinical Differences Between Upper and Lower Motor Neuron Lesions	
Sign	Upper Motor Neuron Lesion	Lower Motor Neuron Lesion
Paralysis	Spasticity present	Flaccid
Muscle atrophy	Not significant	Marked
Fasciculations and fibrillations	Not present	Present
Reflexes	Hyperreflexia	Hyporeflexia
Babinski reflex	Present	Not present
Clonus	Present	Not present

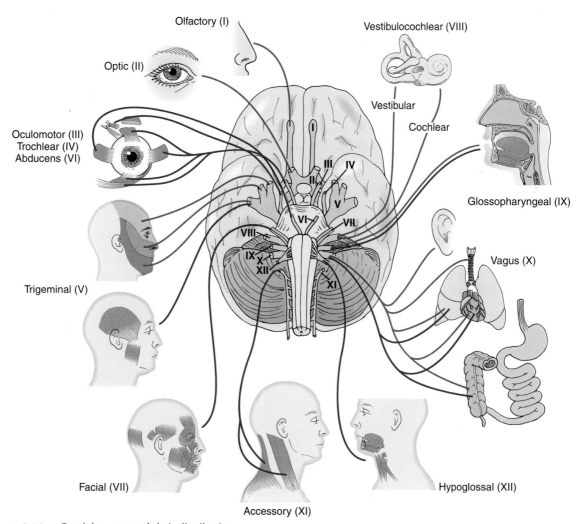

Figure 6-16.   Cranial nerves and their distributions.

Table 6-2	Cranial Nerves			
Number	Name	Type	Function	Mnemonic*
I	Olfactory	Sensory	Smell	On
II	Optic	Sensory	Vision	Old
III	Oculomotor	Motor	Muscles of eye	Olympus
IV	Trochlear	Motor	Muscles of eye	Towering
V	Trigeminal	Mixed	Sensory: Face area Motor: Chewing muscles	Tops
VI	Abducens	Motor	Muscles of eye	A
VII	Facial	Mixed	Sensory: Tongue area Motor: Muscles of facial expression	Finn
VIII	Vestibulocochlear (auditory)	Sensory	Hearing Equilibrium sensation	And
IX	Glossopharyngeal	Mixed	Sensory: Taste, pharynx, middle ear Motor: Muscles of pharynx	German
X	Vagus	Mixed	Sensory: Heart, lungs, GI tract, ear Motor: Heart, lungs, GI tract	Viewed
XI	Spinal accessory	Motor	Sternocleidomastoid and trapezius muscles, swallowing	Some
XII	Hypoglossal	Motor	Muscles of tongue	Hops

* A mnemonic (pronounced "neh-mon-ik") is a learning aid. In this case, the first letter of each word of the saying is also the first letter of the cranial nerve.

innervate all muscles and skin areas not innervated by the posterior ramus, which is the anterior and lateral trunk and all the extremities. Located just peripheral to the posterior ramus is a branch to the autonomic nervous system (sympathetic trunk). It is involved with such functions as blood pressure regulation. Although these functions are vital, they will not be discussed here. Instead, we emphasize the motor functions that occur mostly via the anterior ramus. In the thoracic region, the spinal nerves form the intercostal nerves.

Dermatomes

The area of skin supplied with the **sensory fibers** of a spinal nerve is called the **dermatome** (Fig. 6-19). Contiguous dermatomes often overlap. Complete anesthesia of the area will not occur unless more than

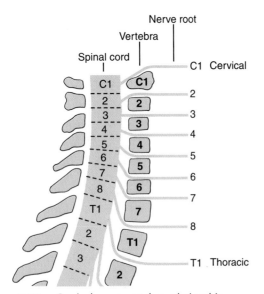

Figure 6-17. Cervical nerve-vertebra relationship.

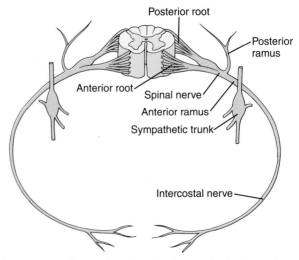

Figure 6-18. Formation of a spinal nerve. In the thoracic region, the spinal nerves form the intercostal nerves.

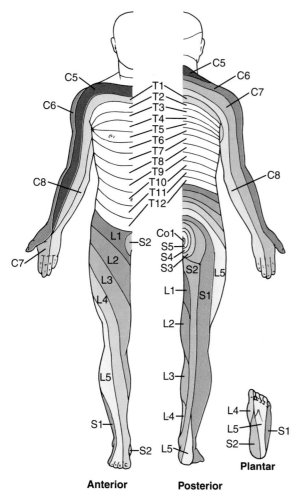

Figure 6-19. Dermatomes: segmental areas of innervation of the skin.

Functional Significance of Spinal Cord Level

Remember that the spinal nerves in the cervical region exit the spinal cord *above* the vertebra (see Fig. 6-17). The C8 spinal nerve comes out *below* the C7 vertebra, because there is one more cervical nerve than there are vertebrae. Starting with the T1 spinal nerve, all spinal nerves below T1 come out below the same numbered vertebra.

In Figure 6-20, one can gain an appreciation for the general innervation level of major muscles. It should be noted that most muscles take innervation from more than one spinal level. Therefore, an injury at one spinal level may weaken a muscle, but some function will remain. For example, the elbow flexors receive innervation from the C5 and C6 spinal level. An injury at the C5 vertebral level will weaken elbow flexion, but function will not be completely lost. This is because the C5 spinal nerve exits the spinal cord above the C5 vertebra while the C6 spinal nerve exits below the C5 vertebra. Therefore, the C5 spinal nerve may not be injured, allowing the elbow flexors to continue to receive partial innervation.

Although there is slight variation among individuals, some general statements can be made about the level of function at various levels of the spinal cord. A person with a spinal cord injury at C3 or above would not have the function of the diaphragm and would be unable to breathe without assistance. Below that level, although breathing would be compromised, a person would probably be able to breathe without assistance. With C5 spinal cord involvement, some innervation of the shoulder abductors and elbow flexors may be present, allowing some function of the upper extremities. The wrist extensors receive innervation from C6 to C8, whereas the triceps are innervated at C7 to C8. The intrinsic muscles of the hand are the lowest to be innervated in the upper extremity at C8 to T1.

In the thoracic level, muscles receive innervation at each spinal level. Because the intercostal and erector spinae muscles receive innervation throughout the thoracic region, the lower the level of injury, the more muscles remain intact. The abdominal muscles receive innervation from the lower thoracic levels.

The muscles of the lumbar and sacral regions are controlled by plexus innervation, so once again the level of injury will be important in knowing which muscles are functioning. The hip flexors and knee extensors are innervated between L2 and L4. Next are the hip adductors at L2 to L3 and the hip abductors at L4 to L5. The hip extensors and knee flexors are innervated at L5 through S2. The ankle motions are innervated between

two spinal nerves have lost function. If an injury involves only one spinal nerve, sensation will be decreased or altered, but it will not be lost.

Thoracic Nerves

There are 12 pairs of thoracic nerves. With the exception of T1, which is part of the brachial plexus, thoracic nerves maintain their segmental relationship and do not join with the other nerves to form a plexus. As described, each nerve branches into a posterior and anterior ramus (see Fig. 6-18). The posterior rami innervate the muscles of the back (motor) and the overlying skin (sensory). The anterior rami become **intercostal nerves,** innervating the anterior trunk and intercostal muscles (motor) as well as the skin of the anterior and lateral trunk (sensory).

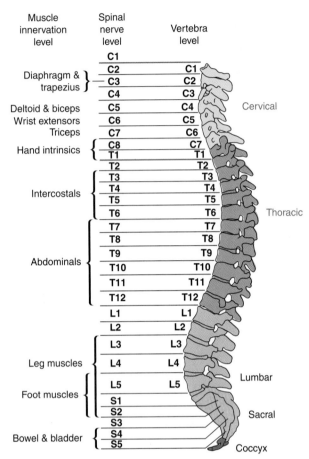

Muscle innervation level	Spinal nerve level	Vertebra level	
	C1		
Diaphragm & trapezius	C2	C1	
	C3	C2	
	C4	C3	
Deltoid & biceps	C5	C4	Cervical
Wrist extensors	C6	C5	
Triceps	C7	C6	
Hand intrinsics	C8	C7	
	T1	T1	
	T2	T2	
	T3	T3	
Intercostals	T4	T4	
	T5	T5	
	T6	T6	Thoracic
	T7	T7	
	T8	T8	
Abdominals	T9	T9	
	T10	T10	
	T11	T11	
	T12	T12	
	L1	L1	
	L2	L2	
Leg muscles	L3	L3	
	L4	L4	
Foot muscles	L5	L5	Lumbar
	S1		
	S2		Sacral
	S3		
Bowel & bladder	S4		
	S5		Coccyx

Figure 6-20. General innervation levels of major muscles. Lateral view of vertebral column.

L4 and S2. Last to receive innervation is bowel and bladder control at S4 to S5.

Sensation changes as one proceeds down the spinal cord. Figure 6-19 shows the sensory innervation (dermatomes) at various levels. A person with a C3 spinal cord injury will have sensation only from the top of the head to the neck. At T3, the entire upper extremity and chest, level with the axilla, are innervated. An injury at L3 would show muscle innervation in an irregular pattern to approximately the midthigh level.

Plexus Formation

Except for the thoracic nerves, the anterior rami of the spinal nerves will join together and/or branch out, forming a network known as a **plexus.** There are three major plexuses (Fig. 6-21):

1. The cervical plexus, made up of C1 through C4 spinal nerves, innervates the muscles of the neck.
2. The brachial plexus, made up of C5 through T1, innervates muscles of the upper limb.

3. The lumbosacral plexus, made up of L1 through S5, innervates muscles of the lower limb.
   a. The lumbar portion, L1 through L4, supplies mostly muscles of the thigh.
   b. The sacral portion, L5 through S3, supplies mostly muscles of the leg and foot.

Cervical Plexus

The anterior rami of the first four cervical nerves (C1 to C4) split and join together in a specific pattern to form the **cervical plexus** (see Fig. 6-21). This plexus will not be described in detail, because only a few muscles covered in this text receive their innervation from the cervical plexus.

A branch from C2 goes to the sternocleidomastoid, and branches from C3 and C4 supply the trapezius. The levator scapula receives innervation from C3 through C5. The anterior scalene gets some innervation from C4, and the middle scalene gets innervation from C3 and C4. Perhaps one of the most significant nerves of the cervical plexus is the *phrenic nerve,* which is formed by branches of C3 through C5 and innervates the diaphragm.

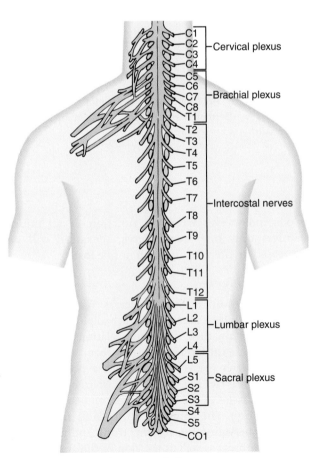

Figure 6-21. Spinal nerves and plexuses.

Brachial Plexus

The **brachial plexus** is formed by the anterior rami of C5 through T1 spinal nerves (see Fig. 6-21). It splits and joins several times before ending in five main peripheral nerves. Its network arrangement consists of roots, trunks, divisions, cords, and peripheral (terminal) nerves, as shown in Figure 6-22.

There are five roots made up of the anterior rami of C5, C6, C7, C8, and T1. These roots join together, forming three **trunks.** The three trunks, named for their position relative to each other, are the following:

1. The superior trunk coming from C5 and C6
2. The middle trunk coming from C7
3. The inferior trunk coming from C8 and T1

Each trunk splits into an anterior and posterior **division,** named for their position relative to each other.

Next are the three **cords,** named according to their relationship to the axillary artery. They are formed by the joining of trunk divisions. The lateral cord is formed by the anterior division of the superior and middle trunks. The posterior cord originates from the posterior divisions of all three trunks, and the medial cord comes from the anterior division of the inferior trunk. The five **peripheral nerves,** which are branches of the cords, form the terminal nerves of the plexus as follows:

1. Musculocutaneous nerve: from the lateral cord
2. Axillary nerve: a branch of the posterior cord

3. Radial nerve: a branch of the posterior cord
4. Median nerve: from the lateral and medial cords
5. Ulnar nerve: from the medial cord

This network arrangement provides muscles with innervation from more than one level. In the event of trauma or disease, perhaps not all levels of innervation will be involved. Therefore, a muscle may be weakened but not completely paralyzed.

For the most part, these five peripheral nerves innervate the muscles of the upper limb; however, some muscles receive innervation from nerves that have branched off the plexus superior to the formation of the peripheral nerves (not shown). The dorsal scapular nerve comes off the anterior ramus of C5 and innervates the rhomboids and levator scapulae muscles. The suprascapular nerve comes off the superior trunk and innervates the supraspinatus and infraspinatus muscles. The medial pectoral nerve comes off the medial cord and innervates the pectoralis major and minor muscles, while the lateral pectoral nerve comes off the lateral cord to provide additional innervation to the pectoralis major. The subscapular nerve comes off the posterior cord and innervates the subscapularis and teres major muscles. The thoracodorsal nerve also comes off the posterior cord to innervate the latissimus dorsi. All other muscles of the upper extremity receive innervation from the five terminal nerves described below.

Terminal Nerves of the Brachial Plexus

The five terminal, or peripheral, nerves of the brachial plexus have been summarized according to the following:

1. The segment, or root, of the spinal cord from which they originate
2. The major muscles they innervate
3. The major sensory distribution
4. The main motor impairments that would be seen following damage to the nerve

Axillary Nerve (Fig. 6-23)

Spinal cord segment	C5, C6
Muscle innervation	Deltoid, teres minor
Sensory distribution	Lateral arm over lower portion of deltoid
Clinical motor features of paralysis	Loss of shoulder abduction
	Weakened shoulder lateral rotation

Musculocutaneous Nerve (Fig. 6-24)

Spinal cord segment	C5, C6
Muscle innervation	Coracobrachialis, biceps, brachialis

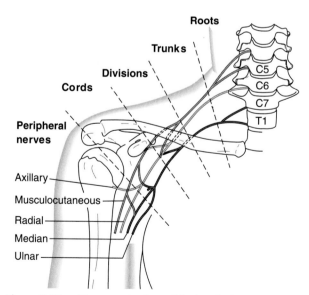

Figure 6-22.   The organization of the brachial plexus from the nerve roots to the peripheral nerves. Some lesser motor and sensory nerves have been omitted.

Sensory distribution
  Anterior lateral surface of forearm

Clinical motor features of paralysis
  Loss of elbow flexion, weakened supination

Radial Nerve (Fig. 6-25)

Spinal segment C6, C7, C8, T1

Muscle innervation Triceps; anconeus; brachioradialis; supinator; wrist, finger, and thumb extensors

Sensory distribution Posterior arm, posterior forearm, and radial side of posterior hand

Clinical motor features of paralysis Loss of elbow, wrist, finger, and thumb extension (commonly called "wrist drop")

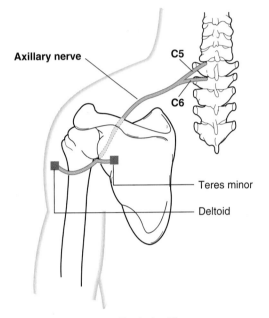

Posterior View

Figure 6-23. The axillary nerve.

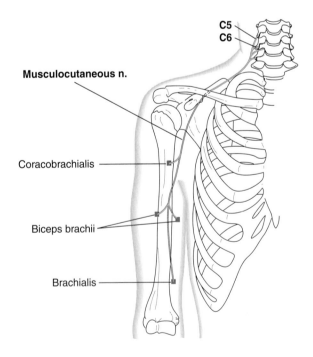

Anterior View

Figure 6-24. The musculocutaneous nerve.

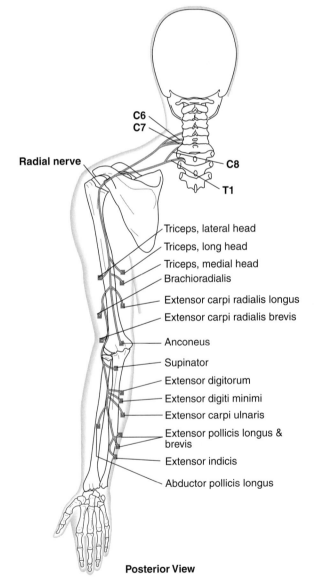

Posterior View

Figure 6-25. The radial nerve.

Median Nerve (Fig. 6-26)

Spinal cord segment	C6, C7, C8, T1
Muscle innervation	Pronators
	Wrist and finger flexors on radial side
	Most thumb muscles
Sensory distribution	Palmar aspect of thumb, second, third, fourth (radial half) fingers
Clinical motor features of paralysis	Loss of forearm pronation
	Loss of thumb opposition, flexion, and abduction ("ape hand"), weakened wrist flexors (radial side), weak-ened wrist radial deviation
	Weakened second and third finger flexion ("pope's blessing" or "hand of benediction")

Ulnar Nerve (Fig. 6-27)

Spinal cord segment	C8, T1
Muscle innervation	Flexor carpi ulnaris
	Flexor digitorum profundus (medial half)
	Interossei
	Fourth and fifth lumbricales

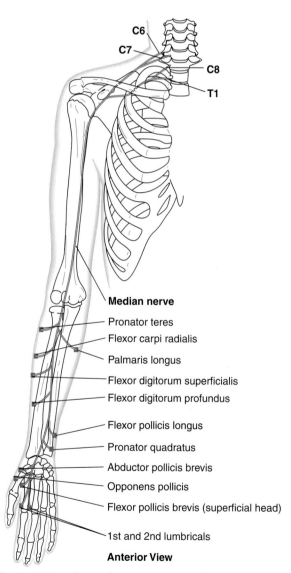

Median nerve
- Pronator teres
- Flexor carpi radialis
- Palmaris longus
- Flexor digitorum superficialis
- Flexor digitorum profundus
- Flexor pollicis longus
- Pronator quadratus
- Abductor pollicis brevis
- Opponens pollicis
- Flexor pollicis brevis (superficial head)
- 1st and 2nd lumbricals

Anterior View

Figure 6-26.   The median nerve.

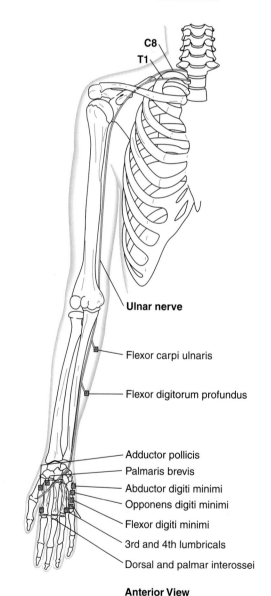

Ulnar nerve
- Flexor carpi ulnaris
- Flexor digitorum profundus
- Adductor pollicis
- Palmaris brevis
- Abductor digiti minimi
- Opponens digiti minimi
- Flexor digiti minimi
- 3rd and 4th lumbricals
- Dorsal and palmar interossei

Anterior View

Figure 6-27.   The ulnar nerve.

Sensory distribution	Fourth finger (medial portion), fifth finger
Clinical motor features of paralysis	Loss of wrist ulnar deviation
	Weakened wrist, finger flexion
	Loss of thumb adduction
	Loss of most intrinsics ("claw hand")

Lumbosacral Plexus

The lumbosacral plexus is formed by the anterior rami of L1 through S3 (Fig. 6-28). Some sources will separate this into a **lumbar plexus** (L1 through L4), which innervates most muscles of the thigh, and a **sacral plexus** (L5 through S3), which innervates mostly muscles of the leg and foot. Because there are several muscles of the lower limb that receive innervation from both plexuses, they will be discussed here as one plexus.

The lumbosacral plexus does not have as much dividing and joining of nerve fibers as does the brachial plexus, although there are some. It has eight roots that each divide into an upper and lower branch. L3 is the only root that does not divide. Most of these branches divide into an anterior and posterior division. These divisions join in a specific pattern to form the six main peripheral nerves.

The upper branch of L1 divides into the iliohypogastric and ilioinguinal nerve fibers. The lower branch of L1 and the upper branch of L2 form the genitofemoral nerve. These three nerves are primarily sensory in nature and will not be discussed in detail.

The anterior divisions of L2, L3, and L4 form the **obturator nerve.** Posterior divisions of the same roots form the **femoral nerve.** The posterior divisions of L4 through S1 form the **superior gluteal nerve,** and the posterior divisions of L5 through S2 make up the **inferior gluteal nerve.** The **sciatic nerve** is made up of branches from L4 through S3. It is actually the tibial and common peroneal nerves joined by a common sheath, and it separates into the two nerves just above the knee. The **common peroneal nerve** comes from L4 through S2, while the **tibial nerve** is made up of anterior divisions of L4 through S3. If all of this is confusing, perhaps the illustrations in Figures 6-29 through 6-33, plus the summary that follows, will provide some clarity. This summary is similar to the one provided for the brachial plexus.

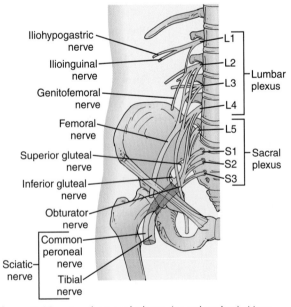

Figure 6-28. Lumbosacral plexus (anterior view). Note that anterior divisions are in yellow and posterior divisions are in green. Some lesser motor and sensory nerves have been omitted.

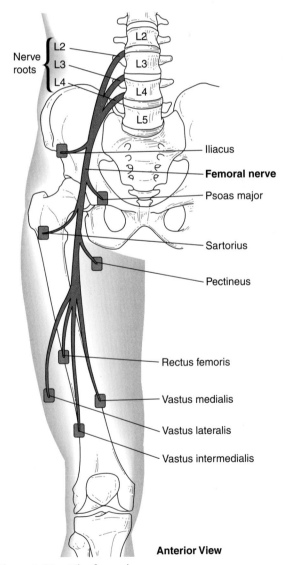

Figure 6-29. The femoral nerve.

Terminal Nerves of the Lumbosacral Plexus

Like the nerves of the upper extremity, the nerves of the lower extremity have been summarized according to the following:

1. The segment, or root, of the spinal cord from which they come
2. The major muscles they innervate
3. The major sensory distribution
4. The main motor impairments that would be seen following damage to the nerve

Femoral Nerve (Fig. 6-29)

Spinal cord segment	L2, L3, L4
Muscle innervation	Iliopsoas (iliacus and psoas major), sartorius, pectineus, quadricep femoris
Sensory distribution	Anterior and medial thigh, medial leg, and foot
Clinical motor features of paralysis	Weakened hip flexion Loss of knee extension

Obturator Nerve (Fig. 6-30)

Spinal cord segment	L2, L3, L4
Muscle innervation	Hip adductors Obturator externus
Sensory distribution	Middle part of medial thigh
Clinical motor features of paralysis	Loss of hip adduction Weakened hip lateral rotation

Sciatic Nerve (Made up of Tibial and Common Peroneal Nerves; Fig. 6-31)

Spinal segment	L4, L5, S1, S2, S3
Muscle innervation	Hamstring muscles
Sensory distribution	None
Clinical motor features of paralysis	Weakened hip extension Loss of knee flexion

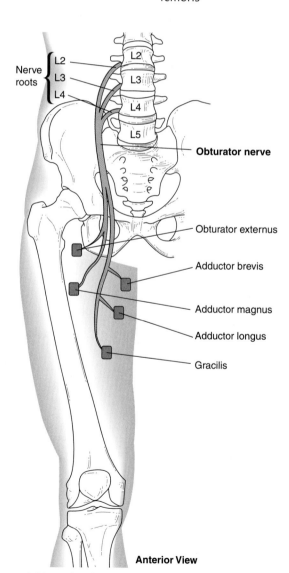

Nerve roots
L2
L3
L4

L2
L3
L4
L5

Obturator nerve

Obturator externus

Adductor brevis

Adductor magnus

Adductor longus

Gracilis

Anterior View

Figure 6-30. The obturator nerve.

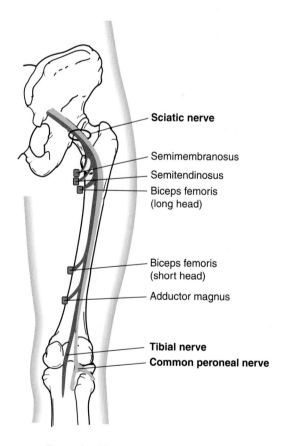

Sciatic nerve

Semimembranosus

Semitendinosus

Biceps femoris (long head)

Biceps femoris (short head)

Adductor magnus

Tibial nerve

Common peroneal nerve

Posterior View

Figure 6-31. The sciatic nerve.

Tibial Nerve (Divides into the Medial and Lateral Plantar Nerves; Fig. 6-32)

Spinal cord segment	L4, L5, S1, S2, S3
Muscle innervation	Popliteus
	Ankle plantar flexors
	Tibialis posterior
	Foot intrinsics (medial and lateral plantar)
Sensory distribution	Posterior lateral leg, lateral foot
Clinical motor features of paralysis	Loss of ankle plantar flexion
	Weakened ankle inversion
	Loss of toe flexion

Common Peroneal Nerve (Divides into Superficial and Deep Peroneal Nerves; Fig. 6-33)

Spinal segment	L4, L5, S1, S2
Muscle innervation	Peroneals (mostly superficial peroneal)
	Tibialis anterior (deep peroneal)
	Toe extensors (deep peroneal)
Sensory distribution	Anterior lateral aspect of leg and foot
Clinical motor features of paralysis	Loss of ankle dorsiflexion ("foot drop")
	Loss of toe extension
	Loss of ankle eversion

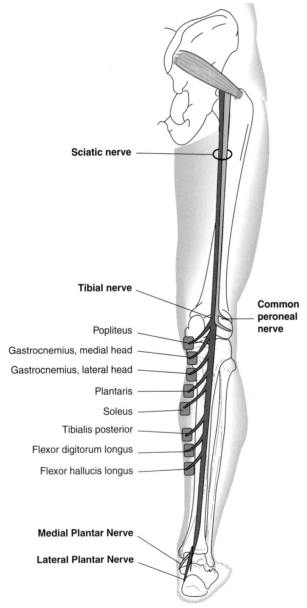

Figure 6-32. The tibial nerve. It divides into the medial and lateral plantar nerves.

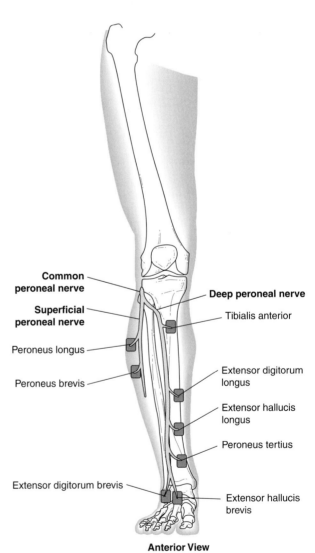

Figure 6-33. The peroneal nerves. The common peroneal nerve divides into the superficial and deep peroneal nerves.

Common Pathologies of the Central and Peripheral Nervous Systems

The following is a very incomplete list of common central and peripheral nerve system pathologies. The very brief description focuses on the anatomical location or the functional implications of the defect or disease.

Common Pathologies of the Central Nervous System

Congenital Defects

Spina bifida is a congenital defect in which the posterior segments of the vertebra fail to close during embryo development. There are three types, ranging from few or no signs and symptoms to quite severe symptoms. With **spina bifida occulta,** a small bony defect is present, but the spinal cord and nerves are usually normal. With **meningocele,** there is a bony defect through which the meninges protrude. There is usually little or no nerve damage. With **myelomeningocele,** the most severe form of spina bifida, the meninges and spinal nerves come through the bony defect. This causes nerve damage and severe disability.

Hydrocephalus, once called "water on the brain," is a congenital or acquired defect involving cerebrospinal fluid (CSF) production, absorption, and flow through the ventricles and subarachnoid space. An excessive accumulation of CSF results in an abnormal widening of the ventricles, which creates potentially harmful pressure on the brain tissues.

Cerebral palsy is a term used to describe a group of nonprogressive disorders of the brain that result from damage in utero, at birth, or soon after birth. It is not always congenital. The signs and symptoms of cerebral palsy are variable and depend upon the area of the brain that is damaged.

Spinal Cord Trauma

Spinal cord injury (SCI) can take many forms, depending on (1) the spinal level and (2) the area of the damage. These injuries usually result in loss of sensation and muscle function. SCIs are divided into two categories, based on level. *Quadriplegia,* which refers to all four extremities, involves T1 and above. *Paraplegia* refers to lower extremity involvement of T2 and below.

An incomplete SCI can result when only part of the cord is damaged. **Central cord syndrome** is associated with greater loss of upper limb function compared to the lower limbs. **Brown-Séquard's syndrome** results from injury to one side of the spinal cord, causing weakness and loss of proprioception on the side of the injury and loss of pain and thermal sensation on the opposite side. **Anterior cord syndrome** occurs when the injury affects the anterior spinal tracts. Because the posterior part of the cord is spared, proprioception that is carried in that part of the cord is preserved, but muscle function, pain sensation, and thermal sensation are lost.

Autonomic dysreflexia, also known as **hyperreflexia,** is a serious and potentially life-threatening complication associated with spinal cord injuries at or above T10. It is usually triggered by a noxious stimulus below the level of injury, such as a distended bladder. Symptoms include severe headache, sudden hypertension, facial flush, sweating, and gooseflesh. Blood pressure may rise to dangerous levels; untreated, it can lead to stroke or death.

Disorders of Muscle and the Neuromuscular Junction

Myasthenia gravis is a disease that involves a defect at the neuromuscular junction, where the terminal axon synapses with the receptor site of muscles. This results in weakness and fatigue of skeletal muscles.

Muscular dystrophy is a hereditary and progressive disease of the muscle tissue. It is characterized by weakness of proximal muscles, followed by progressive involvement of distal muscles.

Degenerative Diseases

Amyotrophic lateral sclerosis is a degenerative motor disease involving both upper and lower motor neurons. It is also know as Lou Gehrig's disease.

Alzheimer's disease is an irreversible, progressive brain disorder causing dementia and loss of cognitive functioning. It eventually destroys a person's ability to function.

Demyelinating Diseases

Multiple sclerosis is characterized by a breaking down of the myelin sheath around axons. This will interfere with normal nerve transmission. *Sclerosis* refers to scars or lesions in the white matter of the brain and spinal cord.

Common Pathologies of Peripheral Nerves

Neuropathy of a peripheral nerve is usually accompanied by neurological deficits along the nerve pathway. They are usually classified according to cause or anatomical location. Sensory distribution and clinical motor features of paralysis have been described earlier, with the individual nerves. The following is a very brief description of some of the more common peripheral nerve conditions.

Typical muscle paralysis patterns can be seen depending on the peripheral nerve involved and the level at which it is injured. **Bell's palsy** involves the facial nerve (cranial nerve VII), which controls movement of facial muscles. The condition is usually temporary and typically affects only one side of the face.

The following conditions commonly affect the upper extremities. **Scapular winging** occurs when an injury to the long thoracic nerve weakens or paralyzes the serratus anterior muscle, causing the medial border of the scapula to rise away from the rib cage.

There are three well-known conditions involving the brachial plexus. **Thoracic outlet syndrome** is a group of disorders that occur when the nerves of the brachial plexus and/or the subclavian artery and vein become compressed in the thoracic outlet—the space between the clavicle and first rib and possibly the scalene muscles. **Burner, or stinger, syndrome** can occur following a stretch or compression injury to the brachial plexus from a blow to the head or shoulder. This is relatively common in football players and is also seen in wrestlers and gymnasts. Symptoms include immediate burning pain, prickly paresthesia radiating from the neck, numbness, and even brief paralysis of the arm. These symptoms should resolve within minutes, although shoulder weakness and muscle tenderness of the neck may continue for a few days. **Erb's palsy** (sometimes known as *tip position*) is a traction injury to a baby's upper brachial plexus and occurs most commonly during a difficult childbirth. The affected arm hangs in shoulder extension and medial rotation, elbow extended, forearm pronated, and wrist flexed.

There are two conditions that affect the radial nerve in approximately the same location but have different causes. **Saturday night palsy** occurs when the radial nerve becomes compressed as it spirals around the mid-humerus. The name derives from the nature of the injury—the person, often intoxicated, falls asleep with his or her arm over the back of a chair. **Wrist drop** (loss of wrist extension) and a weakened ability to release objects (finger extension) will result from a high radial nerve injury, which is often a complication of a mid-humeral fracture.

Carpal tunnel syndrome is the result of compression on the median nerve as it passes within the carpal tunnel. The tunnel is formed by the transverse carpal ligament superficially and the bony floor of the carpal bones deep. A similar condition called **cubital tunnel syndrome** occurs when the ulnar nerve crosses the medial border of the elbow as the nerve runs through a bony passageway called the *cubital tunnel.* When you "hit your funny bone" and have tingling in the small and ring fingers, you are hitting the ulnar nerve at the cubital tunnel. The ulnar nerve can also be compressed distally by sustained pressure on the hypothenar eminence such as leaning on handle bars during long bicycle rides.

The following conditions describe hand positions that result from specific nerve damage. Loss of thumb opposition *(median nerve injury)* is referred to as **ape hand,** because, like apes, the person is unable to oppose the thumb. Inability to flex the thumb, index, and middle fingers (also median nerve) gives the appearance of the **pope's blessing,** or **hand of benediction.** Loss of the intrinsic muscles due to ulnar nerve damage results in a **claw hand.** The proximal phalanges are hyperextended, and the middle and distal phalanges are in extreme flexion.

The following conditions commonly affect the lower extremity. **Sciatica** is caused by irritation on the sciatic nerve roots, with pain radiating down the back of the leg. It is often caused by compression from a herniated lumbar disc.

Damage to the common peroneal nerve can result in **foot drop.** It is often caused by cast pressure at the head of the fibula, where the nerve is quite superficial as it lies over the bony fibular head.

Morton's neuroma is an enlarged nerve and usually occurs between the third and fourth toes (branches of the tibial nerve). The enlargement usually involves nerve compression in a confined space. This could be from a flattening of the metatarsal arch; wearing high heels, which transfers weight forward, putting more pressure on the metatarsal arch area; or wearing a shoe with a tight toe box, creating compression on the nerves as they pass between the metatarsals.

Review Questions

1. The spinal cord extends to about what vertebral level?

2. What makes up gray matter? White matter?

3. Name the bony, membranous, and fluid features that protect the brain from trauma.

4. What are the differences between upper and lower motor neurons?

5. How do thoracic nerves differ from cervical or lumbar nerves?

6. What is the difference between an afferent and an efferent nerve fiber?

7. In an individual who has lost the ability to oppose the thumb, what nerve is involved? What is a common term for this condition?

8. In an individual who has lost the ability to pick up the toes (ankle dorsiflexion), what nerve is involved? What is a common term for this condition?

9. Claw hand involves the loss of what muscle group? What nerve is primarily involved?

10. If a person had a subdural hematoma from a blow to the head, where would that hematoma be located?

11. If a person had pressure on a nerve root, what bony area is likely to be involved?

12. If a person has a spinal cord injury at L4, would it be considered an upper or lower motor neuron lesion?

13. Would the spinal cord injury at L4 show clinical signs more like a spinal cord lesion or a peripheral nerve lesion? Why?

14. Does a motor nerve send impulses from the periphery to the spinal cord or from the spinal cord to the periphery?

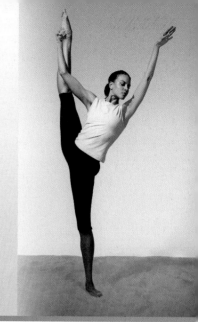

CHAPTER 7
Circulatory System

Cardiovascular System

   Heart

   Blood Vessels

Lymphatic System

   Functions

   Drainage Patterns

Common Pathologies

Review Questions

   Cardiovascular System

   Lymphatic System

The circulatory system includes two types of transport systems: (1) the cardiovascular system and (2) the lymphatic system.

The **cardiovascular system,** which includes the blood vessels (arteries and veins) and the heart, transports blood throughout the body. Arteries and veins transport blood from the capillaries in the lungs—where carbon dioxide is exchanged for oxygen—to capillaries throughout the body, where oxygen is exchanged for carbon dioxide. The heart is the pump that pushes blood through the arteries and veins. Blood and lymph are the liquid mediums in which the materials are transported.

Linked directly to the circulatory system and the immune system, the **lymphatic system** is made up of lymph vessels and nodes. It collects excess extracellular fluid as lymph and transports it from the periphery to the venous system, thereby helping the cardiovascular system maintain adequate blood volume and pressure. In addition, the lymphatic system helps the immune system by filtering bacteria, viruses, waste products, and other foreign matter and by producing specific antibodies that help the immune system fight infection and defend against invasion by foreign material.

Cardiovascular System

Because blood never leaves the body's network of arteries, veins, and capillaries, the cardiovascular system is considered a closed system. It operates two different and distinct circuits, or loops—the pulmonary circuit and the systemic circuit (Fig. 7-1). The **pulmonary circuit** transports oxygen-depleted blood (shown in blue) from the body through the right side of the heart (right atrium and right ventricle) to the lungs via the pulmonary arteries. When blood reaches the lungs, carbon dioxide is exchanged for oxygen before returning to the left side of the heart via pulmonary veins. The **systemic circuit** loops through the left side of the heart (left atrium and

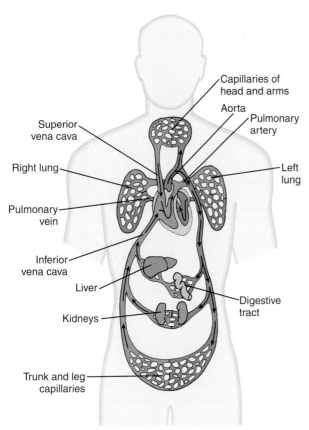

Figure 7-1. Pulmonary and systemic circulation (anterior view).

left ventricle), out to the rest of the body via the aorta and branching arteries, and then to capillary beds. It is here in the capillary beds that oxygenated blood (shown in red) is exchanged for deoxygenated blood, which then returns to the heart through a series of veins.

Heart

Unlike most other muscles discussed in this book, the heart is largely an involuntary muscle. For example, you cannot consciously decide whether to contract your heart muscle like you do, say, the biceps brachii muscle. This is a good thing. Imagine if you got busy doing a task and forgot to contract your heart, or if you went to sleep and didn't tell your heart to contract. In other words, the heart must be under involuntary control, because it needs to work constantly all day and all night. You can learn to control heart rate to some extent, but you cannot stop or start your heart.

How much does the heart work? Assume that your heart contracts 72 times per minute. At 60 minutes per hour, 24 hours per day, and 365 days per year, your heart contracts around 38 million times per year. If

you live to the age of 80, your heart will contract over 3 trillion times without stopping.

The heart's function is to provide the pumping force to move blood though blood vessels (arteries, capillaries, and veins). It is not directly responsible for the exchange of oxygen and carbon dioxide. That function is carried out in the lungs.

Location

The heart is approximately the size of the body's closed fist. It is contained in the middle portion of the thoracic cavity known as the **mediastinum** (Fig. 7-2), with about two-thirds of its mass to the left of midline. The thoracic cavity also contains the left and right lungs, which lie on either side of the heart. All of the chest organs except the lungs are contained within the mediastinum, including the heart, aorta, thymus gland, chest portion of the trachea, esophagus, lymph nodes, and vagus nerves.

The heart lies between the sternum and the vertebral column (Fig. 7-3). Manual, rhythmic pressing and releasing on the sternum creates pressure differences within the thoracic cavity that allows blood to be pumped through the heart. This is the basis for cardiac compression applied during cardiopulmonary resuscitation (CPR).

Chambers

The heart is made up of four separate chambers and is divided into right and left halves. Each half is again divided into an upper and lower part. The two top chambers are called **atria** (singular is *atrium*), and the two bottom chambers are called **ventricles** (Fig. 7-4). The atria, which receive blood from veins, have relatively thin muscular walls, because they are required to

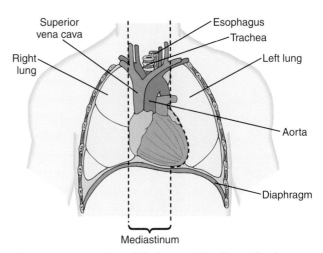

Figure 7-2. Location of the heart within the mediastinum—that area in the chest cavity between the two lungs.

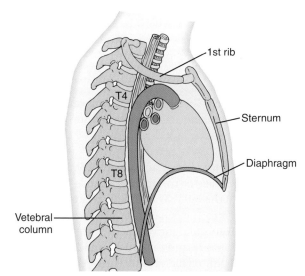

Figure 7-3.   The position of the heart between two hard surfaces (sternum and vertebral column) within the thoracic cavity allows one to apply cardiac compression (of CPR) that will create pressure differences in the heart that will continue pumping blood to the brain.

propel blood only into the ventricles. Larger than the atria, the ventricles have thicker walls that provide a greater pumping force. The left ventricle is approximately three times thicker than the right ventricle. This thickness is necessary to withstand the greater pumping force that is needed to push blood out to all areas of the body, as opposed to just pumping blood from the heart to the lungs.

Valves

Heart valves function by allowing blood to flow through the heart in only one direction. Just as there are four heart chambers, there are four heart valves. These valves lead into and out of the ventricles. Two **atrioventricular** (AV) valves lie between the atria and the ventricles, and two **semilunar** (SL) valves lie between the ventricles and the arteries leading out of the heart (see Fig. 7-4).

When shut, AV valves prevent the backflow of blood from the ventricles into the atria. Because the AV valve between the right atrium and ventricle has three flaps, it is called the **tricuspid valve.** The AV valve between the left atrium and ventricle is called the **bicuspid valve** and has only two flaps. It is also referred to as the **mitral valve,** because it resembles the ceremonial headdress, consisting of two like parts (miter), worn by bishops and certain other clergy.

The SL valve located between the right ventricle and the pulmonary arteries leading to the lungs is also called the **pulmonic,** or **pulmonary, valve.** The valve between the left ventricle and the aorta is the **aortic valve.** These valves prevent blood from flowing backward into the heart.

Blood Flow Through the Heart

Deoxygenated blood (high in carbon dioxide and low in oxygen) from the peripheral tissues of the body returns to the heart via the superior and inferior vena cavae and enters the right atrium. It then passes through the right AV (tricuspid) valve into the right ventricle. Blood continues out of the right ventricle and through the pulmonic

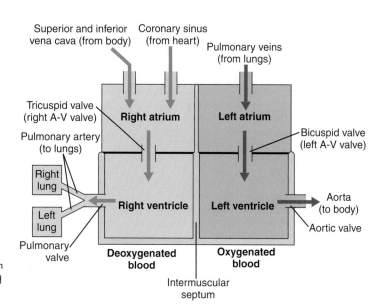

Figure 7-4.   Schematic illustration of heart chambers, valves, and blood flow through the heart. Note that blood vessels have been shown in different positions within the chambers compared to a real heart.

valve into the pulmonary trunk, which branches into the right and left pulmonary arteries and then on to the lungs. It is in the lungs that carbon dioxide is exchanged for oxygen. Oxygenated blood leaves the lungs via the pulmonary veins and enters the heart's left atrium. From there, blood passes through the left AV (bicuspid) valve and into the left ventricle. The left ventricle pumps blood out of the heart through the aortic valve, into the aorta, and then out to the entire body, including the heart muscle itself (Fig. 7-5). Blood leaving the left ventricle is under the greatest pressure due to the powerful contraction needed to push blood throughout the body. In summary, the right side of the heart pumps deoxygenated blood to the lungs, and the left side pumps oxygenated blood throughout the body.

Heart Sounds

Heart sounds, which result when the heart valves close, can be heard with a stethoscope. These sounds are often described as *lub-dub*. The right and left atria contract together, followed by contraction of the right and left ventricles. As stated above, blood returns to the atria, the AV valves (tricuspid and bicuspid) open, the atria contract, and blood flows into the ventricles. When the ventricles are full, the AV valves close, making the first heart sound (*lub*). Next, the SL valves open, the ventricles contract, and blood is pumped to the aortic and pulmonary arteries. The SL valves then close to prevent

blood from flowing back into the ventricles when the ventricles relax. This is when the second heart sound (*dub*) is heard. The cycle starts again and repeats itself approximately 72 times per minute.

Cardiac Cycle

The **cardiac cycle** is a series of mechanical events that we will begin tracing in the right atrium. When the right atrium relaxes, blood rushes out of the superior and inferior vena cavae and into the right atrium. Once filled, the atrium suddenly and sharply contracts, greatly reducing the size of the chamber. Since there are no valves between the vena cavae and the atrium, blood can go backward into the vena cavae or forward, through the opening into the right ventricle. Since the ventricle is relaxed and empty, and the superior and inferior vena cavae are still full of blood wanting to enter the right atrium, the path of least resistance is through the opening between the atrium and the ventricle. Therefore, contraction of the atrium drives the blood into the right ventricle.

As the ventricle fills, the AV valve closes and the blood cannot flow backward into the atrium. Once full, the ventricle contracts and forces the blood out of the heart, through the pulmonic valve, and into the pulmonary arteries. The pulmonary arteries are already full of blood, but the force of the contraction pushes the blood in the pulmonary arteries along to all other vessels

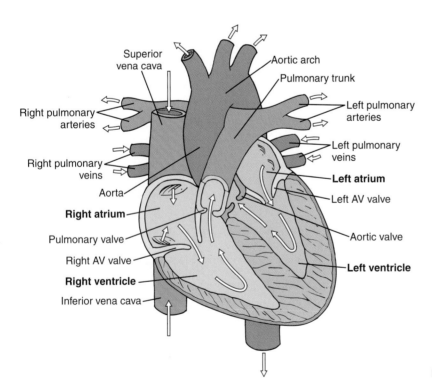

Figure 7-5. Blood flow through heart.

"downstream" and eventually into the lung capillaries. The blood already in the capillaries is pushed onward into the pulmonary veins, and blood flow continues toward the left side of the heart.

What occurs on the right side of the heart also occurs *at the same time* on the left side. Blood enters the left atrium through the pulmonary veins. Once filled, the left atrium contracts, greatly reducing the size of its chamber. The blood takes the path of least resistance and enters the empty and relaxed left ventricle. When the left ventricle is full, the AV valve closes. The ventricle contracts and pushes the blood through the aortic valve into the aorta. The aorta is already full of blood, but the force of the contraction pushes it into the aorta, along to all the other vessels "downstream," and eventually into the capillaries throughout the body. Blood already in the body's capillary beds is pushed into the veins and continues through the venous system toward the right side of the heart.

Blood Vessels

Types of Blood Vessels

There are three basic types of blood vessels: arteries, veins, and capillaries. The walls of arteries and veins are three layers thick. The outermost layer is called the *tunica adventitia,* which is made up of connective tissue; the middle layer is the *tunica media,* which is composed of smooth muscle and elastic fibers; and the innermost layer is the *tunica intima,* which is made up of endothelium. Capillaries are essentially one-layer endothelial tubes.

By definition, **arteries** carry blood away from the heart and to the rest of the body's tissues. The largest artery is the **aorta,** and the smallest ones are called **arterioles.** Because arteries carry blood *away* from the heart, that blood tends to be rich in oxygen. The exceptions are the pulmonary arteries, which carry deoxygenated blood away from the heart and to the lungs, where it is exchanged for oxygen-rich blood. Arterial walls must be very strong, muscular, and elastic to withstand the great pressure to which arteries are subjected.

Veins carry blood *toward* the heart. The largest are the superior and inferior **vena cavae,** and the smallest are **venules.** With the exception of the pulmonary veins, all veins carry deoxygenated blood (rich in carbon dioxide and poor in oxygen) toward the heart. The pulmonary veins carry blood to the heart, but the blood is high in oxygen. Veins tend to be larger in diameter, have thinner walls, and are less elastic than arteries. Veins that carry blood against the force of gravity usually contain valves to prevent backflow. For this reason, valves are more common in the lower extremity than in the upper extremity. They are also more common in the deeper veins than in the superficial ones. The valves are actually folds in the inner layer of the veins, usually arranged in two cusps. The valves allow blood to flow toward the heart, but they fill and come together to occlude the vessel when blood tries to reverse its direction of flow.

Generally speaking, veins are paired with arteries and share the same name. For example, there are the axillary artery and vein, and the femoral artery and vein. Of course, there are exceptions. For example, the carotid artery and the jugular vein run together in the neck. (Some of these exceptions will be noted later in the chapter when describing the blood supply to various areas.) It is important to remember that while arteries and veins may parallel each other, blood is flowing in *opposite* directions.

Capillaries (capillary beds) form the link between arterioles and venules. They are microscopic, with walls only one endothelial cell layer thick. All exchange of oxygen and carbon dioxide occurs in the capillaries.

The cardiovascular system has many general similarities to a highway system. Both systems are involved in orderly two-way transport. Just like freeways, arteries and veins tend to run together throughout the body but in opposite directions—arteries move blood *away* from the heart, and veins move blood *toward* the heart. Visualize driving around the city on a freeway that leads to various destinations. There are many exits (branches and divisions) from the freeway that lead to smaller roads and streets (arteries) until you turn into the driveway (arteriole) of your destination (capillary bed). Once there, you unload the groceries (oxygen) and pick up the recycling (carbon dioxide). You then retrace your route, driving up increasingly larger streets (venules to veins to vena cava) until you return to where you began (the heart).

Arteries and veins generally run parallel throughout the body, connected with a weblike network of capillaries. This two-way transport system goes to every part of the body. To appreciate how vast, dense, and delicate this network of blood vessels is, consider the human body dissected of everything except blood vessels. What remains is a dense, meshlike form of the body (Fig. 7-6).

Regardless of where in the body blood travels after leaving the heart, it gets there through a series of ever smaller arteries and returns via a series of ever larger veins. This anatomical concept is the key to understanding many clinical conditions. For example, a clot that formed in the heart due to turbulent blood flow from a faulty heart valve would travel through the heart and out into the arterial system until it reached an

If a clot dislodges from a vein, it will travel along the venous system, passing through ever larger vessels, through the right side of the heart, and end up in the pulmonary artery system. Why? The clot travels until it reaches a vessel small enough to block further passage. In the venous system, vessel diameter increases along the passageway to the heart. The heart is basically a hollow organ through which blood is pumped. Vessel diameter decreases in size along the arterial system, in this case the pulmonary arteries to the lungs.

Pulse and Blood Pressure

A pulse is an important clinical feature of arteries. It is the "throbbing" that can be felt at various locations in the body, caused by the contraction and expansion of an artery as a wave of blood passes by a particular spot. A pulse can be palpated anywhere that an artery can be compressed against a bone and that is near enough to the surface to be felt. Common sites for feeling a pulse are at the wrist (radial artery), at the neck (carotid artery), and atop the ankle (dorsalis pedis artery, a branch of the posterior tibial artery). Figure 7-7 shows these and other sites where a pulse can be detected. The pulse is usually an accurate measure of heart rate. An average pulse is about 72 beats per minute.

Another important clinical feature of arteries is the measurement of **blood pressure.** You can "hear" your heart in action with a stethoscope. Heart ventricles work together and have two phases. When they contract, they send blood either to the lungs (from the right ventricle) or to the rest of the body (from the left ventricle). Blood

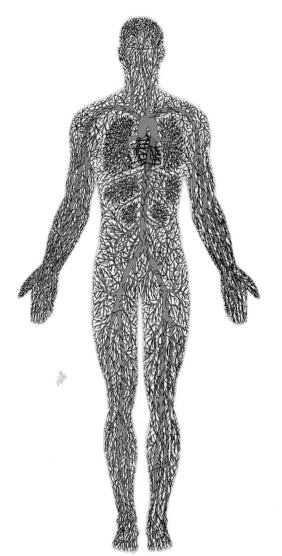

Figure 7-6. The body's vast system of blood vessels creates a dense and delicate web that mirrors the shape of the body.

artery that was too small to allow the clot to travel any farther. There the clot would either decrease the flow of blood beyond that point or block it completely. A clot that originates on the heart's right side will end up in the pulmonary artery system. A clot that originates on the heart's left side will travel through the aorta and end up in a smaller artery somewhere in the body, depending on which branch of the aorta it travels. It could end up in the brain, in an extremity, or in an organ. It could enter one of the coronary arteries, the first branch off of the aorta. How far along the pathway it travels depends on the clot's size. The smaller the clot, the farther along the arterial system it will travel before becoming wedged.

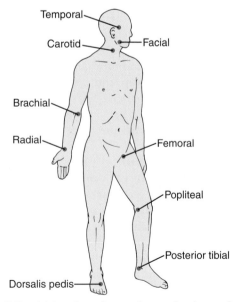

Figure 7-7. Major sites where pulse can be detected.

pressure is highest during the contraction phase (systole) and lowest when the ventricles relax and fill with blood (diastole). Both phases of blood pressure can be measured using a sphygmomanometer (blood pressure cuff). Systolic pressure is the highest pressure in an artery at the moment when the heart beats and pumps blood through the body. This is the first sound heard through the stethoscope as the pressure cuff deflates. Diastolic pressure is the lowest pressure in an artery between successive heartbeats, when heart sounds cannot be heard.

The average systolic pressure is about 120 mm mercury, and an average diastolic pressure is about 80 mm mercury. Because systolic pressure is always recorded first, this would be recorded as 120/80.

Pathways

In the following section, the main arteries are described as they branch and divide, followed by a similar description of the main veins. Keep in mind that arteries and veins often run parallel to each other and often have the same name. However, it is important to remember that blood in these vessels is traveling in opposite directions. In arteries, blood travels *away* from the heart; in veins, blood travels *toward* the heart. Table 7-1 summarizes the major arteries, the main branches described in this chapter, and the area they supply. Table 7-2 summarizes the major veins, the veins they empty into, and the region drained.

The first pathway to be described leads from the heart to the beginning of the lower extremity. The aorta leaves the left ventricle of the heart, passes upward (**ascending aorta**), and arches above the heart (Fig. 7-8). Immediately branching off the ascending aorta are the right and left **coronary arteries,** which supply blood to the heart muscle (myocardium) itself. The cardiac veins, which essentially parallel the coronary arteries, are the tributaries that drain most of the myocardium, emptying into the coronary sinus. The coronary sinus is the largest venous vessel of the heart and empties directly into the right atrium.

The **arch** of the aorta contains three branches: the brachiocephalic, the left common carotid, and the left subclavian arteries. The **brachiocephalic trunk** (from the Latin *brachium,* meaning "arm" and *cephalicus,* meaning "head") is the major blood source for the right arm and right side of the head. This artery is very short, but its pathway allows the right-side arteries to cross over the heart to the body's right side, where it divides into the right common carotid and right subclavian arteries. The second and third branches off the aortic arch are the left common carotid and the subclavian arteries, respectively. The carotid artery travels up the neck, while the subclavian artery goes to the upper extremity.

Table 7-1   Summary of Major Arteries

Name	Main Branches	Area Supplied
Ascending aorta	Coronary	Heart
Aortic arch	Brachiocephalic	
	Left subclavian	Upper extremity—left
	Left common carotid	Neck—left side
Brachiocephalic	Right subclavian	Upper extremity—right
	Right common carotid	Neck—right side
Common carotid	Internal carotid	Brain
	External carotid	External head
Subclavian	Vertebral	Brain
	Axillary	Upper extremity
Axillary	Brachial	Arm
Brachial	Radial and ulnar	Forearm and hand
Descending aorta	Renal	Kidneys
	Common iliac	Lower abdomen
Common iliac	Internal iliac	Pelvic region
	External iliac	Lower extremity
External iliac	Femoral	Thigh
Femoral	Popliteal	Knee
Popliteal	Anterior and posterior tibial	Leg and foot

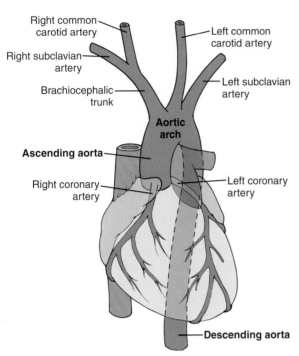

Figure 7-8. Main parts of aorta: ascending aorta, aortic arch, and descending aorta.

After these branches, the aorta turns downward and becomes the **descending aorta.** The aorta's huge diameter largely protects it from blockage by clots, although high pressure within it can make it susceptible to an aneurysm. The descending aorta runs down through the trunk to supply the lower extremities, branching off in many places along the way. At approximately the fourth lumbar vertebra, it divides into the right and left **common iliac** arteries (Fig. 7-9), which in turn divide into **external and internal iliac** arteries. The external iliac arteries supply the lower limbs, while the internal iliac arteries supply the viscera and pelvis.

On the venous side, the **inferior vena cava** travels with the descending aorta through the trunk. Remember that blood flows away from the heart in the aorta and toward the heart in the vena cava. The inferior vena cava is formed at approximately the fifth lumbar vertebra by the confluence of the **right and left common iliac veins** (see Fig. 7-9). These common iliac veins are formed by the merging of the external and internal iliac veins. The **external iliac vein** receives blood flow from the abdominal wall. It also receives blood from the lower extremity via the **femoral vein.** The internal iliac vein receives blood from the viscera and the pelvic region.

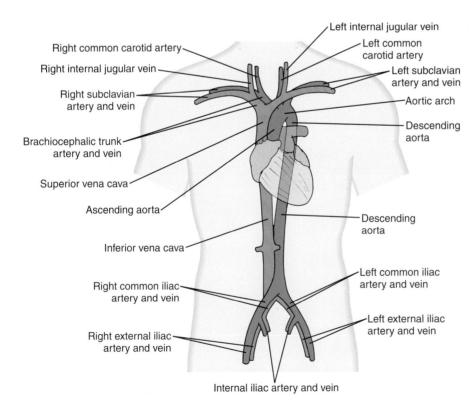

Figure 7-9. Major branches of aorta and vena cavae.

Table 7-2	Summary of Major Veins		
Vein	**Vein Joined**	**Region Drained**
Trunk		
Brachiocephalic	Superior vena cava	Upper body
Renal	Inferior vena cava	Kidneys
Hepatic	Inferior vena cava	Liver
Internal iliac	Common iliac	Pelvic region
External iliac	Common iliac	Lower extremity
Common iliac	Inferior vena cava	Lower extremity and abdomen
Lower Extremity		
Anterior and posterior tibial	Popliteal	Leg and foot
Popliteal	Femoral	Knee
Small saphenous	Popliteal	Superficial leg and foot
Great saphenous	Femoral	Superficial lower extremity
Femoral	External iliac	Thigh
Head and Neck		
Cranial venous sinuses	Internal jugular	Brain (including reabsorbed cerebral spinal fluid)
Internal jugular	Brachiocephalic	Neck
External jugular	Subclavian	Face and neck
Subclavian	Brachiocephalic	Shoulder
Brachiocephalic	Superior vena cava	Upper body
Superior vena cava	Right atrium	Upper body
Upper Extremity		
Radial and ulnar	Brachial	Forearm and hand
Cephalic	Axillary	Superficial arm and forearm
Basilic	Axillary	Superficial arm
Median cubital	Basilic and cephalic	Cubital fossa
Brachial	Axillary	Arm
Axillary	Subclavian	Axilla
Subclavian	Brachiocephalic	Shoulder

Circulation of the lower extremity begins as the external iliac artery and vein pass under the inguinal ligament and become the **femoral artery and vein** (Fig. 7-10). Because the artery is fairly superficial in this area, the femoral pulse can be felt (see Fig. 7-7). This area, which is bordered by the inguinal ligament superiorly, by the sartorius laterally, and by the adductor longus medially, is called the **femoral triangle** (Fig. 7-11). In addition to the femoral artery and vein, the femoral nerve, numerous lymph nodes, and the terminal portion of the great saphenous vein lie in this triangle.

The femoral artery runs deep along the length of the thigh, passes posteriorly through an opening in the insertion of the adductor magnus muscle, and enters the popliteal fossa on the back of the knee. Here, its name changes to the **popliteal artery.** The popliteal pulse can be felt in the middle of the popliteal space (see Fig. 7-7).

Just distal to the knee, the popliteal artery divides into the **anterior and posterior tibial arteries** (see Fig. 7-10A). As their names imply, these arteries run down the anterior and posterior aspects of the tibia, branching off in numerous places. At the ankle on the dorsum of the foot, a branch called the **dorsalis pedis artery** can be palpated and a pulse felt (see Fig. 7-7).

Traveling in the opposite direction in the lower extremity are two main venous systems: the deep and superficial systems (see Fig. 7-10B). Deep veins tend to parallel arteries of the same name. The **anterior and posterior tibial veins** drain the foot and lower leg before emptying into the popliteal vein. The **popliteal vein** drains the knee region before becoming the

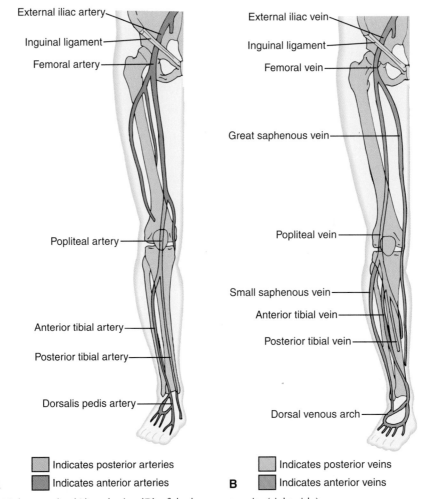

Figure 7-10. Major arteries **(A)** and veins **(B)** of the lower extremity (right side).

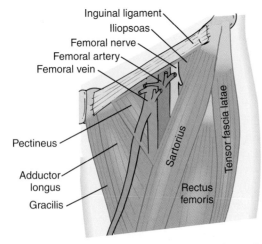

Figure 7-11. Femoral triangle, containing the femoral artery, vein, and nerve (right side).

femoral vein. The **femoral vein** drains the thigh area and joins the external iliac vein as it passes under the inguinal ligament. The two main superficial veins of the lower extremities are the saphenous veins. The **great saphenous vein,** the longest vein in the body, runs superficially along most of the length of the lower extremity on the medial side before emptying into the femoral vein. The **small saphenous vein** runs superficially from the lateral side of the foot and up the posterior lower leg to empty into the popliteal vein.

This next pathway off the aorta describes the circulatory pathway to the upper extremities. The **subclavian artery** delivers arterial blood to the upper extremity, chest wall, and neck. The right subclavian artery comes off the aortic arch via the short brachiocephalic trunk, while the left subclavian artery comes directly off the aortic arch. The subclavian artery is clinically important when it becomes compressed between the clavicle and first rib in a crowded space called the *thoracic outlet,* producing symptoms.

At the lateral border of the first rib, the subclavian artery becomes the **axillary artery** (Fig. 7-12A). It runs through the axilla to the proximal end of the arm, where it becomes the **brachial artery** and runs the length of the arm. At the anterior elbow, the brachial artery is often used to measure blood pressure and is where it divides into the **radial and ulnar arteries.** These arteries run down the forearm on the radial and ulnar sides, respectively. Each artery has many branches in the forearm, and they all terminate by forming two arches in the palmar side of the hand.

Similar to the lower extremity, the upper extremity has both deep and superficial veins (Fig. 7-12B). The deep veins of the upper extremity eventually drain into the **subclavian vein,** which parallels the artery of the same name. The **radial and ulnar veins** drain the lateral and medial forearm and hand, respectively, and then join the **brachial vein,** which drains the upper arm. In addition to these deep veins, three superficial veins are worth noting. Draining the forearm is the **cephalic**

vein, which runs laterally to empty into the axillary vein. The **basilic vein** runs medially up the forearm to empty into the brachial vein. Anteriorly in the cubital fossa is the **median cubital vein,** which unites the basilic and cephalic veins. It is here in the cubital fossa that one of these three veins is commonly used for drawing blood.

The description of the circulatory pathway to the head and neck will begin with the **common carotid artery.** It runs up each side of the neck beside the trachea, where its pulse can be palpated. The left common carotid artery arises directly from the aortic arch, while the right common carotid artery comes off the brachiocephalic trunk of the aortic arch (Fig. 7-13). At about the level of the jaw, each common carotid artery divides into the external and internal carotid arteries (Fig. 7-14A). The **external carotid artery** supplies the external head—the face, jaw, scalp, and skull. The **internal carotid artery** continues upward and enters the cranium through the carotid canal in the temporal bone, primarily supplying the anterior portion of the brain. Several venous sinuses within the layers of the dura mater receive blood from the brain.

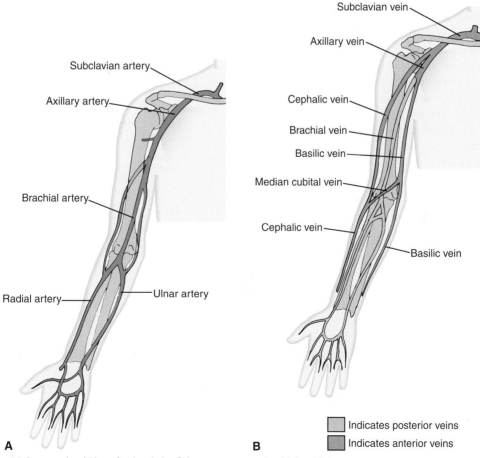

Figure 7-12.   Major arteries **(A)** and veins **(B)** of the upper extremity (right side).

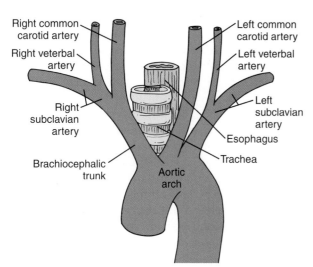

Figure 7-13.   Branches of the aortic arch.

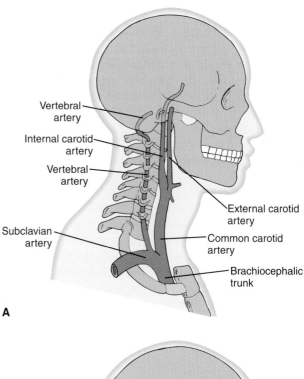

A

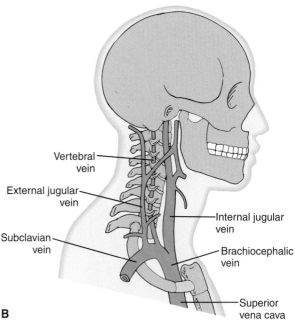

B

Figure 7-14.   Main arteries **(A)** and veins **(B)** of the neck (right side).

Eventually all of these sinuses drain into the internal jugular vein. Paralleling the carotid arteries and draining the head and neck regions are the **internal and external jugular veins** (Fig. 7-14B).

The **vertebral artery** is the first and largest branch of the subclavian artery (see Fig. 7-13). It runs upward in the cervical region, through the transverse foramen of the cervical vertebrae (see Fig. 7-14A). It then enters the base of the brain through the foramen magnum, supplying the posterior portion of the brain. The right and left vertebral arteries supply blood to the medulla and cerebellum before joining together to form the **basilar artery** on the underside of the brainstem, which supplies parts of the cerebellum, pons, and midbrain. The **vertebral vein** parallels the vertebral artery in the neck and within the skull (see Fig. 7-14B).

Blood Supply

At the base of the brain, the internal carotid arteries (anteriorly) and the basilar artery (posteriorly) are joined by communicating arteries, forming a circle that is often referred to as the **circle of Willis** (Fig. 7-15), after the English physician Thomas Willis, who first described this interconnection. Immediately upon entering the cranium, the internal carotid artery branches into the middle and anterior cerebral arteries. The **middle cerebral artery** supplies the lateral cerebral hemispheres. The **anterior cerebral arteries** supply the medial surface of the brain. The basilar artery divides to form the **posterior cerebral arteries,** which supply the occipital lobes and part of the temporal lobes.

The anterior cerebral artery (from the internal carotid) and the posterior cerebral artery (from the basilar) are joined at the base of the brain by the **posterior communicating artery.** The right and left anterior cerebral arteries are joined by the **anterior communicating artery.** The design of this circle is to ensure continued blood flow to the brain area should one of these major arteries fail. However, the circle of Willis is not always completely developed, so it does not ensure continued blood flow to the brain in every individual.

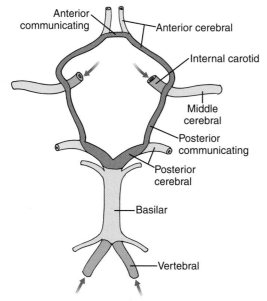

Figure 7-15.   Circle of Willis.

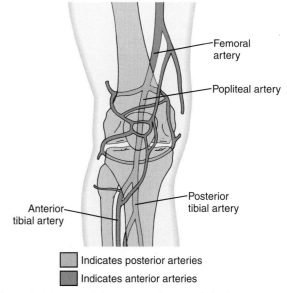

Indicates posterior arteries

Indicates anterior arteries

Figure 7-16.   Arterial anastomosis around the knee.

Clinical Significance of Anastomosis

An **anastomosis** is a joining of (or communication between) like vessels, such as artery to artery or vein to vein. The purpose for this structural connection is to provide alternate circulation if one of the vessels becomes blocked. This helps ensure that blood will get to its intended destination (i.e., arterial blood will get to capillaries for exchange of oxygen and carbon dioxide, and venous blood will get back to the heart).

Within each extremity, smaller anastomosing branches are commonly found around each joint. These smaller alternative arterial pathways allow the distal part of the limb to receive vital oxygenated blood should a main artery in an area become blocked. With time, these communicating branches may become large enough to meet the needs of the area involved. In Figure 7-16, note that there are several smaller branches off the femoral artery around the knee. Many of these branches join with either the anterior or posterior tibial artery distal to the knee. There are also anastomoses between the major cerebral arteries.

Lymphatic System

The lymphatic system is linked to the cardiovascular system and the immune system. Lymphatic vessels collect fluid and proteins that have leaked out of the blood capillaries and return them back to the venous system as lymph. Knowing the lymphatic structures and how they drain into the cardiovascular system helps one understand the treatment of certain pathological conditions.

The lymphatic organs serve as staging areas for defense against infection from microbes and other foreign particles. En route to the venous system, lymph fluid filters through lymph nodes and other lymphatic tissue, where microbes are detected and an immune system attack can be launched.

Whereas the circulatory system is a closed system of veins and arteries, the lymphatic system is a partially open system that moves fluids only from the periphery to the subclavian veins. The blood vascular system is an ongoing circular loop (i.e., arteries to capillaries to veins, etc.). However, the lymphatic system begins as capillaries in the tissues and ends as major ducts emptying into the subclavian vein. Unlike the two-way cardiovascular system, the lymphatic system is a one-way route from the periphery to the venous system.

Functions

The vast network of lymphatic vessels has four main functions: (1) collecting lymph from the body's interstitial (intercellular) spaces, (2) filtering the lymph through lymph nodes, (3) detecting and fighting infection in the lymph nodes, and (4) returning the lymph to the bloodstream.

Lymph Collection

Blood capillaries generally deliver more fluid to peripheral tissues than they carry away. A certain amount of fluid leaks out of the capillaries into the tissue spaces (interstitial spaces). The lymphatic system collects this excess fluid and returns it to the venous system. In doing that, it plays a vital role in maintaining normal blood volume and blood pressure within the circulatory system.

Similar to blood capillaries in structure, lymph capillaries begin in the intercellular spaces of most tissues. These intercellular spaces are also referred to as **interstitial spaces,** or tissue spaces—the spaces between cells (Fig. 7-17). To better visualize this arrangement, think of your body as a vase full of marbles. The marbles are tissue cells, and the spaces between the marbles are interstitial spaces. If you pour water (interstitial fluid) into the container, you fill all the spaces. Removing this fluid requires a vast network of minute lymph capillaries woven throughout most of the body. Lymph capillaries act as if their walls have one-way valves. When pressure outside the lymph capillary is greater, the cells allow the interstitial fluid to seep in. When the pressure within the lymph capillary becomes greater, the cell walls stop allowing fluid into the lymph capillaries. Once inside the lymph capillary, the interstitial fluid is called **lymph.**

Lymph originates as plasma—the fluid portion of blood. As arterial blood enters the capillary bed, it slows down. This allows the plasma to move into the tissues, where it is called **intercellular** (or **interstitial**) **fluid.** Oxygen and nutrients are delivered to the cells. When the fluid leaves the cells, it collects waste products. Most of this fluid (approximately 90%) returns to blood circulation through the venules as plasma. The remaining 10% is now known as lymph, which is rich in protein. Approximately 2 liters of lymph flow into blood circulation daily.

Transport

The lymphatic system begins as minute capillaries in the tissues. These initial lymph vessels, or **lymph capillaries,** form a vast network throughout most of the body. Lymph capillaries are not found in the central nervous system, bones, teeth, epidermis, certain types of cartilage, or any avascular tissue.

Lymphatic capillaries join together into larger lymph vessels. Think of the leaves of a tree as the interstitial spaces. The leaves connect to the small branches that begin the drainage system. The branches join together on larger branches. Large branches join onto larger limbs, which then join the main trunk of the tree. This same idea of smaller vessels joining together on larger vessels is true of the lymphatic system. As lymph capillaries become larger and collect more lymphatic fluid, they are referred to as **lymph vessels.**

Lymph vessels are wider than veins, have thinner walls and more valves, and contain kidney bean–shaped sacs called **lymph nodes** that are located in various places along the route. The function of these nodes will be discussed later in this chapter.

While the cardiovascular system has the heart to pump blood along in the blood vessels, the lymphatic system has no such pump. Lymph is propelled through lymph vessels in several ways by actions both within and outside the lymphatic system. Like veins, lymphatic vessels have valves that prevent any backward flow of fluid. Between valves is a segment of lymph vessel called an **angion.** Smooth muscles in the walls of the lymphatic vessels cause a stretch reflex of the lymph angions (Fig. 7-18), resulting in sequential contractions that are activated by the nerves that encircle the angions. The continuing chain reaction of contracting and stretching assists the onward flow of lymph from one angion to the next in a peristalsis-like movement controlled mainly by the filling state of each lymph angion. The pulsation helps move lymph onward from one lymph angion to the next. The

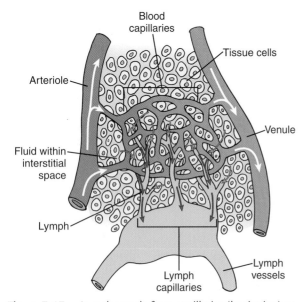

Figure 7-17.   Lymph vessels from capillaries (beginning) to subclavian vein (end).

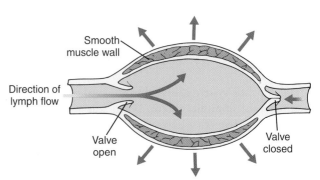

Figure 7-18.   Stretch mechanism of a lymph angion.

motion is similar to the "wave" often done by the stadium crowd at sporting events.

There are also more subtle actions external to the lymphatic system that influence the movement of lymph within lymph vessels. The squeezing of the surrounding skeletal muscles assists in moving lymph along, much like the way blood is moved along in veins. This is especially true in the extremities during the pumplike movement of contracting and relaxing muscles. The movement of the diaphragm and the changes in thoracic cavity pressure during the phases of breathing—especially abdominal breathing (see Chapter 16)—can provide a subtle "pumping" effect on the lymphatic vessels within the trunk. Maintenance of good posture (see Chapter 21) allows more efficient abdominal breathing, hence greater pumping effect on the lymphatic vessels.

Filtration and Protection

As mentioned earlier, lymph passes through lymph nodes en route to its end point, the subclavian vein. Lymph nodes are frequently arranged in groups along the pathways of lymph vessels. The first node of a group is called the **sentinel node,** which can be considered the first line of defense. Lymph nodes filter out bacteria, cell debris, and other foreign particles from the lymph.

The lymph enters a node through several **afferent lymph vessels** and exits through one or two **efferent lymph vessels** (Fig. 7-19). Therefore, an efferent lymph vessel of one lymph node becomes an afferent lymph vessel of another lymph node in a chain. As a general rule, lymph travels through one or more lymph nodes before entering the bloodstream.

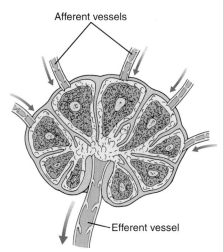

Figure 7-19.   Lymph node and vessels.

As lymph passes through a lymph node, bacteria and other foreign particles are intercepted, engulfed, and digested by white blood cells (macrophages and lymphocytes). When infection is present, nodes enlarge and become tender to the touch as the accumulating bacteria and an increasing number of lymphocytes cause them to swell.

Lymph nodes are often erroneously called *lymph glands.* A distinguishing feature of a gland is secretion. For example, the pituitary gland secretes growth hormone, the pancreas secretes insulin, sweat glands secrete sweat, and salivary glands secrete saliva. Lymph nodes filter lymph as it passes through, but they don't secrete anything. Therefore, they are not considered glands.

There are a multitude of lymph nodes throughout the body; one estimate states there are 500 to 1,000. Most nodes are concentrated in the cervical, axillary, and inguinal areas. Lymph nodes are able to increase or decrease in size, but a damaged or destroyed node cannot regenerate.

Drainage Patterns

Since lymph is really transported only from the periphery to the subclavian veins and not back to the periphery, one should think of lymph **drainage** rather than lymph circulation. There is a fairly predictable pattern of lymph drainage from tissues and organs, although some variation can be expected. Understanding these patterns is key to knowing the location of an infection or tumor and determining treatment.

Superficial lymph vessels drain the skin and subcutaneous tissue, forming a vast network that eventually drains into the deep lymph vessels. Deep lymph vessels drain the deeper structures. They tend to accompany the major blood vessels in the various regions.

While there are lymph nodes throughout the body, there are three main groups of regional nodes: cervical (neck), axillary (upper extremity), and inguinal (lower extremity). These regional nodes are located at the junctions of the head and extremities with the trunk (Fig. 7-20). The cervical, axillary, and inguinal nodes drain into the jugular, subclavian, and lumbar **lymphatic trunks,** respectively.

These lymphatic trunks, plus those in the abdominal and chest area, drain in turn into one of two ducts that empty into the venous system (Fig. 7-21). The **right lymphatic duct** is by far the smaller of the two ducts. It is only about 1 to 2 inches long and is located at the base of the neck on the right side. Only the right head and neck, the right upper extremity, and the right upper trunk empties into this duct, which then empties into the right subclavian vein.

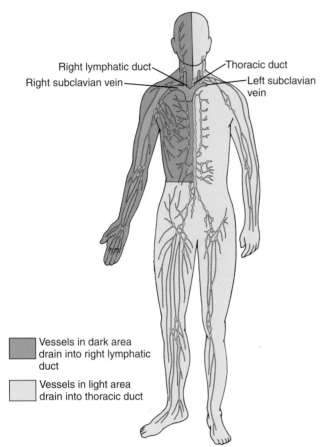

Figure 7-20.   Regional lymph nodes and drainage watersheds.

Vessels in dark area
drain into right lymphatic
duct

Vessels in light area
drain into thoracic duct

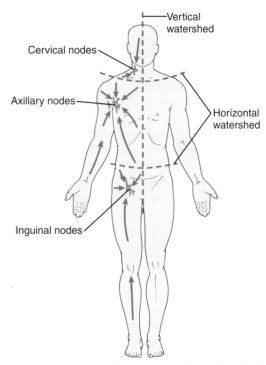

Figure 7-21.   Lymphatic drainage into the two lymph ducts:
the right lymphatic duct and the thoracic duct. Note that the
superficial vessels are shown on the right side and the deep
vessels on the left side.

The rest of the body's lymph empties into the **thoracic duct.** For the most part, this includes the entire left side of the body as well as the right side below the diaphragm. All deep lymphatics in the thorax, abdomen, pelvis, perineum, and lower extremities enter the thoracic duct. To complete this lymph drainage, the thoracic duct enters the venous circulation at the left subclavian vein.

In addition, the body has three main **watersheds** that separate the areas of lymph drainage (see Fig. 7-20). Visualize a mountain ridge; water will flow in opposite directions down each side of the ridge. The body has one vertical line at the midline that drains the right and left sides, and it has two horizontal lines, one at the level of the clavicle and the other at the level of the umbilicus. Lymph vessels draining above the clavicle enter the cervical lymph nodes. Those draining between the clavicle and the umbilicus enter the axillary nodes, while those draining below the umbilicus enter the inguinal nodes. The lymph collectors start at the watersheds and travel toward the regional lymph node bed. Because there are lymphatic capillary anastomoses between all the watersheds, this allows some crossover, if needed, to support drainage. The fact that this crossover is even possible is an important concept in the treatment of lymphedema.

Common Pathologies

Hemorrhage (bleeding) occurs when a break in a blood vessel allows blood to leak out of the closed system. A **cerebral hemorrhage** is particularly serious because it occurs within the confines of the bony skull. With nowhere for the blood to go, it can quickly put pressure on vital structures within the brain, causing a **stroke** or even death. It can also be serious if a hemorrhage occurs in an unconfined area like the abdomen, where blood loss volume can be great. Hemorrhage that occurs from head trauma tends to be either epidural (between the skull and the dura mater) or subdural (under the dura mater). **Epidural bleeds** occur in arteries; therefore, symptoms develop more quickly due to higher pressure within the vessel. **Subdural bleeds** occur in veins, which are under less pressure, so symptoms tend to develop more slowly.

Congestive heart failure is a condition in which the heart can't pump strongly enough to push an adequate supply of blood out to the various parts of the body. As blood flowing from the heart slows, blood returning to the heart through the veins backs up, causing congestion in the body's tissues. This often results in edema, especially in the feet, ankles, and lungs.

A **heart murmur** is an extra or unusual heart sound in addition to the normal *lub-dub* sounds heard during a heart contraction. The *whooshing* that can be heard through a stethoscope is usually turbulent blood backflow. It may be normal for that individual or a sign of valve pathology that allows blood to flow in the wrong direction.

If an artery becomes narrow, blood flow will slow or stop. This can be from a blood clot traveling through an artery or from deposits within an artery. Another condition that will slow blood flow is **arteriosclerosis,** or "hardening" of the arteries. It is especially a problem in the legs and feet. The vessel wall becomes less elastic and cannot dilate to allow greater blood flow when needed. **Atherosclerosis,** a type of arteriosclerosis, is when fatty deposits in the artery wall cause narrowing or blockage of the vessel. The site of the blockage will determine the problem. For example, a partial blockage that occurs and slows blood flow in a **coronary artery,** which supplies blood to the heart muscle, can cause **ischemia,** resulting in chest pain **(angina).** If the blockage is complete, it can cause a heart attack **(myocardial infarction).** If it occurs in an artery to or in the brain, it can cause a stroke **(cerebrovascular accident).** If it occurs in a leg artery, it can cause ischemia, **pain,** and possible **occlusion.** These same conditions caused by fatty deposits in the artery wall can occur with a blood clot.

If a vein loses elasticity, it will stretch. As the vein enlarges, the valve flaps will no longer meet properly and blood that should be flowing toward the heart will flow backward. **Varicose veins** occur as the blood pools in the vein, enlarging it even more. This condition is more common in superficial veins of the leg, because standing subjects them to higher pressure. Deep veins tend to be surrounded by muscles that, as they contract, assist the veins in pumping the blood onward.

Phlebitis is an inflammation of a vein. **Thrombosis** is the formation of a blood clot that may partially or totally block a blood vessel (artery or vein). **Thrombophlebitis** (often shortened to *phlebitis*) occurs when a clot causes inflammation in a vein. **Embolism** is a blood clot (or other foreign matter, such as air, fat, or tumor) that becomes dislodged and travels to another part of the body through ever smaller vessels until becoming wedged, causing an obstruction.

An **aneurysm** is an abnormal outward bulging or ballooning that is often caused by a weakened area in the wall. An aneurysm may go undetected until it ruptures.

Thoracic outlet syndrome is a group of disorders involving compression of the brachial plexus and/or the subclavian artery and vein within in the spaced called the *thoracic outlet*. Various vascular, neurological, and muscular symptoms may result.

Why are drainage patterns important? When lymphatic tissue or nodes have been damaged, destroyed, or removed, lymph cannot drain normally from the involved area. This will result in an accumulation of excess lymph and swelling, a condition known as **lymphedema,** and most commonly involves the arms or legs. Treatment of lymphedema is often based on the patterns of lymph drainage.

Review Questions

Cardiovascular System

1. The right atrioventricular (AV) valve is also referred to as the _____ valve.

2. The left AV valve has two other names.
   a. Referring to the number of flaps, it is called the _____ valve.
   b. Referring to its shape, it is called the _____ valve.

3. The semilunar valve located at the exit of the right ventricle is also called the _____ valve. The valve located at the exit of the left ventricle is called the _____ valve.

4. The blood vessels that transport blood from the heart to the lungs are the _____. Those that transport blood from the lungs to the heart are the _____.

(continued on next page)

Review Questions—cont'd

5. a. Veins carry which type of blood? (oxygenated/deoxygenated)
   b. What is the exception?
   c. Arteries carry which type of blood? (oxygenated/deoxygenated)
   d. What is the exception?

6. a. The first heart sound (*lub*) is heard when which valves close?
   b. The second heart sound (*dub*) is heard when which valves close?

7. If a clot breaks loose in a leg artery, where will it end up?

8. If a clot breaks loose in a leg vein, where will it end up?

9. At the inguinal ligament, the main artery and vein change name from _____ (proximally) to _____ (distally).

10. The head and neck regions are drained mostly by what two veins?

11. The pulse of which artery can be felt in the neck?

12. Name the 10 structures that a clot would travel through on its way from the left femoral vein (1) to the lung (10).

13. a. Which pressure is lowest in an artery? When does it occur?
    b. Which pressure is highest in an artery? When does it occur?

Lymphatic System

1. Does the lymph in an afferent or efferent lymph vessel contain more impurities?

2. At what point does lymph drain into the vascular system?

3. Lymph capillaries are found in
   a. brain.
   b. bone.
   c. muscle.
   d. all of the above.

4. Name five mechanisms that help move lymph from the periphery to the venous system.

5. Superficial lymph drainage goes into what three regional lymph node groups?

6. Which lymph duct drains a larger area of the body?

7. What are the three main functions of lymph vessels?

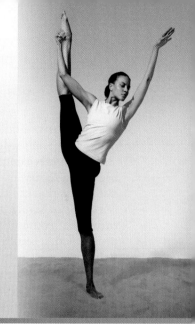

CHAPTER 8
Basic Biomechanics

Laws of Motion

Force

Torque

Stability

Simple Machines

Levers

Pulleys

Wheel and Axle

Inclined Plane

Points to Remember

Review Questions

The human body, in many respects, can be referred to as a living machine. It is important when learning about *how* the body moves (kinesiology) to also learn about the forces placed on the body that *cause* the movement. As illustrated in Figure 8-1, **mechanics** is the branch of physics dealing with the study of forces and the motion produced by their actions. **Biomechanics** involves taking the principles and methods of mechanics and applying them to the structure and function of the human body. As mentioned in Chapter 1, mechanics can be divided into two main areas: statics and dynamics. **Statics** deals with factors associated with nonmoving or nearly nonmoving systems. **Dynamics** involves factors associated with moving systems and can be divided into kinetics and kinematics. **Kinetics** deals with forces causing movement in a system, whereas **kinematics** involves the time, space, and mass aspects of a moving system. Kinematics can be divided into osteokinematics and arthrokinematics. **Osteokinematics** focuses on the manner in which bones move in space without regard to the movement of joint surfaces, such as shoulder flexion/extension. **Arthrokinematics** deals with the manner in which

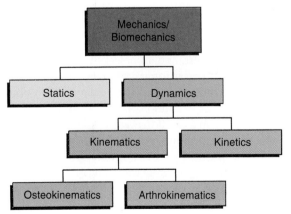

Figure 8-1. Mechanics/biomechanics relationship flowchart.

adjoining joint surfaces move in relation to each other—that is, in the same or opposite direction.

Various mechanical terms must be defined before beginning to discuss these topics. **Force** is a push or pull action that can be represented as a vector. A **vector** is a quantity having both magnitude and direction. For example, if you were to push a wheelchair, you would push it with a certain speed and in a certain direction. **Velocity** is a vector that describes speed and is measured in units such as feet per second or miles per hour.

A **scalar** quantity describes only magnitude. Common scalar terms are *length, area, volume,* and *mass.* Everyday examples would be units such as 5 feet, 2 acres, 12 fluid ounces, and 150 pounds. **Mass** refers to the amount of matter that a body contains. In this example, the amount of matter within and making up the body is the mass. **Inertia** is the property of matter that causes it to resist any change of its motion in either speed or direction. Mass is a measure of inertia—its resistance to a change in motion.

Kinetics is a description of motion with regard to what causes motion. **Torque** is the tendency of force to produce rotation around an axis. Muscles within the body produce motion around joint axes. **Friction** is a force developed by two surfaces, which tends to prevent motion of one surface across another. For example, if you slide across a carpeted floor in your stocking feet, there will be so much friction between the two surfaces that you won't slide very far. However, if you slide across a highly polished hardwood floor in your stocking feet, there will be very little friction between these two surfaces and you will have a good slide.

Laws of Motion

Motion is happening all around you—people walking, cars traveling on highways, airplanes flying in the air, water flowing in rivers, balls being thrown, and so on. Isaac Newton's three laws explain all types of motion. Newton's first law of motion states that an object at rest tends to stay at rest, and an object in motion tends to stay in motion. This is sometimes referred to as the **law of inertia,** because inertia is the tendency of an object to stay at rest or in motion. To demonstrate this law, consider riding in a car. If the car moves forward quickly from a starting position, your body pushes against the back of the seat and your neck probably hyperextends. Your body was at rest before the car moved, and it tended to stay at rest as the car started to move. If the car is moving and then stops suddenly, your body is thrown forward and your neck goes into extreme flexion, because your body was in motion and tended to stay in motion when the car stopped. Unfortunately, many of the people with neck injuries from automobile accidents have demonstrated this law.

A force is needed to overcome the inertia of an object and cause the object to move, stop, or change direction. The object's acceleration depends on the strength of the force applied and the object's mass. For example, kick a soccer ball and it will roll along the grass. If no forces act on it, the ball will roll forever. However, the force of friction acting on the ball causes the ball to eventually stop. There is friction between any two surfaces. In this case, it is the friction of the grass on the surface of the ball that causes the ball to stop rolling.

A soccer ball can also be used to demonstrate Newton's second law. First, mildly kick the ball and notice how far it travels. Next, kick the ball about twice as hard as the first kick. Notice that the ball will travel approximately twice as far. **Acceleration** is any change in the velocity of an object. The soccer ball is accelerating when it starts moving. If you were to kick the ball again even harder, it would travel proportionately farther. This is Newton's second law of motion, the **law of acceleration:** The amount of acceleration depends on the strength of the force applied to an object. Acceleration can also deal with a change in direction. Force is needed to change direction; according to the law, the change in an object's direction depends on the force applied to it.

Another part of Newton's second law deals with the mass of an object. *Mass* is the amount of matter in an object. Acceleration is inversely proportional to the mass of an object. If you apply the same amount of force to two objects of differing mass, the object with greater mass will accelerate less than the object with less mass. You can demonstrate this by first rolling a soccer ball, then rolling a bowling ball with the same amount of force. The heavier bowling ball will not travel nearly as far.

Newton's third law of motion, the **law of action-reaction,** states that for every action there is an equal and opposite reaction. The strength of the reaction is always equal to the strength of the action, and it occurs in the opposite direction. This can be demonstrated by jumping on a trampoline. The action is you jumping down on the trampoline. The reaction is the trampoline pushing back with the same amount of force. This causes you to rebound up in the opposite direction that you jumped. The harder you jump, the higher you rebound.

As stated, no motion can occur without a force. There are basically two types of force that will cause the body to move. Forces can be internal, such as muscular contraction, ligamentous restraint, or bony support. Forces can also be external, such as gravity or any externally applied resistance such as weight, friction, and so on.

Force

Force is one of those concepts that everyone understands but is difficult to define. To create a force, one object must act on another. Force can be either a push, which creates compression, or a pull, which creates tension. Movement occurs if one side pushes (or pulls) harder than the other.

Forces are vector quantities. A vector quantity describes both magnitude and direction. A person pulling a heavy load with a rope is an example of a vector. The tension in the rope represents the vector's magnitude, and the direction of the pull on the rope represents the vector's direction.

A vector force can be shown graphically by a straight line of appropriate length and direction. Figure 8-2 shows two people (representing forces) pushing on the chest of drawers, but at right angles to each other. The characteristics of force include the following:

1. Magnitude (each person is pushing equally in this case)
2. Direction (shown by the arrow)
3. Point of application (the same for both people)

Forces can be described by the effect they produce. A **linear force** results when two or more forces are acting along the same line. Figure 8-3A shows two people pulling a boat with the same rope in the same direction. Figure 8-3B shows two people pulling on the same rope but in opposite directions. **Parallel forces** occur in the same plane and in the same or opposite direction. An

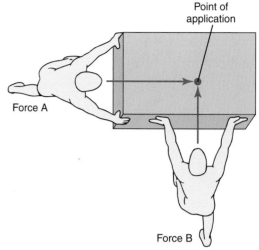

Figure 8-2. Concurrent force system. Two people pushing at different angles to each other through a common point of application.

example of parallel forces would be the three-point pressures of bracing (Fig. 8-4). Two forces—in this case, X and Y—are parallel to each other and pushing in the same direction, while a third parallel force (Z), the back brace, is pushing against them. This middle force must always be located between the two parallel forces. To be effective, the middle force must be of sufficient strength to resist the other two forces. You could also say that the two forces must be of sufficient strength to resist the middle force.

To produce **concurrent forces,** two or more forces must act on a common point but must pull or push in

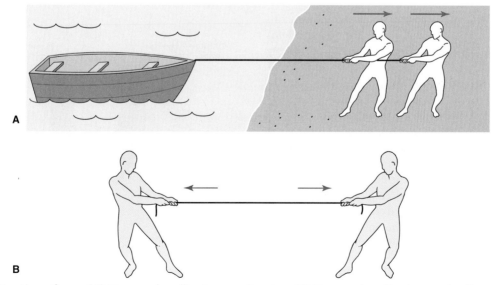

Figure 8-3.   Linear forces. **(A)** Two people pulling in same direction. **(B)** Two people pulling in opposite directions.

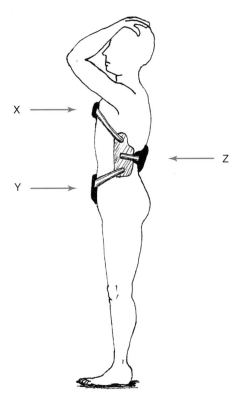

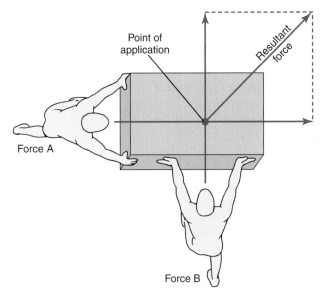

Figure 8-5.   A parallelogram shows graphically the resultant force of two concurrent forces pushing on a chest of drawers.

Figure 8-4.   Parallel forces of body brace. Forces X and Y are parallel in the same direction, while force Z is parallel but in the opposite direction. Force Z must be between forces X and Y to provide stability. If force Z was at either end, instead of in the middle, motion would occur.

different directions, such as the two people pushing on the cabinet in Figure 8-5. The overall effect of these two different forces is called the **resultant force** and lies somewhere in between.

Because forces can be represented as vectors, they can be shown graphically using what is called the **parallelogram method.** Using Figure 8-5 as an example, first draw in vectors for the two forces (solid lines). Secondly, complete the parallelogram using dotted lines. Next, draw in the diagonal of the parallelogram (middle line and arrow). This diagonal line represents the resultant force.

An example of resultant force in the body is the anterior and posterior parts of the deltoid muscle (Fig. 8-6). Although both parts have a common attachment (the insertion), they pull in different directions. When both parallel forces are equal, the resultant force causes the shoulder to abduct. If the pull of the two forces were not equal (i.e., if the pull of the anterior deltoid were stronger than that of the posterior), the resultant force would produce motion more in the direction of the anterior deltoid (Fig. 8-7). The shoulder would flex and abduct diagonally in a forward and outward direction.

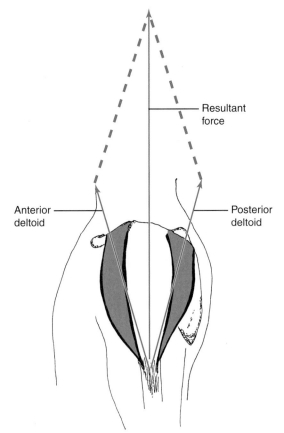

Figure 8-6.   Resultant force of equal forces of anterior and posterior deltoid muscles.

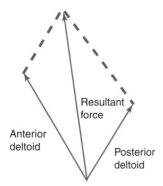

Figure 8-7. Resultant force of unequal forces moves toward the stronger force.

A **force couple** occurs when two or more forces act in different directions, resulting in a turning effect. In Figure 8-8, notice that the upper trapezius pulls up and in, the lower trapezius pulls down, and the serratus anterior pulls out. The combined effect is that the scapula rotates.

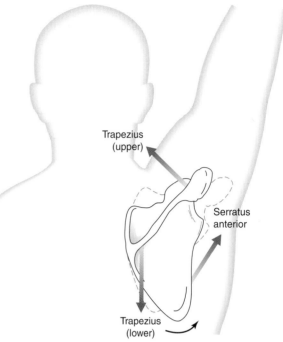

Figure 8-8. Force couple of muscles rotating the scapula.

Torque

Torque, also known as **moment of force,** is the ability of force to produce rotation around an axis. It can be thought of as rotary force. The amount of torque a lever has depends on the amount of force exerted and the distance it is from the axis. Use of a wrench demonstrates torque. The twisting force (torque) exerted by the wrench can be increased either by

1. increasing the force applied to the handle, or
2. increasing the length of the handle.

Torque is also the amount of force needed by a muscle contraction to cause rotary joint motion.

How much torque can be produced depends upon the strength of the force (magnitude) and its perpendicular distance from the force's line of pull to the axis of rotation. That perpendicular distance is called the **moment arm,** or *torque arm* (Fig. 8-9). Therefore, the moment arm of a muscle is the perpendicular distance between the muscle's line of pull and the center of the joint (axis of rotation). Torque is greatest when the angle of pull is at 90 degrees (Fig. 8-10A), and it decreases as the angle of pull either decreases (Fig. 8-10B) or increases (Fig. 8-10C) from that perpendicular position.

No torque is produced if the force is directed exactly through the axis of rotation. Although this is not quite possible for a muscle, it comes very close. For example, if the biceps contracts when the elbow is nearly or completely extended, there is very little torque produced (see

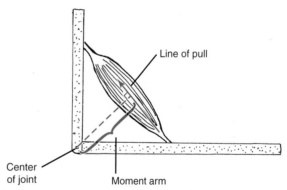

Figure 8-9. Moment arm of biceps is the perpendicular distance between the muscle's line of pull and the center of the joint.

Fig. 8-10B). This is because the perpendicular distance between the joint axis and the line of pull is very small. Therefore, the force generated by the muscle is primarily a **stabilizing force,** in that nearly all of the force generated by the muscle is directed back into the joint, pulling the two bones together.

Contrary to that, when the angle of pull is at 90 degrees (see Fig. 8-10A), the perpendicular distance between the joint axis and the line of pull is much larger. Therefore, the force generated by the muscle is primarily an **angular force,** or movement force, in that most of the force generated by the muscle is directed at rotating, not stabilizing, the joint.

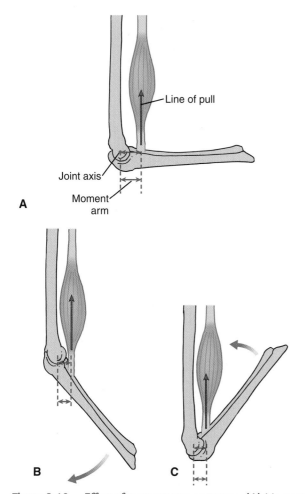

Figure 8-10.   Effect of moment arm on torque. **(A)** Moment arm and angular force are greatest at 90 degrees. **(B)** As joint moves toward 0 degrees, moment arm decreases and stabilizing force increases. **(C)** As joint moves beyond 90 degrees and toward 180 degrees, moment arm decreases and dislocating force increases.

As a muscle contracts through its range of motion (ROM), the amount of angular or stabilizing force changes. As the muscle increases its angular force, it decreases its stabilizing force and vice versa. At 90 degrees, or halfway through its range, the muscle has its greatest angular force. Past 90 degrees, the stabilizing force becomes a **dislocating force,** because the force is directed away from the joint (see Fig. 8-10C). In Figures 8-10B and C, when the stabilizing and dislocating forces are increasing, the angular (rotating) force is decreasing. Stated another way, a muscle is most efficient at moving, or rotating, a joint when the joint is at or near 90 degrees. It becomes less efficient at moving or rotating when the joint angle is at the beginning or near the end of the joint range. Some muscles have a much greater stabilizing force than angular force

throughout the range, and therefore are more effective at stabilizing the joint than moving it. The coraco-brachialis of the shoulder joint is a good example (see Fig. 10-17). Its line of pull is mostly vertical and quite close to the axis of the shoulder joint. Therefore, it has a very short moment arm, which makes this muscle more effective at stabilizing the head of the humerus in the shoulder joint than at moving the shoulder joint.

The angular force of the quadriceps muscle is increased by the presence of the patella. The patella, a sesamoid bone encapsulated in the tendon, increases the moment arm of the quadriceps muscle by holding the tendon out and away from the femur. This changes the angle of pull, allowing the muscle to have a greater angular force (Fig. 8-11A). Without a patella, the moment arm is smaller, making the muscle's line of pull more vertical, and much of the force of the quadriceps is directed back into the joint (Fig. 8-11B). Although this is good for stability, it is not effective for motion. To have effective knee motion, it is vital that the quadriceps provide a strong angular force.

In summary, if the moment arm is greater, then the angular force (torque) is also greater. Moment arm is determined by measuring the perpendicular distance between the joint axis and the muscle's line of pull. If the joint angle is near 0 degrees (almost straight), the moment arm is small and the force is a stabilizing action that moves the two bones of the joint together. If the joint angle is nearer 180 degrees (completely bent), the moment arm is small and the force is dislocating,

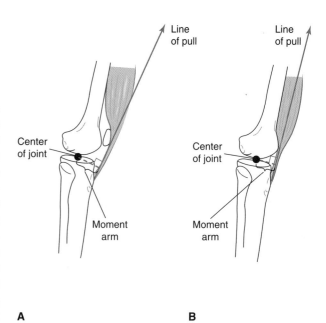

Figure 8-11.   Moment arm of quadriceps muscle with a patella **(A)** and without a patella **(B).**

pulling the two bones away from each other. If the joint angle is in the midrange of motion, the moment arm is greatest, and the ability to move the joint is strongest. Moment arm, size of the muscle, and contractile strength of the muscle all determine how effective a muscle is in causing joint motion.

Stability

When an object is balanced, all torques acting on it are even and it is in a **state of equilibrium.** How secure or precarious this state of equilibrium is depends primarily on the relationship between the object's center of gravity and its base of support. To understand the principles of stability, certain terms must be defined. **Gravity** is the mutual attraction between the earth and an object. **Gravitational force** is always directed vertically downward, toward the center of the earth. Practically speaking, gravitational force is always directed toward the ground. **Center of gravity** (COG) is the balance point of an object at which torque on all sides is equal. It is also the point at which the planes of the body intersect, as shown in Figure 8-12.

In the human body, the COG is located in the midline at about the level of, though slightly anterior to, the second sacral vertebra of an adult. Because body proportions change with age, the COG of a child is higher than that of an adult. To demonstrate this, move your right arm up over your head and touch your left ear (Fig. 8-13A). Now, ask a 3-year-old to do the same. You will notice that while you can easily touch your ear, the child's hand reaches only to about the top of the head (Fig. 8-13B). The child's head is much larger in proportion to the arms and rest of the body.

As a point of interest, height-arm span is a body proportion made famous by the illustration of Leonardo da Vinci. The length of an adult's outstretched arms is equal to his or her height (Fig. 8-14).

Base of support (BOS) is that part of a body that is in contact with the supporting surface. If you outlined the surface of the body in contact with the ground, you would have identified the BOS. **Line of gravity** (LOG) is an imaginary vertical line passing through the COG toward the center of the earth. These are shown in Figure 8-15.

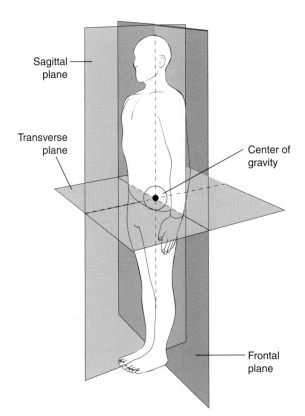

Figure 8-12. The center of gravity is the point at which the three cardinal planes intersect.

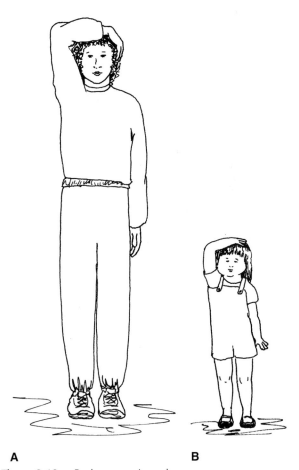

A   **B**

Figure 8-13. Body proportions change as a person grows. **(A)** Adult can reach over top of head to touch opposite ear. **(B)** Child can reach over head only part way.

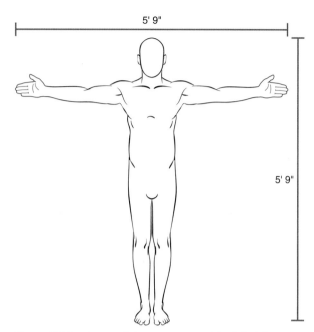

5' 9"

5' 9"

Figure 8-14. In an adult, arm span and body height are equal.

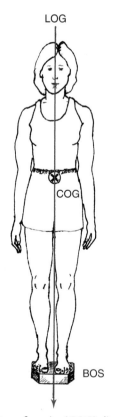

LOG

COG

BOS

Figure 8-15. Center of gravity (COG), line of gravity (LOG), and base of support (BOS).

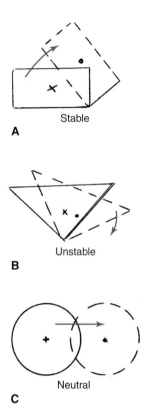

Stable

A

Unstable

B

Neutral

C

Figure 8-16. Three states of equilibrium: **(A)** stable, **(B)** unstable, and **(C)** neutral.

There are basically three states of equilibrium (Fig. 8-16). **Stable equilibrium** occurs when an object is in a position where disturbing it would require its COG to be raised. A simple example is that of a brick. When the widest part of the brick is in contact with the surface (BOS), it is quite stable (Fig. 8-16A). To disturb it, the brick would have to be tipped up in any direction, thus raising its COG. The same could be said of a person lying flat on the floor. **Unstable equilibrium** occurs when only a slight force is needed to disturb an object. Balancing a pencil on its pointed end is a good example. A similar example is that of a person standing on one leg. Once balanced, it takes very little force to knock over the pencil or person (Fig. 8-16B). **Neutral equilibrium** exists when an object's COG is neither raised nor lowered when it is disturbed. A good example is a ball. As the ball rolls across the floor, its COG remains the same (Fig. 8-16C). A person moving across the room while seated in a wheelchair demonstrates neutral equilibrium.

The following principles demonstrate the relationships between balance, stability, and motion:

1. The lower the COG, the more stable the object. In Figure 8-17, both triangles have the same base of support. However, the triangle on the left is taller, has a higher COG, and thus is more unstable

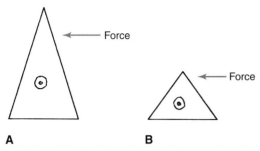

Figure 8-17. Relationship of height of center of gravity to stability. **(A)** Higher COG is less stable. **(B)** Lower COG is more stable.

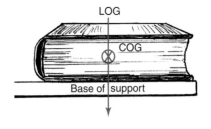

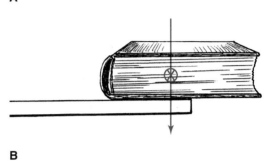

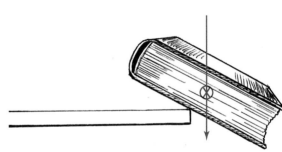

Figure 8-18. Relationship of COG to BOS. **(A)** The book is very stable because its COG is in the middle of its BOS. **(B)** The book is less stable because its COG is near the edge of its BOS. **(C)** The book is unstable and will fall because its COG is beyond its BOS.

than the triangle on the right. It would take less force to disturb the taller triangle.

2. The COG and LOG must remain within the BOS for an object to remain stable. (Keep in mind that the LOG passes through the COG. Therefore, what can be said of one can be said of the other. For the purpose of clarity, from this point forward, the term COG will be used.) The wider the BOS, the more stable the object. In the example in Figure 8-18A, the book is resting entirely on its BOS (tabletop) and is quite stable. As you push it off the edge (Fig. 8-18B), it becomes less stable. When its COG is no longer over its BOS (Fig. 8-18C), the book will fall.

   Another example is a woman standing upright on both feet (Fig. 8-19A). Her COG lies at or near the center of the base of support. As she leans to the side (Fig. 8-19B), her COG moves toward the border of her BOS. As soon as her COG passes beyond the BOS, she becomes unstable, and if her posture is not corrected or if her BOS is not widened, she will fall. To lean farther without losing her balance, she could either raise her opposite arm or widen her stance. In either case, her COG would move back over her BOS.

3. Stability increases as the BOS is widened in the direction of the force. A person standing at a bus stop on a very windy day would be more stable when facing into the wind and placing one foot behind the other, thus widening the BOS in the direction of the wind (Fig. 8-20).

4. The greater the mass of an object, the greater its stability. This concept is observed by looking at the size of players on a football team. Linebackers are traditionally heavier, and thus harder to push over, but they are not particularly fast. Halfbacks, whose job is to run with the ball, are much lighter (and easier to push over). It can be said that what is gained in stability is lost in speed and vice versa.

5. The greater the friction between the supporting surface and the BOS, the more stable the body will be. Walking on an icy sidewalk is a slippery experience, because there is essentially no friction between the ice and the shoe. Sanding the sidewalk increases the friction of the icy surface, thus improving traction. Having a surface with a great deal of friction is not always desirable. Pushing a wheelchair across a hardwood floor is much easier than pushing one across a carpeted floor. The carpet creates more friction, making it harder to push the wheelchair.

6. People have better balance while moving if they focus on a stationary object rather than on a moving object. Therefore, people learning to walk with crutches will be more stable if they focus on an object down the hall rather than look down at their moving feet or crutches.

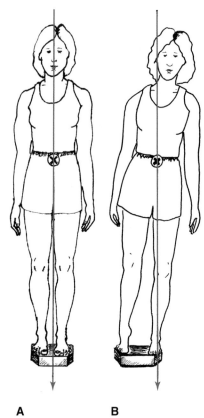

A   **B**

Figure 8-19. Relationship of COG to BOS. **(A)** She is stable—her COG is in the middle of her BOS. **(B)** She is less stable because her COG is near the edge of her BOS.

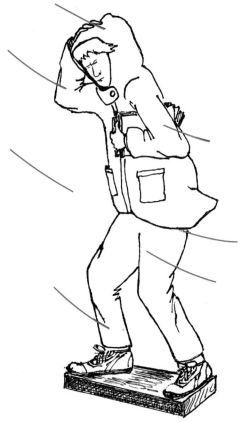

Figure 8-20. Wider base of support in direction of force increases stability.

Simple Machines

In engineering, various machines are used to change the magnitude or direction of a force. The four simple machines are the lever, the pulley, the wheel and axle, and the inclined plane. Examples of each of these machines, except for the inclined plane, can be found in the human body. The lever, the wheel and axle, and the inclined plane allow a person to exert a force greater than could be exerted by using muscle power alone; the pulley allows force to be applied more efficiently. This increase in force is usually at the expense of speed and can be expressed in terms of mechanical advantage, which will be described later.

Levers

There are three classes of levers, each with a different purpose and a different mechanical advantage. We use levers daily to help us accomplish various activities. Usually a lever will favor either power or distance (range of motion), but not both. However, the basic rule of all simple machines is that the advantage gained in power is lost in distance. Sometimes, a great deal of power is needed, such as moving a heavy rock. Other times, distance (range of motion) is needed, such as swinging a tennis racket. Wheelbarrows, crowbars, manual can openers, scissors, golf clubs, and playground seesaws are but a few examples of levers. Different types of levers can also be found in the human body. Each type of lever will favor power or distance, but not both.

To understand the structure and function of levers, you should be familiar with certain terms. A **lever** is rigid and can rotate around a fixed point when a force is applied. A bone is an example of a lever in the human body. The fixed point around which the lever rotates is the **axis (A),** sometimes referred to as the *fulcrum*. In the body, the joint is the axis. The **force (F),** sometimes called the *effort,* that causes the lever to move is usually muscular. The **resistance (R),** sometimes called the *load,* that must be overcome for motion to occur can include the weight of the part being moved (arm, leg, etc.), the pull of gravity on the part, or an external weight being moved by the body part. When determining a muscle's role (force or resistance), it is important to use the point of attachment to the bone, not the muscle belly, as the point of reference. When determining the resistance of the part, use its COG.

The **force arm (FA)** is the distance between the force and the axis, while the **resistance arm (RA)** is the distance between the resistance and the axis (Fig. 8-21). The arrangement of the axis *(A)* in relation to the force *(F)* and the resistance *(R)* determines the type of lever. The longer the FA, the easier it is to move the part. Conversely, the longer the RA, the harder it is to move the part. Remember, there is always a trade-off. With the longer FA, the part will be easier to move, but the FA will have to move a greater distance. When the RA is longer, it won't have to move as far, but it will be harder to move.

Classes of Levers

In a **first-class lever,** the axis is located between the force and the resistance:

First-class lever F ———————— R
A

If the axis is close to the resistance, the RA will be shorter and the FA will be longer. Therefore, it will be easy to move the resistance. If the axis is close to the force, just the opposite will occur; it will be hard to move the resistance.

Try this with a pencil (axis), a ruler (force), and a fairly heavy book (resistance). Something small that doesn't roll easily would make a better axis; otherwise, have someone hold the pencil in place. The ruler—or even another long pencil—can be used, but it must be a rigid bar. Place the ruler about 2 inches under the book so it will stay under the book as the book is raised. Place the pencil perpendicularly under the ruler near the book (Fig. 8-22A). You have created a long FA and a short RA. Push down on the outer end of the ruler and notice two things: (1) how easy it is to raise the book, and (2) how far down you have to push the ruler. Next, move the pencil (axis) out toward the other end of the ruler, and push down on the ruler (Fig. 8-22B). This time you should notice that it is harder to raise the book, but you didn't

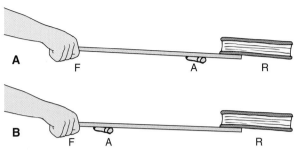

Figure 8-22. First-class lever. FAR (F = force; A = axis; R = resistance). **(A)** A is closer to R. **(B)** A is closer to F.

have to push the ruler down very far. You have just demonstrated that with a longer FA (or a shorter RA),

1. It is easy to move the resistance (book),
2. The resistance is moved only a short distance, and
3. The force has to be applied through a long distance.

However, with a shorter FA (or a longer RA),

1. It is harder to move the resistance,
2. The resistance moves a longer distance, and
3. The force is applied through a short distance.

This is an example of a first-class lever, because the axis is in the middle, with the force on one side and resistance on the other. By placing the axis close to the resistance, you have a lever that favors force. By placing the axis close to the force, you have a lever that favors distance (range of motion) and speed. If you place the axis midway between the force and the resistance (assuming they are the same weight), the lever favors balance.

Figure 8-23 shows a worker carrying two bundles of hay. Each bundle (one is force and the other is resistance)

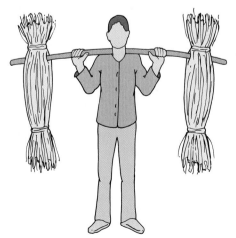

Figure 8-23. First-class lever. The two loads (F and R) are balanced on the shoulders.

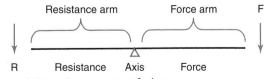

Figure 8-21. Components of a lever.

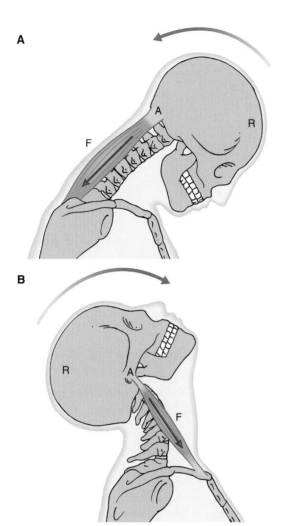

Figure 8-24. Head moving on neck demonstrates a first-class lever. In **(A)**, the axis is the head posteriorly moving on the vertebral column and is located between force (the extensor muscles), and resistance (weight of the head itself). In **(B)**, the axis is the head moving anteriorly on the vertebral column and is located between the force (flexor muscles) and the resistance (weight of head).

is approximately the same weight and distance from the axis. The shoulder is the axis. If one bundle is heavier, it would have to be moved closer to the axis to keep the overall load balanced.

An example of a first-class lever in the human body is the head sitting on the first cervical vertebra, moving up and down in cervical flexion and hyperextension. The vertebra is the axis, the resistance is the weight on one side of the head, and the force is the muscle pulling down on the opposite side of the head. The force and resistance will change places, depending on which way the head is tipped. For example, as shown in Figure 8-24A, if your head is tipped toward your chest and you want to return to the upright position, your posterior neck muscles

(force) must contract to pull the weight of your head up against gravity (resistance). If you look up to the sky, your head would rock back and you would use your anterior neck muscles to pull your head into the upright position (Fig. 8-24B). Although force and resistance may change places, depending on the motion, the axis is always in the middle of a first-class lever.

In a **second-class lever,** the resistance is in the middle, with the axis at one end and the force at the other end:

$$\text{Second-class lever} \quad \frac{\quad \overset{R}{\quad} \quad \overset{F}{\quad} \quad}{A}$$

The wheelbarrow is an example of a second-class lever (Fig. 8-25). The wheel at the front end is the axis, the wheelbarrow contents are the resistance, and the person pushing the wheelbarrow is the force. If we assume that the wheelbarrow is carrying a load of heavy bricks, we can apply the earlier statement that *the longer the FA, the easier it is to move the part* and *the longer the RA, the harder it is to move the part.* If we put all the bricks as close to the

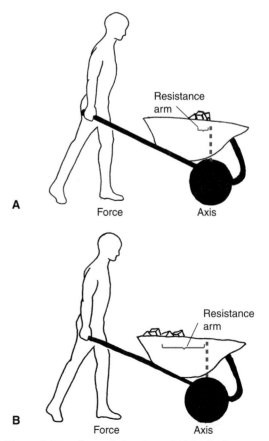

Figure 8-25. Second-class lever. **(A)** RA is shorter. **(B)** RA is longer.

wheel as possible (Fig. 8-25A), we now have a long FA and a short RA. The wheelbarrow should be fairly easy to move. However, if we move the bricks to the other end of the wheelbarrow (Fig. 8-25B), the FA remains the same length, but the RA is longer. The wheelbarrow is now harder to move because we have lengthened the RA.

There are relatively few examples of second-class levers in the body; however, the action of the ankle plantar flexor muscles when a person stands on tiptoe is one (Fig. 8-26). In this case, the axis is the metatarsophalangeal (MTP) joints in the foot, the resistance is the tibia and the rest of the body weight above it, and the force is provided by the ankle plantar flexors. Therefore, the resistance (body weight) is between the axis (MTP joint) and the force (plantar flexors). The RA is only slightly shorter than the FA. This lever favors power because a relatively small force (the muscle) can move a large resistance (the body). However, the body can be raised only a fairly short distance. This again proves the basic rule of simple machines—what is gained in power (raising the body weight) is lost in distance (the body can't be raised very far).

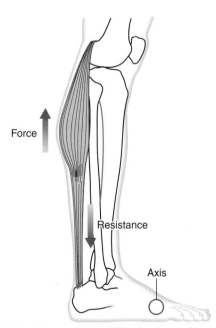

Figure 8-26. Plantar flexors lifting body weight demonstrates a second-class lever.

A **third-class lever** has force in the middle, with resistance and the axis at the opposite ends:

$$\text{Third-class lever} \frac{\text{F} \quad \text{R}}{\text{A}}$$

An example of this type of lever is a person moving one end of a boat either toward or away from a dock (Fig. 8-27). The axis is the front of the boat tied to the dock. The force is the person pushing on the boat, and the resistance is the weight of the boat. If the person pushes close to the front of the boat as in Fig. 8-27A, it will be harder to move the boat but the back of the boat will swing farther away from the dock. Conversely, if the person pushes farther back on the boat as in Fig. 8-27B, the boat stern won't swing away from the dock as far, but it will be easier to move. In this case, the RA doesn't change, but the FA does. When the FA is shorter, the boat is hard to push but moves a greater distance. When the FA is lengthened, the boat is easier to push but doesn't move as far. In other words, any gain in distance is lost in power.

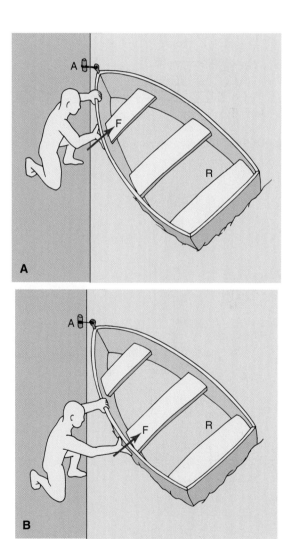

Figure 8-27. Moving boat tied to dock demonstrates a third-class lever (axis, force, resistance). A is the point where the boat is held against the dock. F is where the person pushes (or pulls) the boat away (toward) the dock, and R is the weight of the boat. In **(A)**, it will be easier to move the boat, while in **(B)** it will be harder.

The advantage of the third-class lever is speed and distance. This is, by far, the most common lever in the body. In the example of elbow flexion (Fig. 8-28), the axis is the elbow joint, the biceps muscle exerts the force, and the resistance is the weight of the forearm and hand. For the hand to be truly functional, it must be able to move through a wide range of motion. The resistance, in this case, will vary depending on what, if anything, is in the hand.

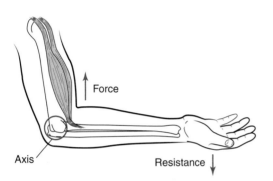

Axis

Force

Resistance

Figure 8-28. The biceps demonstrating a third-class lever.

Why are there so many third-class levers (which favor speed and distance) and so few second-class levers (which favor power) in the body? Probably because the advantage gained from increased speed and distance is more important than the advantage gained from increased power. Examine the roles of the biceps and the brachioradialis muscles in elbow flexion (Fig. 8-29). They both cross the elbow but attach to the radius at very different places. The biceps muscle attaches to the proximal end of the radius, while the brachioradialis muscle attaches to the distal end. The biceps muscle acts as the force in a third-class lever because it attaches between the axis (elbow) and the resistance (COG of forearm/hand; Fig. 8-29A). The brachioradialis muscle is the force in a second-class lever (Fig. 8-29B) because it attaches at the end of the forearm, putting the resistance (COG of forearm/hand) in the middle. For example, say that each muscle is capable of contracting approximately 4 inches. Remember that a muscle can shorten to half of its resting length. Therefore, the brachioradialis muscle will be able to move the distal end of the forearm and, subsequently, the hand approximately 4 inches, because its attachment is near the distal end. The biceps muscle, with its attachment at the

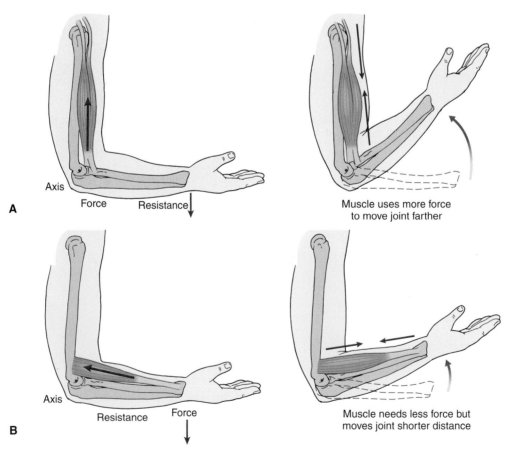

Axis

Force   Resistance

A

Muscle uses more force
to move joint farther

Axis

Resistance   Force

B

Muscle needs less force but
moves joint shorter distance

Figure 8-29. Third-class levers favor distance **(A),** and second-class levers favor force **(B).**

proximal end, will move the proximal end of the forearm approximately 4 inches, which will move the hand at the distal end much farther, say 12 inches. Because the main function of the upper extremity is to allow the hand to move through a wide range, it makes sense that most muscles act as third-class levers, favoring range of motion.

Factors That Change Class

Under certain conditions, a muscle may change from a second-class (axis-resistance-force) to a third-class lever (axis-force-resistance), and vice versa. For example, the brachioradialis has been described as a second-class lever, with the weight of the forearm and hand being the resistance. Using the middle of the forearm as its COG, the weight of the forearm and hand (R) is located between the axis (elbow joint) and the force (distal muscle attachment), as shown in Figure 8-30A. However,

if you put a weight in the hand, the COG of the resistance is now located farther from the axis than the force (muscle), as depicted in Figure 8-30B. Therefore, the brachioradialis is now working as a third-class lever.

The direction of the movement in relation to gravity is another factor that will affect lever class. For example, the biceps illustrated in Figure 8-31A is a third-class lever because it contracts concentrically to flex the elbow. The muscle is the force and the forearm is the resistance. The force is between the axis and the resistance; therefore, it is a third-class lever. If you put a weight in the hand, it will still be a third-class lever. However, if the muscle contracted eccentrically, it will become a second-class lever. What has changed? As the elbow extends, moving the same direction as the pull of gravity, the biceps must contract eccentrically to slow the pull of gravity. Gravity and its pull on the forearm becomes the force. The biceps becomes the resistance slowing elbow extension (Fig. 8-31B). With the resistance now in the middle between the force and the axis, the biceps becomes a second-class lever.

There are many applications of leverage in rehabilitation. The importance of levers can be seen in such things as saving energy or making tasks possible when

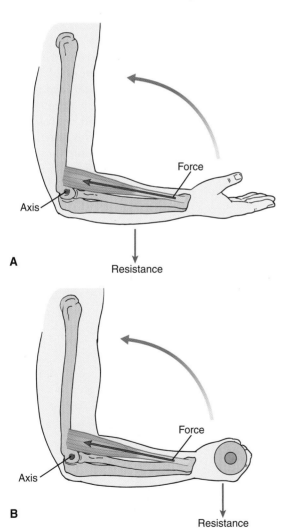

Figure 8-30. **(A)** The brachioradialis as a second-class lever. **(B)** It becomes a third-class lever when a weight is placed in the hand.

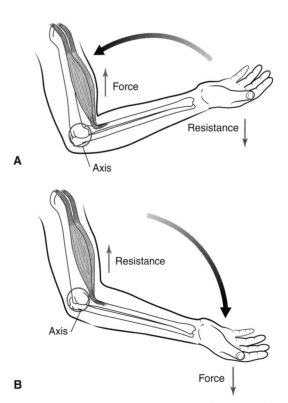

Figure 8-31. The biceps acts as a third-class lever when contracting concentrically **(A)**, and a second-class lever when contracting eccentrically **(B)**.

strength is limited. To summarize, less force is required if you put the resistance as close to the axis as possible and apply the force as far from the axis as possible.

Pulleys

A **pulley** consists of a grooved wheel that turns on an axle with a rope or cable riding in the groove. Its purpose is to either change the direction of a force or to increase or decrease its magnitude. A **fixed pulley** is a simple pulley attached to a beam. It acts as a first-class lever with F on one side of the pulley (axis) and R on the other. It is used only to change direction. Clinical examples of this can be found in overhead and wall pulleys (Fig. 8-32) and in home cervical traction units. In the body, the lateral malleolus of the fibula acts as a pulley for the tendon of the peroneus longus and changes its direction of pull (Fig. 8-33). Another example of a pulley is a Velcro strap on a shoe. The strap passes through a slot and folds over on itself.

A **movable pulley** has one end of the rope attached to a beam; the rope runs through the pulley to the other end where the force is applied. The load (resistance) is suspended from the movable pulley (Fig. 8-34). The purpose of this type of pulley is to increase the mechanical advantage of force. **Mechanical advantage** is the number of times a machine multiplies the force. The load is

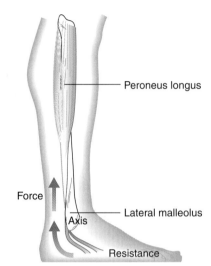

Figure 8-33. The lateral malleolus acts as a pulley, allowing the peroneus longus to change its direction of pull.

supported by both segments of the rope on either side of the pulley so it has a mechanical advantage of 2. It will require only half as much force to lift the load because the amount of force gained has doubled. Although only half of the force is needed to lift the load, the rope must be pulled twice as far. In other words, it is easier to pull the rope, but the rope must be pulled a much farther distance. The human body has no examples of a movable pulley.

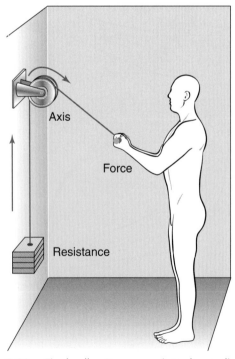

Figure 8-32. Fixed pulley. Its purpose is to change direction.

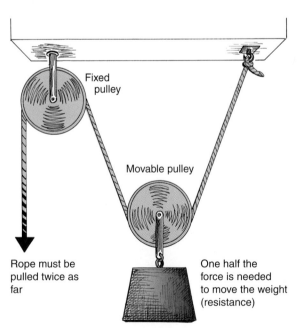

Figure 8-34. A movable pulley has a mechanical advantage for force.

Wheel and Axle

The **wheel and axle** is another type of simple machine. It is actually a lever in disguise. The wheel and axle consists of a wheel, or crank, attached to and turning together with an axle. In other words, it is a large wheel connected to a smaller wheel and typically is used to increase the force exerted. Turning around a larger wheel or handle requires less force, whereas turning around a smaller axle requires a greater force. An example of a wheel and axle is a faucet handle (Fig. 8-35). The handle is the wheel and the stem is the axle. Turning the faucet requires a certain amount of force made easier by a longer force arm (wheel radius; Fig. 8-36A). However, take off the handle and you are left with only the axle (Fig. 8-36B). Try turning it and you will realize that a great deal more strength is needed to do so. Simply stated, the larger the wheel (handle) in relation to the axle, the easier it is to turn the object. Just like the lever—in which the longer the FA, the greater the force—the wheel and axle provides greater force with a larger wheel.

Assume that you are treating a person who has severe arthritis in the hands and is unable to turn faucet handles easily. If you replace the handle (Fig. 8-37A) with a long, lever-type handle (Fig. 8-37B), you still have a wheel and axle. Visualize the handle as one spoke of the wheel with the rest of the spokes missing. The longer faucet handle is easier to turn (force advantage), but the handle must be turned a greater distance.

To give an example of a wheel and axle in the human body, think of performing passive shoulder rotation on a patient. It can best be visualized by looking down on

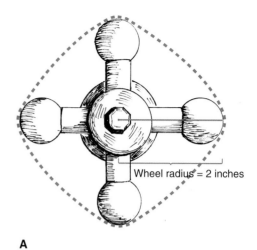

Wheel radius = 2 inches

A

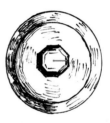

Axle radius = 1/8 inch

B

Figure 8-36. The wheel of the faucet handle **(A)** has a longer radius than the axle **(B)**. Therefore, the larger wheel is easier to turn than the smaller axle.

the shoulder from a superior view (Fig. 8-38). The shoulder joint serves as the axle, and the forearm serves as the wheel. With the elbow flexed, the wheel is much longer than the axle and thus much easier to turn.

Inclined Plane

Although there are no examples of an inclined plane in the human body, the concept of wheelchair accessibility

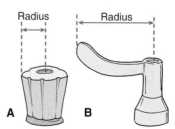

Radius | Radius

A **B**

Figure 8-37. Typical faucet handles. Note that **(A)** has a shorter radius and requires more force to turn the wheel than **(B)**.

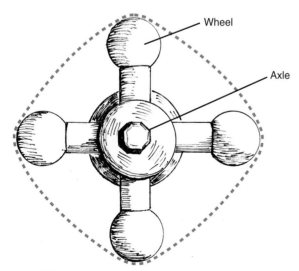

Wheel

Axle

Figure 8-35. A faucet handle demonstrates a wheel and axle.

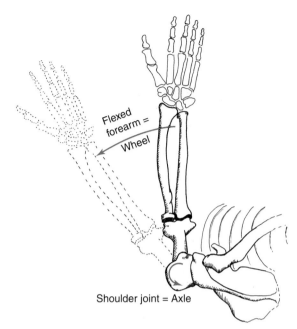

Figure 8-38.   The upper extremity acting as a wheel and axle.

often depends on this type of simple machine. An **inclined plane** is a flat surface that slants. It exchanges increased distance for less effort. The longer the length of a wheelchair ramp, the greater the distance the wheelchair must travel; however, it requires less effort to propel the chair up the ramp, because the ramp's incline is less. For example, if a porch is 2 feet from the ground

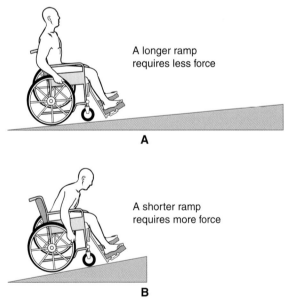

Figure 8-39.   Inclined plane as a wheelchair ramp. A longer ramp **(A)** requires less force but greater distance to reach a certain height. A shorter ramp **(B)** requires more force but less distance to reach same height.

and the ramp is 24 feet long, it would be fairly easy to propel the wheelchair up this long ramp (Fig. 8-39A). If the ramp is only 12 feet long, it would be much steeper. The person would not have to propel the wheelchair as far but would have to use more force to do so (Fig. 8-39B). Repeating the basic rule of simple machines: the advantage gained in force (decreased effort needed) is lost in distance (longer ramp needed).

Points to Remember
- The effect of forces can be linear, parallel, or concurrent.
- A force couple occurs when forces act together but in opposite directions to provide the same motion.
- A scalar quantity describes magnitude, whereas vector also includes direction.
- Forces can be stabilizing, angular, or dislocating.
- Gravity has an effect on all objects, and its force is always downward.
- Stability is affected by an object's COG and BOS.
- The three classes of levers have different purposes and mechanical advantages, depending on the relationship of the axis, the force, and the resistance.
- Changing the length of the FA or RA will make the part easier or harder to move.
- Fixed pulleys in the human body change the direction of a muscle's force.
- The wheel and axle, much like the lever, can increase the force.
- Inclined planes can exchange increased distance for decreased effort.

Review Questions

1. Putting a weight cuff in which position would require more effort at the shoulder joint to move the weight cuff through shoulder range of motion? Explain your answer.
   a. Cuff positioned at the wrist
   b. Cuff positioned at the elbow

2. Two people have the same weight and BOS, but one is on stilts. Which person is more stable? Why?
   a. The person on stilts
   b. The person not on stilts

3. What is the resultant force of the following muscles?
   a. Two heads of the gastrocnemius

   b. Sternal and clavicular portions of the pectoralis major

4. You are given two different sets of instructions. The first instruction tells you to run 5 miles, and the second instruction tells you to walk 30 feet to the north. Circle the correct answer.
   a. Running 5 miles is a vector/scalar quantity.
   b. Walking 30 feet to the north is a vector/scalar quantity.

5. A delivery person has several boxes stacked on a hand truck. Would the person have to use more force to push the hand truck when the hand truck is more horizontal or more vertical? Why?

6. Compare the push rims of a standard wheelchair and a racing wheelchair. Note that the racing wheelchair has much smaller push rims. What is the advantage of smaller push rims to a wheel chair racer?

7. Label the BOS, COG, and LOG for the object shown here. The object is of uniform density throughout its shape. Can this object remain upright without support? Why?

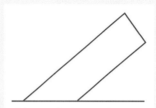

8. In terms of BOS, why is it more difficult for a person in a wheelchair to balance on only the back wheels ("wheelie") rather than on all four wheels?

9. Two people are standing on the same side of a patient's bed. They plan to move the patient toward them by pulling on the draw sheet. This move would be what type of force: linear, parallel, concurrent, or force couple?

10. Prior to moving the patient, what can the people do to increase their own stability?

11. When cracking an almond with a nutcracker, will the almond be easier to crack if it is closer to the axis or closer to the end of the handles? Why?

12. Does the figure below represent forces that are linear, parallel, or concurrent? Why?

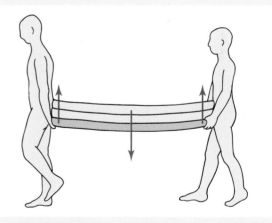

13. Give an example of bony structures at the knee acting as a pulley to increase the angle of pull.

14. Explain why a person leans to the right when carrying a heavy suitcase in the left hand. If the suitcase was very heavy, what might the person do with her right arm? Why?

15. Why are rubber tips put on the ends of crutches?

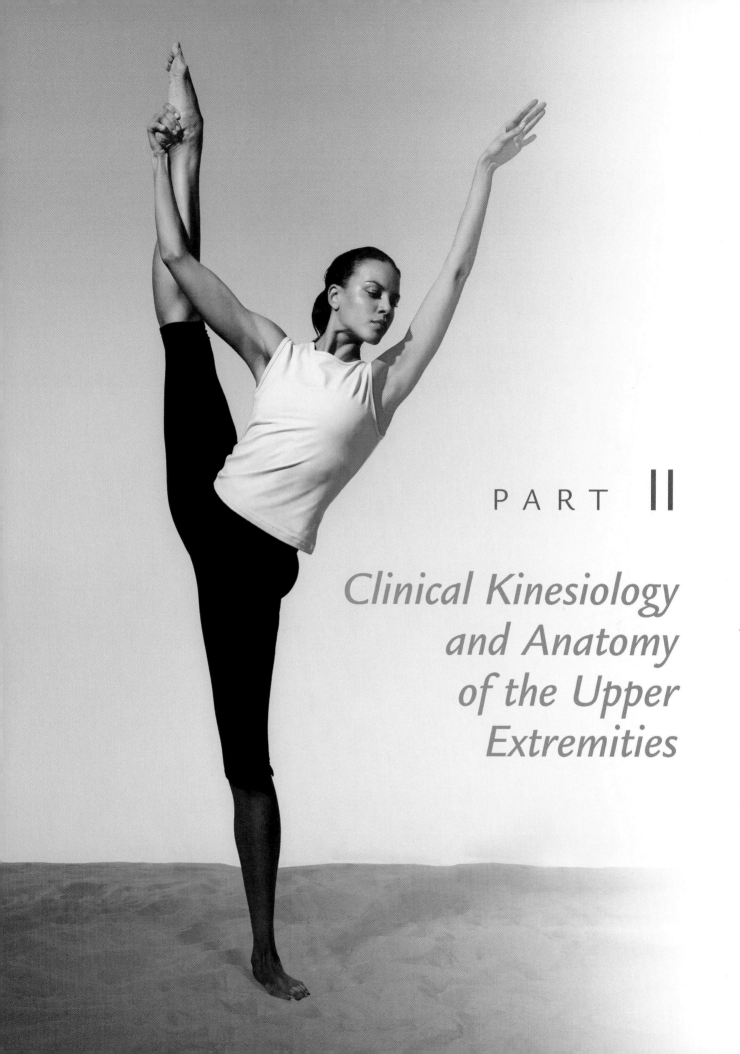

PART **II**

*Clinical Kinesiology
and Anatomy
of the Upper
Extremities*

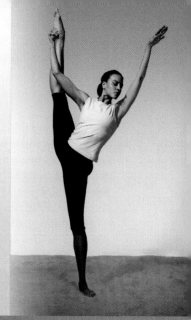

CHAPTER 9
Shoulder Girdle

Clarification of Terms

Bones and Landmarks

Joints and Ligaments

Joint Motions

    *Companion Motions of the Shoulder Joint
and Shoulder Girdle*

    Scapulohumeral Rhythm

    Angle of Pull

Muscles of the Shoulder Girdle

    Muscle Descriptions

    Anatomical Relationships

    Force Couples

    Reversal of Muscle Action

    Summary of Muscle Innervation

Points to Remember

Review Questions

    General Anatomy Questions

    Functional Activity Questions

    Clinical Exercise Questions

Clarification of Terms

The purpose of the shoulder and the entire upper extremity is to allow the hand to be placed in various positions to accomplish the multitude of tasks it is capable of performing. The shoulder, or glenohumeral joint, is the most mobile joint in the body and is capable of a great deal of motion. However, in talking about shoulder motion, we must recognize that motion also occurs at three other joints, or areas. *Shoulder complex* is a term that is sometimes used to include all of the structures involved with motion of the shoulder. The **shoulder complex** consists of the scapula, clavicle, sternum, humerus, and rib cage, and includes the sternoclavicular joint, acromioclavicular joint, glenohumeral joint, and "scapulothoracic articulation" (Fig. 9-1). In other words, it includes the shoulder girdle (scapula and clavicle) and the shoulder joint (scapula and humerus). The **scapulothoracic articulation** is not a joint in the pure sense of the word. Although

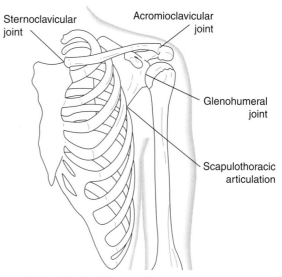

Figure 9-1. The shoulder complex (anterior view).

115

the scapula and thorax do not have a point of fixation, the scapula does move over the rib cage of the thorax. The scapula and thorax are not directly attached but are connected indirectly by the clavicle and by several muscles. The scapulothoracic articulation does provide motion and flexibility to the body.

Shoulder girdle is a term often used to discuss the activities of the scapula and clavicle and, to a lesser degree, the sternum. The sternoclavicular and acromioclavicular joints allow shoulder girdle motions, including elevation and depression, protraction and retraction, and upward and downward rotation. Five muscles attach to the scapula, the clavicle, or both, providing motion of the shoulder girdle.

The **shoulder joint,** also called the *glenohumeral joint,* consists of the scapula and humerus. The motions of the shoulder joint are flexion, extension and hyperextension, abduction and adduction, medial and lateral rotation, and horizontal abduction and adduction. Because the shoulder joint is so mobile, it has few ligaments. The nine muscles that cross the shoulder joint are the prime movers in shoulder joint motion.

Now that the various terms connected with the shoulder complex have been defined, the shoulder girdle will be discussed in more detail. The shoulder joint will be addressed in the Chapter 10.

Bones and Landmarks

The scapula, a triangular-shaped bone located superficially on the posterior side of the thorax, and the clavicle make up the shoulder girdle. The scapula attaches to the trunk indirectly through its ligamentous attachment to the clavicle. It is slightly concave anteriorly and glides over the convex posterior rib cage. Many muscles also connect the scapula to the trunk.

In the resting position, the scapula is located between the second and seventh ribs, with the vertebral border approximately 2 to 3 inches lateral from the spinous processes of the vertebra. The spine of the scapula is approximately level with the spinous process of the third and fourth thoracic vertebrae (Fig. 9-2).

Figures 9-1 and 9-2 show the position of the scapula on the body from an anterior and posterior view, respectively. In terms of shoulder girdle function, the important bony landmarks of the scapula (Fig. 9-3) are the following:

Superior Angle
Superior medial aspect, providing attachment for the levator scapula muscle

Inferior Angle
Most inferior point and where vertebral and axillary border meet. This point determines scapular rotation.

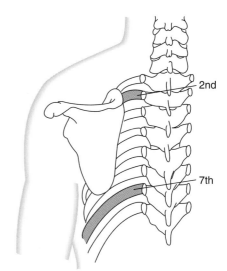

Figure 9-2.   Resting position of the scapula on the thorax (posterior view).

Vertebral Border
Between superior and inferior angles medially, and attachment of the rhomboid and serratus anterior muscles

Axillary Border
The lateral side between glenoid fossa and inferior angle

Spine
Projection on posterior surface, running from medial border laterally to the acromion process. It

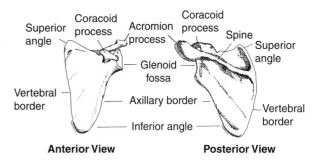

Anterior View   **Posterior View**

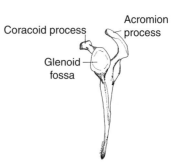

Lateral View

Figure 9-3.   Bony landmarks of the left scapula.

provides attachment for the middle and lower trapezius muscles.

Coracoid Process

Projection on anterior surface, providing attachment for the pectoralis minor muscle

Acromion Process

Broad, flat area on superior lateral aspect, providing attachment for the upper trapezius muscle

Glenoid Fossa

Slightly concave surface that articulates with humerus on superior lateral side above the axillary border and below the acromion process

The **clavicle** is an S-shaped bone that connects the upper extremity to the axial skeleton at the sternoclavicular joint. Figure 9-1 shows the position of the clavicle in relation to the sternum, scapula, and rib cage. For shoulder girdle function, the important bony landmarks of the clavicle (Fig. 9-4) are as follows:

Sternal End

Attaches medially to sternum

Acromial End

Attaches laterally to scapula and provides attachment for the upper trapezius muscle

Body

Area between the two ends

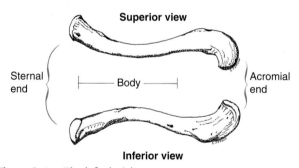

Figure 9-4. The left clavicle.

The **sternum** is a flat bone located in the midline of the anterior thorax (Fig. 9-5). The position of the sternum in relation to the rib cage and the clavicles is shown in Figure 9-1. At its superior end, the sternum provides attachment for the clavicle, followed beneath by attachments for the costal cartilages of the ribs. It is divided into three parts:

Manubrium

The superior end, providing attachment for the clavicle and the first rib

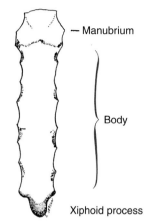

Figure 9-5. The sternum (anterior view).

Body

The middle two-thirds of the sternum, providing attachment for the remaining ribs

Xiphoid Process

Meaning "sword-shaped," the inferior tip

Joints and Ligaments

The **sternoclavicular joint** (Fig. 9-6) provides the shoulder girdle with its only direct attachment to the trunk. This plane-shaped synovial joint has a double gliding motion. Sternoclavicular joint motions include elevation and depression, protraction and retraction, and rotation. Because these motions occur in three planes, the joint has three degrees of freedom. Sternoclavicular joint motions accompany the motions of the shoulder girdle. Although these motions are more subtle than those at most other joints, they are nonetheless important. Basically, the clavicle moves while the sternum remains stationary.

Being a synovial joint, the sternoclavicular joint has a joint capsule. It also has three major ligaments and a

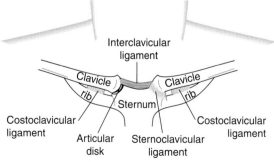

Figure 9-6. Ligaments of the sternoclavicular joint (left side cut away to show the disk; anterior view).

joint disk. The joint capsule surrounds the joint and is reinforced by the anterior and posterior sternoclavicular ligaments. The articular disk has a unique attachment that contributes to the motion of this joint. The upper part of the disk is attached to the posterior superior part of the clavicle, while the lower part is attached to the manubrium and first costal cartilage. This double attachment is much like that of the double hinge found on doors that swing in both directions. During shoulder girdle elevation and depression, motion occurs between the clavicle and the disk. During protraction and retraction, motion occurs between the disk and the sternum. The articular disk also serves as a shock absorber, especially from forces generated by falls on the outstretched hand. The disk and its ligamentous support are so effective that dislocation at the sternoclavicular joint is rare.

The three major ligaments supporting this joint are the sternoclavicular, costoclavicular, and interclavicular ligaments. The **sternoclavicular ligament** connects the clavicle to the sternum on both the anterior and posterior surfaces and is therefore divided into the anterior and posterior sternoclavicular ligaments. These ligaments limit anterior-posterior movement of the clavicle's medial end. The posterior sternoclavicular ligament limits anterior motion and the anterior sternoclavicular ligament limits posterior motion. They both reinforce the joint capsule. The **costoclavicular ligament** is a short, flat, rhomboid-shaped ligament that connects the clavicle's inferior surface to the superior surface of the costal cartilage of the first rib. The primary purpose of this ligament is to limit the amount of clavicular elevation. The **interclavicular ligament** is located on top of the manubrium, connecting the superior sternal ends of the clavicles. Its purpose is to limit the amount of clavicular depression.

The **acromioclavicular joint** (Fig. 9-7) connects the acromion process of the scapula with the lateral end of

the clavicle. It is a plane-shaped synovial joint with three planes of motion. The motions are minimal but important to normal shoulder motion. The joint capsule surrounds the articular borders of the joint. It is quite weak and is reinforced above and below by the superior and inferior **acromioclavicular ligaments.** These ligaments support the joint by holding the acromion process to the clavicle, thus preventing dislocation of the clavicle.

The coracoclavicular ligament and coracoacromial ligaments are two accessory ligaments of the acromioclavicular joint. Although the **coracoclavicular ligament** is not directly located at the joint, it does provide stability to that joint and allows the scapula to be suspended from the clavicle. It connects the scapula to the clavicle by attaching to the inferior surface of the clavicle's lateral end and to the superior surface of the scapula's coracoid process (Fig. 9-7). The ligament is divided into a lateral trapezoid portion and the deeper medial conoid portion. Together they prevent backward motion of the scapula, and individually they limit the rotation of the scapula.

The **coracoacromial ligament** does not actually cross the acromioclavicular joint, but rather forms a roof over the head of the humerus and serves as a protective arch, providing support to the head when an upward force is transmitted along the humerus (Fig. 9-8). It attaches laterally on the superior surface of the coracoid process and runs up and out to the inferior surface of the acromial process.

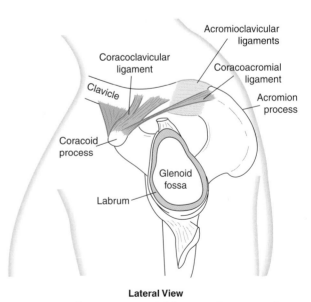

Lateral View

Figure 9-8. The coracoacromial ligament forms a roof over the shoulder joint.

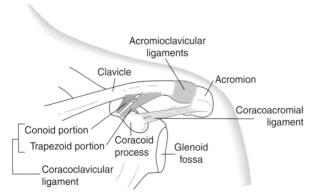

Figure 9-7. Ligaments of the acromioclavicular joint (anterior view).

Joint Motions

As mentioned previously, the motions of the shoulder girdle are elevation and depression, protraction and retraction, and upward and downward rotation (Fig. 9-9). Because these motions can be seen best by looking at the scapula, they are commonly described as either *shoulder girdle* or *scapular motion.* For example, *shoulder girdle protraction and retraction* is synonymous with *scapular abduction and adduction,* and scapular rotation is the same as shoulder girdle rotation.

Elevation/depression and **protraction/retraction** are essentially linear motions. All points of the scapula move up and down along the thorax and away from and toward the vertebral column in parallel lines. Angular motion occurs during upward and downward rotation of the scapula. Because of the scapula's triangular shape, one side moves one way while another side moves in an opposite or different direction. During **upward rotation,** the inferior angle of the scapula rotates up and away from the vertebral column, while **downward rotation** is the return to the resting anatomical position. For example, when the inferior angle rotates up and out, the superior angle moves down and the glenoid fossa moves

up and in. Therefore, it is important to have a point of reference to define this rotation. The inferior angle is that reference point (Fig. 9-10). Note that the downward rotation motion is the return to anatomical position from an upwardly rotated position. The scapula does not move past anatomical position toward the vertebral column.

Another scapular motion should be mentioned—**scapular tilt** (see Fig. 9-9, lower right). Scapular tilt occurs when the shoulder joint goes into hyperextension. The superior end of the scapula tilts anteriorly, and the inferior end tilts posteriorly. Examples of these combined motions are the "windup" or prerelease phase of a softball pitch, a bowling delivery, or a racing dive in swimming.

Because of the complexity of joint shapes and joint interaction in the shoulder complex, some very subtle motions occur that are beyond the scope of this book. One such movement is worthy of mention so as to clarify normal versus abnormal motion. Scapular winging is the posterior lateral movement of the vertebral border of the scapula in the transverse plane. In other words, the vertebral border of the scapula moves away from the rib cage. This motion occurs primarily at the acromioclavicular joint but is seen most often at the scapulothoracic articulation. This can be demonstrated by asking a person with a "normal" shoulder to place his or her hand on the small of the back. The vertebral border of the scapula lifts away from the rib cage. This

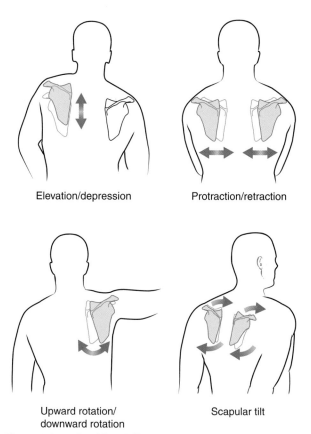

Elevation/depression   Protraction/retraction

Upward rotation/
downward rotation   Scapular tilt

Figure 9-9. Shoulder girdle motions (posterior view).

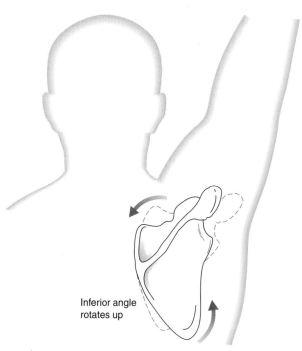

Inferior angle
rotates up

Figure 9-10. Scapular motion during upward rotation.

motion can only be done in combination with several other motions. However, pathological "winging of the scapula" also occurs when the stabilizing muscles around the scapula are weak or paralyzed. A serratus anterior muscle weakness or paralysis is a dramatic example. When a person with that condition pushes against a wall with an outstretched hand (Fig. 9-11), the involved scapula will rise away from the rib cage, standing out like a small wing. A video demonstration of this can be seen at the following website: http://www.shoulderdoc.co.uk/article.asp?section=492. Excessive winging is considered abnormal.

At the sternoclavicular joint during shoulder girdle elevation and depression, the convex surface of the clavicle slides inferiorly and superiorly on the concave manubrium as the clavicle's lateral end moves up and down, respectively. During protraction and retraction, the concave portion of the clavicle slides anteriorly and posteriorly on the convex costal cartilage, respectively, as the clavicle's lateral end moves forward and backward. During rotation, the clavicle spins on the sternum.

At the acromioclavicular joint, the acromion of the scapula is concave, while the lateral end of the clavicle is convex. Therefore, the joint surface of the acromion slides in the same direction as the clavicle during scapular movement.

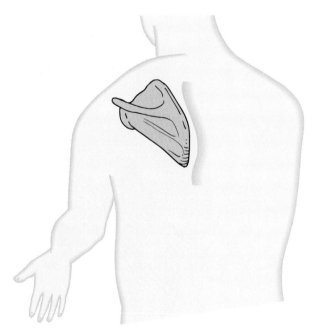

Figure 9-11.   Winging of the scapula (posterior view). This person's left serratus anterior muscle is paralyzed. When pushing against the wall with both hands, the left scapula rises away from the rib cage, standing out like a small wing.

Companion Motions of the Shoulder Joint and Shoulder Girdle

During the linear movements of elevation/depression and protraction/retraction, it is possible to move the shoulder girdle (clavicle and scapula) up, down, forward, or backward without moving the humerus. However, shoulder joint motions must accompany the angular motions of upward and downward rotation. To rotate the scapula upward, you must also flex or abduct the shoulder joint. Stated another way, when there is flexion or abduction of the shoulder joint, the scapula must also rotate upward. When there is extension or adduction of the shoulder joint, the scapula returns to anatomical position, or rotates downward. Because of the complex and interrelated activities of the shoulder girdle and the shoulder joint, it is difficult to discuss the function of one without discussing activities of the other. Impairment at one joint will also impair function at the other. The following list summarizes the shoulder girdle motions that must occur during various shoulder joint motions:

Shoulder Joint	Shoulder Girdle
Flexion	Upward rotation; protraction
Extension	Downward rotation; retraction
Hyperextension	Scapular tilt
Abduction	Upward rotation
Adduction	Downward rotation
Medial rotation	Protraction
Lateral rotation	Retraction
Horizontal abduction	Retraction
Horizontal adduction	Protraction

Scapulohumeral Rhythm

Scapulohumeral rhythm is a concept that further describes the movement relationship between the shoulder girdle and the shoulder joint. The first 30 degrees of shoulder joint motion is pure shoulder joint motion. However, after that, for every 2 degrees of shoulder flexion or abduction that occurs, the scapula must upwardly rotate 1 degree. This 2:1 ratio is known as *scapulohumeral rhythm.*

It is possible to demonstrate that the first part of shoulder joint motion occurs only at the shoulder joint, but further motion must be accompanied by shoulder girdle motion. With a person in the anatomical position, stabilize the scapula by putting the heel of your hand against the axillary border to prevent rotation of the scapula. Instruct the person to abduct the shoulder joint. Notice that the individual is able to abduct only a short distance before shoulder joint motion is impaired.

Angle of Pull

As discussed in Chapter 5, several factors determine the role that a muscle will play in a particular joint motion. Determining whether a muscle has a major role (prime mover), a minor role (assisting mover), or no role at all will depend on such factors as its size, the angle of pull, the joint motions possible, and the location of the muscle in relation to the joint axis. Angle of pull is usually a major factor, because most muscles pull at a diagonal. As discussed in Chapter 8 regarding torque, most muscles have a diagonal line of pull. That diagonal line of pull is the resultant force of a vertical force and a horizontal force. In the case of the shoulder girdle, muscles with a greater vertical angle of pull will be effective in pulling the scapula up or down (elevating or depressing the scapula). Muscles with a greater horizontal pull will be more effective in pulling the scapula in or out (protracting or retracting). Muscles with a more equal horizontal and vertical pull will have a role in both motions (see Fig. 5-12). For example, the levator scapula has a stronger vertical component, the middle trapezius has a stronger horizontal component, and the rhomboids have a more equal pull in both directions. As you will see when these muscles are described later in this chapter, the levator scapula is a prime mover in scapular elevation, the middle trapezius is a prime mover in retraction, and the rhomboids are a prime mover in both elevation and retraction.

Muscles of the Shoulder Girdle

Muscle Descriptions

There are five muscles primarily responsible for moving the scapula. Each muscle will be discussed with particular emphasis on its location and function. This will be followed by a summary of its proximal attachment origin (O), its distal attachment insertion (I), and its joint motions in which it is a prime mover action (A). This listing is given for clarity and is not intended to be the only description. You are encouraged to visualize the attachments and describe them using proper terminology instead of memorizing these listings. The nerve (N) that innervates the muscle, as well as the spinal cord level of that innervation, is also given.

The muscles of the shoulder girdle are the following:

Trapezius
Levator scapula
Rhomboids
Serratus anterior
Pectoralis minor

Trapezius

The **trapezius muscle** (Fig. 9-12) is a large, superficial muscle that appears diamond-shaped when looking at both right and left sides. Functionally, it is usually divided into three parts: upper, middle, and lower. The reason for this separation is that there are three different lines of pull (upward, inward, downward) resulting in different muscle actions.

The **upper trapezius muscle** (Fig. 9-13) originates from the occipital protuberance and the nuchal ligament of the upper cervical vertebrae. The nuchal ligament attaches to the spinous processes of the cervical vertebrae. The upper trapezius inserts on the lateral end of the clavicle and acromion process. Because its diagonal line of pull is more vertical (upward) than horizontal (inward), it is a prime mover in scapular elevation and upward rotation and is only an assisting mover in scapular retraction.

The **middle trapezius muscle** (Fig. 9-14) originates from the nuchal ligament of the lower cervical vertebrae and spinous process of C7 and the upper thoracic vertebrae. It inserts on the medial aspect of the acromion process and along the scapular spine. Its line of pull is horizontal, which makes it very effective at scapular retraction. Because the line of pull passes just above the axis for upward rotation, its role in scapular upward rotation is only assistive.

The **lower trapezius muscle** (Fig. 9-15) originates from the spinous processes of the middle and lower

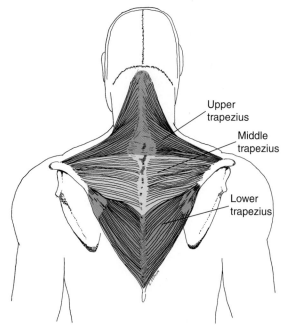

Figure 9-12. The three parts of the trapezius muscle (posterior view).

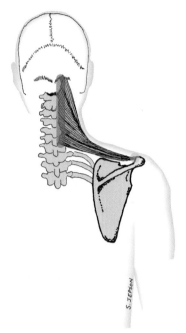

Figure 9-13.   The upper trapezius muscle (posterior view).

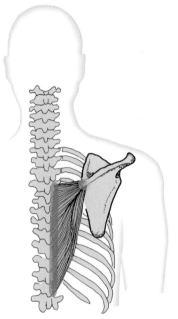

Figure 9-15.   The lower trapezius muscle (posterior view).

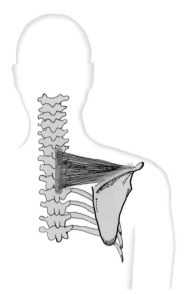

Figure 9-14.   The middle trapezius muscle (posterior view).

thoracic vertebrae and inserts on the base of the scapular spine. Its diagonal line of pull is more downward (vertical) than inward (horizontal), making it effective in depression and upward rotation of the scapula and only assistive in retraction.

Upper Trapezius Muscle

O	Occipital bone, nuchal ligament on upper cervical spinous processes
I	Outer third of clavicle, acromion process
A	Scapular elevation and upward rotation
N	Spinal accessory (cranial nerve XI), C3 and C4 sensory component

Middle Trapezius Muscle

O	Spinous processes of C7 through T3
I	Scapular spine
A	Scapular retraction
N	Spinal accessory (cranial nerve XI), C3 and C4 sensory component

Lower Trapezius Muscle

O	Spinous processes of middle and lower thoracic vertebrae
I	Base of the scapular spine
A	Scapular depression and upward rotation
N	Spinal accessory (cranial nerve XI), C3 and C4 sensory component

All three parts of the trapezius muscle work together (synergists) to retract the scapula. Remember, however, that the middle trapezius muscle is the prime mover and that the upper and lower trapezius muscles can only assist. The upper and lower trapezius muscles are antagonistic to each other in elevation/depression and are agonistic in upward rotation. To visualize the upward rotation component of these muscles, think of the scapula as a steering wheel (Fig. 9-16). In this example, a right scapula is used. Tie a ribbon at the bottom of the wheel to represent the inferior angle of the scapula. Put your right hand at the two o'clock position, representing the upper trapezius attachment; put your left hand at the ten o'clock position, representing the lower trapezius attachment. Turn the wheel to the left and note that the ribbon moves upward toward the right. In the case of the scapula, the upper trapezius muscle (right hand) moves up and in, while the lower trapezius muscle (left hand) moves down and in. This combined effort causes the inferior angle to move up and out (upward rotation).

The **levator scapula muscle** is named for its function of scapular elevation. It is covered entirely by the trapezius muscle. It arises from the transverse processes of C1 through C4 and attaches on the vertebral border of the scapula between the superior angle and the spine (Fig. 9-17). Its diagonal line of pull is mostly vertical. Therefore, it is a prime mover in scapular elevation and only an assisting mover in retraction. It is also a prime mover in downward rotation. Visualize the steering wheel with your left hand in the ten o'clock position. Pull up (turning the wheel to the right) and notice that the inferior angle (ribbon) moves to the left (downward rotation). Keep in mind that downward rotation is the return to anatomical position from an upwardly rotated position.

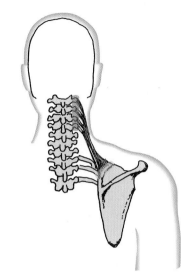

Figure 9-17. The levator scapula muscle (posterior view).

Levator Scapula Muscle

O	Transverse processes of first four cervical vertebrae
I	Vertebral border of scapula between the superior angle and spine
A	Scapular elevation and downward rotation
N	Third and fourth cervical nerves and dorsal scapular nerve (C5)

The **rhomboids** are actually two muscles: rhomboid major and rhomboid minor. They are commonly considered together as one muscle, because it is anatomically difficult to separate them, and functionally they have the same actions. The rhomboids derive their name from their shape. This geometric shape is basically a rectangle that has been skewed so that the sides have oblique angles instead of right angles. The rhomboid muscles lie under the trapezius muscle and can be palpated when the trapezius muscle is relaxed. They originate from the nuchal ligament and spinous processes of C7 through T5, and they insert on the vertebral border of the scapula below the levator scapula muscle between the spine and the inferior angle (Fig. 9-18). Because their oblique line of pull has a good horizontal and vertical component, they are a prime mover in retraction and elevation. Like the levator scapula muscle, the rhomboids rotate the scapula downward.

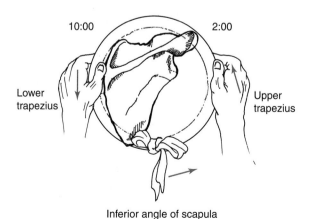

10:00   2:00

Lower trapezius

Upper trapezius

Inferior angle of scapula

Figure 9-16. Rotational movement of the right scapula.

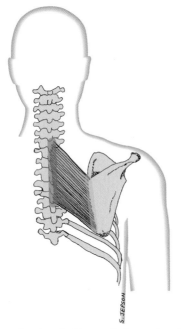

Figure 9-18. The rhomboid muscle (posterior view).

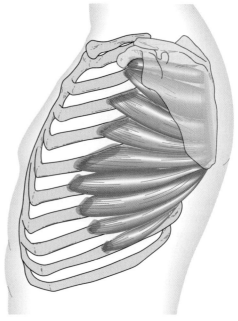

Figure 9-19. The serratus anterior muscle (lateral view).

Rhomboid Muscles

O	Spinous processes of C7 through T5
I	Vertebral border of scapula between the spine and inferior angle
A	Scapular retraction, elevation, and downward rotation
N	Dorsal scapular nerve (C5)

It is impossible to raise your arm above your head without the action of the **serratus anterior muscle.** This muscle gets its name from the serrated, or sawtooth, pattern of attachment on the anterior, lateral side of the thorax. It is superficial at this point and can be palpated when the arm is overhead. The muscle runs posteriorly to pass between the scapula and the rib cage. It attaches on the anterior surface of the scapula along the vertebral border between the superior and inferior angles (Fig. 9-19). Because it has a nearly horizontal line of pull outward, it is a prime mover in scapular protraction. Its lower fibers pulling outward on the lower part of the scapula are effective in rotating the scapula upward. These fibers join with the upper and lower trapezius muscles to form a force couple that rotates the scapula upward. Another function of the serratus anterior muscle is to keep the vertebral border of the scapula against the rib cage. Without this muscle, the vertebral border lifts away from the rib cage, which is called "winging of the scapula" (see Fig. 9-11).

Serratus Anterior Muscle

O	Lateral surface of the upper eight ribs
I	Vertebral border of the scapula, anterior surface
A	Scapular protraction and upward rotation
N	Long thoracic nerve (C5, C6, C7)

The **pectoralis minor muscle** lies deep to the pectoralis major muscle and is the only shoulder girdle muscle located entirely on the anterior surface of the body. It arises from the anterior surface of the third through fifth ribs near the costal cartilages, and it runs upward to its attachment on the coracoid process of the scapula (Fig. 9-20). Its downward diagonal line of pull is mostly vertical, making it a prime mover in scapular depression, downward rotation, and scapular tilt. Although it is rather easy to see the depression action, the downward rotation is less obvious, because the muscle is on the anterior surface while the scapula moves on the posterior surface. Visualize the steering wheel again with the ribbon (inferior angle of the scapula) rotated up to the right. Place your right hand in the two o'clock position (coracoid process) and pull down. Notice that the ribbon (inferior angle) moves downward toward the left (downward rotation). Because the pectoralis minor attaches on the anterior superior surface (coracoid process) of the scapula and moves vertically downward toward its attachment on the ribs, one can

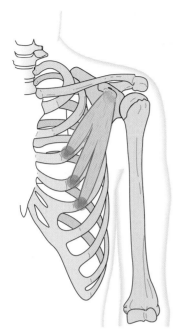

Figure 9-20. The pectoralis minor muscle (anterior view).

visualize the top part of the scapula being pulled down and forward, causing the bottom (inferior angle) to tip "out." In other words, the pectoralis minor causes scapular tilt.

Pectoralis Minor Muscle

O	Anterior surface, third through fifth ribs
I	Coracoid process of the scapula
A	Scapular depression, protraction, downward rotation, and tilt
N	Medial pectoral nerve (C8, T1)

Table 9-1 on page 126 summarizes the actions of the prime movers of the shoulder girdle.

Anatomical Relationships

The shoulder girdle muscles have been described by their attachments to bones, the joint motions that can occur because of these attachments, and their lines of pull. However, the relationship between muscles, whether superficial or deep, anterior or posterior, and so on, must also be described. All five shoulder girdle muscles have their origin on the trunk; three are located posteriorly, one laterally, and one anteriorly. Of the three posterior muscles, the trapezius is the most superficial. The right and left upper, middle, and lower trapezius covers most of the back in the form of a large diamond (see Fig. 9-12). Remove the trapezius, and the

rhomboids and levator scapula lie directly underneath (Fig. 9-21).

The pectoralis minor is on the anterior side of the body but deep to the pectoralis major muscle (Fig. 9-22). The serratus anterior originates anteriorly and runs posteriorly. As it crosses the lateral chest wall in a horizontal direction, it can be seen between the latissimus dorsi (posteriorly) and the pectoralis major (anteriorly), as shown in Figure 9-23.

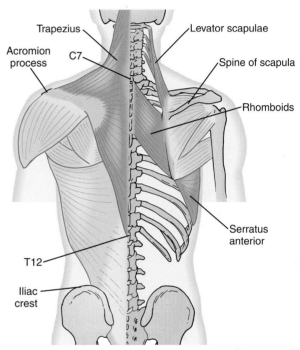

Figure 9-21. Muscles of posterior shoulder girdle.

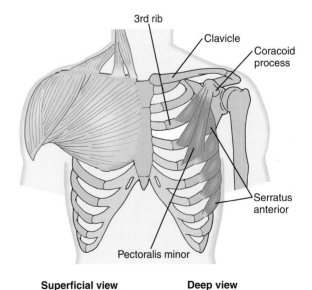

Superficial view   **Deep view**

Figure 9-22. Muscles of anterior shoulder girdle.

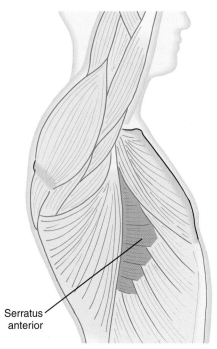

Figure 9-23.   Muscles of lateral shoulder girdle.

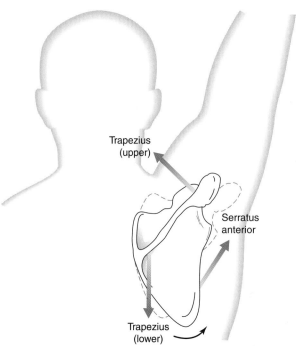

Figure 9-24.   The muscular force couple produces upward rotation of the scapula (posterior view).

Table 9-1	Prime Movers of the Shoulder Girdle
Action	**Muscles**
Retraction	Middle trapezius, rhomboids
Protraction	Serratus anterior, pectoralis minor
Elevation	Upper trapezius, levator scapula, rhomboids
Depression	Lower trapezius, pectoralis minor
Upward rotation	Upper and lower trapezius Serratus anterior (lower fibers)
Downward rotation	Rhomboids, levator scapulae, pectoralis minor
Scapular tilt	Pectoralis minor

Force Couples

A **force couple** is defined as muscles pulling in different directions to accomplish the same motion. In the case of the shoulder girdle, the upper trapezius muscle pulls up, the lower trapezius muscle pulls down, and the lower fibers of the serratus anterior muscle pull outward in a horizontal direction. The net effect is that the scapula rotates upward (Fig. 9-24).

Downward rotation is another example of a force couple. The combined effect of the pectoralis minor muscle pulling down, the rhomboid muscles pulling in, and the levator scapular muscle pulling up is downward rotation of the scapula (Fig. 9-25). This motion is accomplished when the shoulder joint is forcefully extended, as when chopping wood, paddling a canoe, or pulling down on an overhead exercise machine. Downward rotation of the scapula must accompany extension of the shoulder joint.

Reversal of Muscle Action

The actions of the shoulder girdle muscles have been described as moving insertion toward the origin. However, if the insertion is stabilized, the origin will move. As discussed in Chapter 5, this is called **reversal of muscle action.** It allows some of the shoulder girdle muscles to have assistive roles in other joints, primarily the head and neck.

Because of its attachment on the occiput and cervical vertebrae, the upper trapezius plays a role in moving the head and neck. When the shoulder girdle is stabilized, the upper trapezius can assist in extending the head and neck, laterally bending it to the same side (ipsilateral) and rotating it to the opposite side (contralateral).

With the shoulder girdle stabilized, the lower trapezius can reverse its action and assist in elevating the trunk. This is particularly useful during crutch walking.

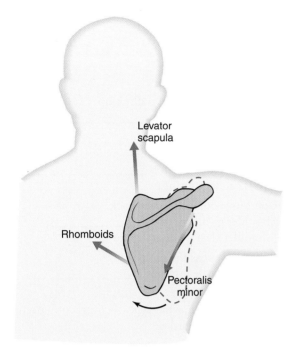

Figure 9-25. The muscular force couple produces downward rotation of the scapula (posterior view).

Table 9-2 Innervation of the Muscles of the Shoulder Girdle

Muscle	Nerve	Spinal Segment
Trapezius*	Cranial nerve XI	C3, C4 (sensory)
Levator scapula	Dorsal scapular	C3, C4, C5
Rhomboids	Dorsal scapular	C5
Serratus anterior	Long thoracic	C5, C6, C7
Pectoralis minor	Medial pectoral	C8, T1

*The 11th cranial nerve provides motor innervation. C3 and C4 are sensory.

Table 9-3 Segmental Innervation of Shoulder Girdle Muscles

Spinal Cord Level	C3	C4	C5	C6	C7	C8	T1
Trapezius	X	X					
Levator scapula	X	X	X				
Rhomboids			X				
Serratus anterior			X	X	X		
Pectoralis minor						X	X

With the crutches planted on the floor in front, the person swings the body through. The lower origin on the vertebral column moves toward the higher attachment on the scapula, thus raising the body as it swings through the crutches.

When the scapula is stabilized, the levator scapula can move the neck. It can assist the splenius cervicis, a neck muscle, in rotating and laterally bending the neck ipsilaterally.

Summary of Muscle Innervation

The shoulder girdle gets its innervation fairly high off the spinal cord from a variety of sources proximal to the terminal nerves of the brachial plexus. The 11th cranial (spinal accessory) nerve innervates the trapezius muscle with sensory innervation from C3 and C4. The third and fourth cervical nerves innervate the levator scapula muscle with partial innervation by the dorsal scapular nerve coming from C5. The serratus anterior muscle is innervated by the long thoracic nerve, which is made up of branches of C5 through C7, and the rhomboid muscles are innervated by the dorsal scapular nerve, a branch of the anterior ramus to C5. The pectoralis minor muscle receives innervation from the medial pectoral nerve, which branches off the medial cord of the brachial plexus. Table 9-2 summarizes the innervation of these muscles, and Table 9-3 gives the spinal cord level of innervation for each muscle.

Points to Remember

- The shoulder girdle has both linear and angular motions.
- The inferior angle is the point of reference for scapular rotation.
- Certain shoulder girdle and shoulder joint motions are connected.
- Scapulohumeral rhythm is an example of the combined motions of these joints.
- Muscles pulling in different directions to accomplish the same motion are a force couple.
- Concentric and eccentric are accelerating and decelerating activities. With isometric, there is no joint motion.
- Kinetic chain movement depends upon whether the distal segment is fixed (closed) or free to move (open).

Review Questions

General Anatomy Questions

1. Identify the structures that make up the shoulder girdle, the shoulder joint, and the shoulder complex.

2. Given that the scapula is shaped somewhat like a triangle,
    a. what landmark is commonly used to determine the direction the scapula is rotating?
    b. what direction is the landmark moving if the scapula is rotating upwardly?

3. Which shoulder girdle motions are mostly linear?

4. Which shoulder girdle motions are mostly angular?

5. What is scapulohumeral rhythm?

6. How is shoulder joint motion affected by the absence of scapulohumeral rhythm?

7. The trapezius muscle is usually referred to and described as consisting of three different muscles. The two rhomboid muscles (major and minor) are referred to and described as one. From a functional perspective,
    a. why is the trapezius muscle separated into three muscles?
    b. why are the rhomboid muscles described as one muscle?

8. Raising your hand over your head requires the combined action of which three shoulder girdle muscles?

9. Name and define the biomechanical term used to describe the combined action in question 8.

10. Starting at the inferior angle and going clockwise, name the shoulder girdle muscles that attach to the posterior surface of the right scapula.

11. The pectoralis minor muscle is deep to what muscle?

12. As you look at the lateral chest wall, the serratus anterior is deep to what two muscles?

Functional Activity Questions

Identify the shoulder girdle motions that occur with the following actions. Accompanying shoulder joint motions have been provided in parentheses.

1. Closing a window by pulling down
    Shoulder girdle motion _____
    (Shoulder extension)

2. Opening a window by pulling up
    Shoulder girdle motion _____
    (Shoulder flexion)

3. Carrying a heavy suitcase
    Shoulder girdle motion _____
    (No shoulder motion)

4. Combing your hair in the back
    Shoulder girdle motion _____
    (Shoulder flexion, lateral rotation)

5. Reaching across the table
    Shoulder girdle motion _____
    (Shoulder flexion)

6. In questions 1–5, what type of contraction occurs at the shoulder girdle?

Clinical Exercise Questions

1. Lie prone on a table with your right arm hanging over the side of the table and holding a weight in your right hand (Fig. 9-26). Using only shoulder girdle motion and no shoulder joint motion, pull the weight straight up from the floor.
    a. What joint motion is occurring at the shoulder girdle?
    b. What muscles are prime movers of this shoulder girdle action?
    c. Is this an open-chain or closed-chain activity?

2. Lie prone on a table with your right arm hanging over the side of the table and holding a weight in your right hand. Move your arm up and out by doing shoulder horizontal abduction.
    a. What shoulder girdle motion is accompanying shoulder horizontal abduction?

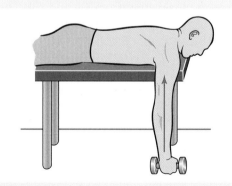

Figure 9-26.   Starting position.

Review Questions—cont'd

    b. What muscles are prime movers in this shoulder girdle motion?

    c. Is this a concentric, eccentric, or isometric contraction?

3. Sit in a chair that has arms; place your hands on the armrests in a position that puts your shoulders in hyperextension. Push down on the armrests and raise your buttocks off the seat of the chair.

    a. What shoulder girdle motion is accompanying the shoulder flexion action (from hyperextension to neutral)?

    b. What muscles are prime movers in this shoulder girdle motion?

    c. Is this a concentric or eccentric activity?

4. Lie in a prone position with your legs together, hands on the table next to your shoulders with your fingers pointing forward (Fig. 9-27). Push up with your hands as far as you can while straightening your elbows, bending your knees, and keeping your back straight.

    a. What shoulder girdle motion is occurring?

    b. What muscles are prime movers in this shoulder girdle motion?

    c. Is this an open-chain or closed-chain activity?

5. Using a lat pull-down machine of the Universal Gym (or some other comparable apparatus), reach up and grasp the handles. Pull down while keeping your arms moving in the frontal plane.

    a. What shoulder girdle motions are accompanying shoulder adduction and lateral rotation?

    b. What muscles are prime movers in these shoulder girdle motions?

    c. Is this a concentric or eccentric activity?

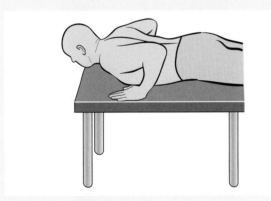

Figure 9-27.　Starting position.

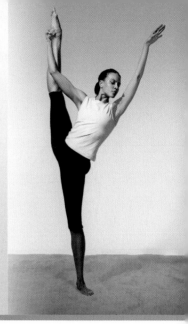

CHAPTER **10**

Shoulder Joint

Joint Motions

Bones and Landmarks

Ligaments and Other Structures

Muscles of the Shoulder Joint

Anatomical Relationships

Glenohumeral Movement

Summary of Muscle Action

Summary of Muscle Innervation

Common Shoulder Pathologies

Points to Remember

Review Questions

General Anatomy Questions

Functional Activity Questions

Clinical Exercise Questions

The **shoulder joint** is a ball-and-socket joint with movement in all three planes and around all three axes (Fig. 10-1). Therefore, the joint has three degrees of freedom. The humeral head articulating with the glenoid fossa of the scapula makes up the shoulder joint. It is one of the most movable joints in the body and, consequently, one of the least stable.

Joint Motions

There are four groups of motions possible at the shoulder joint (Fig. 10-2): (1) flexion, extension, and hyperextension; (2) abduction and adduction; (3) medial and lateral rotation; and (4) horizontal abduction and

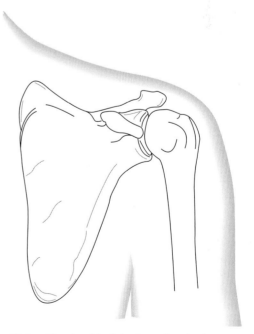

Figure 10-1. The shoulder joint (anterior view).

131

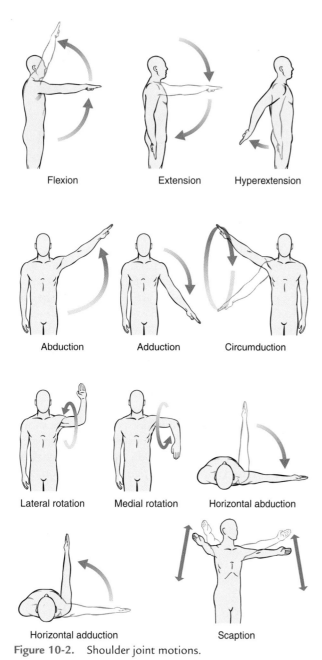

Flexion   Extension   Hyperextension

Abduction   Adduction   Circumduction

Lateral rotation   Medial rotation   Horizontal abduction

Horizontal adduction   Scaption

Figure 10-2.   Shoulder joint motions.

it is possible to move 90 degrees in each direction. **Horizontal abduction** and **horizontal adduction** also occur in the transverse plane around the vertical axis. From an arbitrary starting position for these motions of 90 degrees of shoulder abduction, there would be approximately 30 degrees of horizontal abduction (backward motion) and approximately 120 degrees of horizontal adduction (forward motion). *Circumduction* is a term used to describe the arc or circle of motion possible at the shoulder. Because it is really only a combination of all the shoulder motions, this term will not be used here.

Another term frequently seen in the literature, especially regarding therapeutic exercise for shoulder conditions, is **scaption.** This motion is similar to flexion or abduction but occurs in the **scapular plane** as opposed to the sagittal or frontal plane. The scapular plane is approximately 30 degrees forward of the frontal plane. It is not quite midway between flexion and abduction. With scaption of the shoulder, 180 degrees of up and down motion is possible. Most common functional activities occur in the scaption plane.

The normal end feel for all shoulder joint motions is **soft tissue stretch.** This is due to tension from various ligaments and muscles and from the joint capsule. Reviewing its description from Chapter 4, end feel is the feel at the end of a joint's passive range of motion when slight pressure is applied.

In terms of arthrokinematics, the convex humeral head moves within the concave glenoid fossa. As stated by the concave-convex rule, the convex joint surface (humeral head) moves in a direction opposite to the movement of the body segment (the arm). Therefore, when the shoulder joint flexes or abducts, the humeral head glides inferiorly. In extension and adduction, the humeral head glides superiorly. With medial rotation, the head glides posteriorly, and with lateral rotation, it glides anteriorly. Discussion of this and the muscles involved appears later in the chapter (see "Glenohumeral Movement").

adduction. Flexion, extension, and hyperextension occur in the sagittal plane around the frontal axis. **Flexion** is from 0 to 180 degrees, and **extension** is the return to anatomical position. Approximately 45 degrees of **hyperextension** are possible from the anatomical position. **Abduction** and **adduction** occur in the frontal plane around the sagittal axis with 180 degrees of motion possible. **Medial** and **lateral rotation** occur in the transverse plane around the vertical axis. Sometimes the terms *internal* and *external* are used in place of *medial* and *lateral,* respectively. From a neutral position,

Bones and Landmarks

The **scapula** and many of its landmarks were described in the chapter on the shoulder girdle. The following are landmarks of the scapula that you should know when talking about the shoulder joint (Fig. 10-3).

Glenoid Fossa
A shallow, somewhat egg-shaped socket on the superior end, lateral side; articulates with the humerus

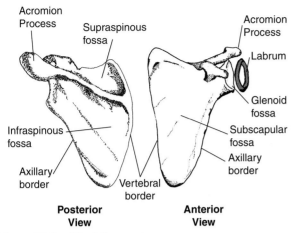

Figure 10-3.   The left scapula.

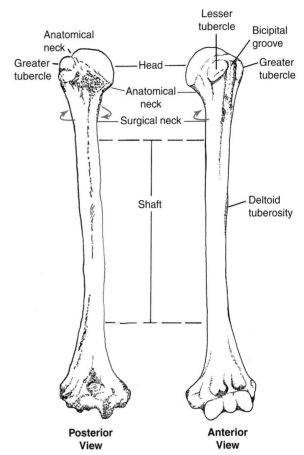

Figure 10-4.   The left humerus.

Glenoid Labrum
Fibrocartilaginous ring attached to the rim of the glenoid fossa, which deepens the articular cavity

Subscapular Fossa
Includes most of the area on the anterior (costal) surface, providing attachment for the subscapularis muscle

Infraspinous Fossa
Below the spine, providing attachment for the infraspinatus muscle

Supraspinous Fossa
Above the spine, providing attachment for the supraspinatus muscle

Axillary Border
Providing attachment for the teres major and teres minor muscles

Acromion Process
Broad, flat area on the superior lateral aspect, providing attachment for the middle deltoid muscle

The **humerus** is the longest and largest bone of the upper extremity (Fig. 10-4). The position of the humerus with the scapula is shown in an anterior view in Figure 10-1. The important landmarks are as follows:

Head
Semirounded proximal end; articulates with the scapula

Surgical Neck
Slightly constricted area just below tubercles where the head meets the body

Anatomical Neck
Circumferential groove separating the head from the tubercle

Shaft
Or "body"; the area between the surgical neck proximally and the epicondyles distally

Greater Tubercle
Large projection lateral to head and lesser tubercle; provides attachment for the supraspinatus, infraspinatus, and teres minor muscles

Lesser Tubercle
Smaller projection on the anterior surface, medial to the greater tubercle; provides attachment for the subscapularis muscle

Deltoid Tuberosity
On the lateral side near the midpoint; not usually a well-defined landmark

Bicipital Groove
Also called the "intertubercular groove"; the longitudinal groove between the tubercles, containing the tendon of the long head of the biceps

Bicipital Ridges

Also called the lateral and medial lips of the bicipital groove, or the crests of the greater and lesser tubercles, respectively. The lateral lip (crest of the greater tubercle) provides attachment for the pectoralis major, and the medial lip (crest of the lesser tubercle) provides attachment for the latissimus dorsi and teres major.

Ligaments and Other Structures

The **joint capsule** is a thin-walled, spacious container that attaches around the rim of the glenoid fossa of the scapula and the anatomical neck of the humerus (Figs. 10-5 and 10-6). The joint capsule is formed by an outer fibrous membrane and an inner synovial membrane. With the arm hanging at the side, the superior portion of the capsule is taut, and the inferior part is slack. When the shoulder is abducted, the opposite occurs: The inferior portion is taut, and the superior part is slack. The superior, middle, and inferior **glenohumeral ligaments** (see Fig. 10-5) reinforce the anterior portion of the capsule. These are not well-defined ligaments but actually pleated folds of the capsule.

The **coracohumeral ligament** attaches from the lateral side of the coracoid process and spans the joint anteriorly to the medial side of the greater tubercle (see Figs. 10-5 and 10-6). It strengthens the upper part of the joint capsule.

The **glenoid labrum** is a fibrous ring that surrounds the rim of the glenoid fossa (see Figs. 10-3 and 10-7). Its function is to deepen the articular cavity.

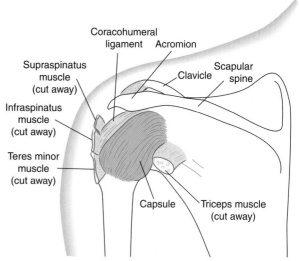

Figure 10-6. Left shoulder joint capsule and coracohumeral ligament. Posterior view, muscles cut away.

There are several bursae in the shoulder joint area. The subdeltoid bursa is large and located between the deltoid muscle and the joint capsule. The subacromial bursa lies below the acromion and coracoacromial ligament, between them and the joint capsule, and is frequently continuous with the subdeltoid bursa.

The **rotator cuff** is the tendinous band formed by the blending together of the tendinous insertions of the subscapularis, supraspinatus, infraspinatus, and teres minor muscles. These muscles help to keep the head of the humerus "rotating" against the glenoid fossa during joint motion. This rotating motion is what inspired the

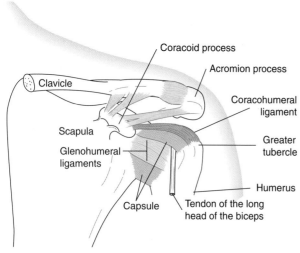

Figure 10-5. The shoulder joint capsule and the ligaments that reinforce it (anterior view).

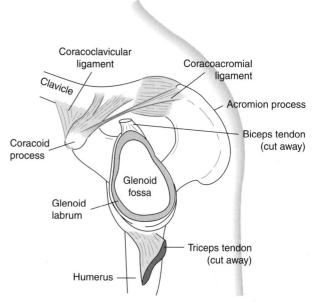

Figure 10-7. The glenoid labrum, lateral view.

term *rotator cuff,* not the muscular action of medial or lateral rotation.

The **thoracolumbar fascia** (lumbar aponeurosis) is a superficial fibrous sheet that attaches to the spinous processes of the lower thoracic and lumbar vertebrae, the supraspinal ligament, and the posterior part of the iliac crest, covering the sacrospinalis muscle (see Fig. 10-19). It provides a very broad attachment for the latissimus dorsi muscle.

As mentioned, the shoulder joint allows a great deal of motion, making it rather unstable. Several features contribute to whatever stability this joint does have. The fairly shallow glenoid fossa is made deeper by the glenoid labrum. The fossa is positioned in an anterior, lateral, and upward direction. This upward direction provides some stability to the joint. The joint is held intact by the joint capsule and is reinforced by the coracohumeral and glenohumeral ligaments. Because the capsule completely surrounds the joint, it creates a partial vacuum, which helps hold the head against the fossa. The rotator cuff muscles hold the joint surfaces together during joint motion. It is mostly the shoulder muscles that keep the joint from subluxing, or partially dislocating. An individual who has had a stroke and has lost function in the involved extremity often develops a subluxed shoulder. The lack of a deep socket for the humeral head to fit into, the loss of muscle tone, the weight of the extremity, and gravity all contribute to joint subluxation.

Muscles of the Shoulder Joint

The muscles that span the shoulder joint are as follows:

Deltoid
Pectoralis major
Latissimus dorsi
Teres major
Supraspinatus
Infraspinatus
Teres minor
Subscapularis
Coracobrachialis
Biceps brachii
Triceps brachii, long head

The **deltoid muscle** is a superficial muscle that covers the shoulder joint on three sides, giving the shoulder its characteristic rounded shape. The name *deltoid* describes its triangular shape (Fig. 10-8). Functionally, this muscle is separated into three parts: anterior, middle, and posterior.

The **anterior deltoid muscle** attaches on the outer third of the clavicle and runs down and out to the deltoid

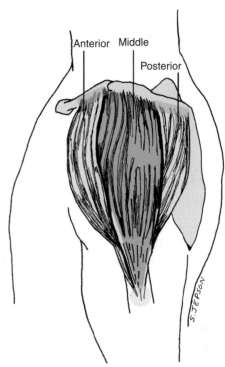

Figure 10-8. The three parts of the deltoid muscle (lateral view).

tuberosity, which is located on the lateral aspect of the humerus near the midpoint. It spans the joint on the anterior surface at an oblique angle. Therefore, it is effective in abduction, flexion, and medial rotation. When the arm is at shoulder level, the line of pull is mostly horizontal and, therefore, an effective horizontal adductor.

The **middle deltoid muscle** attaches on the lateral side of the acromion process and runs directly down to the deltoid tuberosity. Because its vertical line of pull is lateral to the joint axis, it is most effective in abducting the shoulder joint.

The **posterior deltoid muscle** attaches to the spine of the scapula and runs obliquely down to its attachment with the anterior and middle fibers on the deltoid tuberosity. Because its oblique line of pull is posterior to the joint axis, it is strong in shoulder abduction, extension, hyperextension, and lateral rotation. When the arm is at shoulder level, the line of pull is mostly horizontal, making it effective in horizontal abduction.

The "inchworm effect" is a concept that describes the action of the shoulder girdle and the deltoid muscles, especially the middle deltoid muscle, during shoulder abduction. If the humerus moved during abduction, the middle deltoid muscle would quickly run out of contractile power as it approached 90 degrees. However, the middle deltoid muscle is effective throughout the entire range. Remember that for every 2 degrees the shoulder joint abducts, the shoulder girdle upwardly rotates 1 degree (scapulohumeral rhythm; see Chapter 9). With this upward rotation of the scapula, the origin of the deltoid muscle (the acromion process, the lateral end of the clavicle, and the scapular spine) moves away from the insertion on the humerus. This motion lengthens the muscle, restoring its contractile potential, and allows it to continue to effectively contract throughout its entire range.

Anterior Deltoid Muscle

O	Lateral third of the clavicle
I	Deltoid tuberosity
A	Shoulder abduction, flexion, medial rotation, and horizontal adduction
N	Axillary nerve (C5, C6)

Middle Deltoid Muscle

O	Acromion process
I	Deltoid tuberosity (same as anterior deltoid muscle)
A	Shoulder abduction
N	Axillary nerve (C5, C6)

Posterior Deltoid Muscle

O	Spine of scapula
I	Deltoid tuberosity (same as anterior deltoid muscle)
A	Shoulder abduction, extension, hyperextension, lateral rotation, horizontal abduction
N	Axillary nerve (C5, C6)

The **pectoralis major muscle** (Fig. 10-9) is a large muscle of the chest, as its name implies (*pectus* means "breast" or "chest"). It is superficial except for its distal attachment lying under the deltoid muscle. Because this muscle crosses the joint on the anterior surface from medial to lateral, it is effective in adduction and medial rotation of the shoulder joint.

The pectoralis major muscle, because of its proximal attachments and different lines of pull, is often separated into a clavicular and sternal portion. The **clavicular portion** attaches to the medial third of the clavicle. The clavicular portion has a more vertical line of pull when the shoulder is extended, making it very effective at flexing the shoulder during the first part of the range. As the shoulder approaches 90 degrees (shoulder level), the line of pull changes

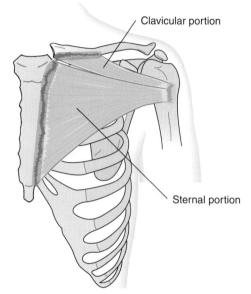

Figure 10-9.   The two parts of the pectoralis major muscle (anterior view).

from vertical to horizontal; thus, this portion of the pectoralis major muscle is no longer effective. It is most effective in the early portion of the range (0–30 degrees) and becomes more ineffective toward the midpoint of the range (90 degrees). Therefore, it is safe to say that the clavicular portion of the pectoralis major acts as a prime mover in the first 60 degrees of shoulder flexion.

The **sternal portion** attaches to the sternum and costal cartilages of the first six ribs. It has a more vertical line of pull when the shoulder is in full flexion and loses effectiveness as the shoulder approaches 90 degrees of extension. Similar to the clavicular portion but in the opposite direction, the sternal portion is most effective in the early part of the range (180–150 degrees). It becomes more ineffective toward the midpoint of the range (90 degrees). Therefore, it is safe to say that the sternal portion of the pectoralis major acts as a prime mover in the first 60 degrees of shoulder extension. Since extension begins from a position of full flexion (180 degrees) and moves to anatomical position (0 degrees), the first 60 degrees of shoulder extension would be from 180 degrees to 120 degrees.

Both portions of the pectoralis major muscle are effective in the first parts of motion in the sagittal plane (clavicular portion for flexion, sternal portion for extension). Therefore, they are antagonistic to each other in flexion and extension, but they are agonists in shoulder adduction, medial rotation, and horizontal adduction.

Pectoralis Major Muscle, Clavicular Portion

O	Medial third of clavicle
I	Lateral lip of bicipital groove of humerus
A	Shoulder flexion—first 60 degrees

Pectoralis Major Muscle, Sternal Portion

O	Sternum, costal cartilage of first six ribs
I	Lateral lip of bicipital groove of humerus (same as clavicular portion)
A	Shoulder extension—first 60 degrees (from 180 degrees to 120 degrees)

Pectoralis Major Muscle, Clavicular and Sternal Portions

A	Shoulder adduction, medial rotation, and horizontal adduction
N	Lateral and medial pectoral nerve (C5, C6, C7, C8, T1)

As its name implies, the **latissimus dorsi muscle** (Fig. 10-10) is a broad, sheetlike muscle located on the back (in Latin, *latissimus* means "widest" and *dorsi* means "back" or "posterior"). It is mostly superficial except for a small portion covered posteriorly by the lower trapezius muscle and covered distally as it passes through the axilla to attach on the proximal, anterior, and medial surfaces of the humerus. Because of its attachment on the ilium and sacrum, it can elevate the pelvis if the arms are stabilized. This action occurs during crutch walking, when the arms are stabilized on the crutch handles. This closed-chain activity is a good example of "reversal of muscle function" where the proximal (origin) attachment pulls toward the distal (insertion) attachment, instead of the more common distal attachment pulling toward the proximal. The latissimus dorsi muscle is a strong agonist in extension, hyperextension, adduction, and medial rotation of the shoulder, because it crosses the shoulder joint inferior and medial to the joint axes.

Latissimus Dorsi Muscle

O	Spinous processes of T7 through L5 (via dorsolumbar fascia), posterior surface of sacrum, iliac crest, and lower three ribs
I	Medial floor of bicipital groove of humerus
A	Shoulder extension, adduction, medial rotation, hyperextension
N	Thoracodorsal nerve (C6, C7, C8)

The **teres major muscle** (Fig. 10-11) has its proximal attachment on the axillary border of the scapula, just

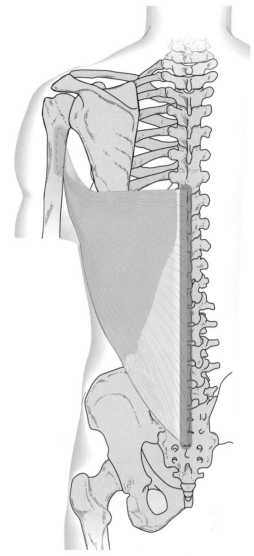

Figure 10-10. The latissimus dorsi muscle (posterior view). Note that the humeral attachment is on the anterior surface, as indicated by the dotted line.

below the teres minor muscle. In Latin, *teres* means "long and round." Both muscles are superficial at this point. The teres major muscle travels with the latissimus dorsi muscle through the axilla to the point where they attach close together on the anterior medial surface of the humerus near the proximal end. The teres major muscle is often referred to as the "little helper" of the latissimus dorsi muscle, because it does everything that the latissimus dorsi muscle does at the shoulder except hyperextension and because it is much smaller in size. Although the teres major muscle is a prime mover in extension, adduction, and medial rotation, its much smaller size makes it less effective than the latissimus dorsi.

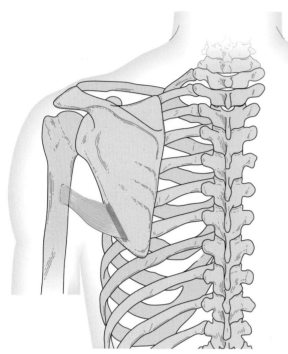

Figure 10-11.   The teres major muscle (posterior view). Note that the humeral attachment is on the anterior surface, as indicated by the dotted line.

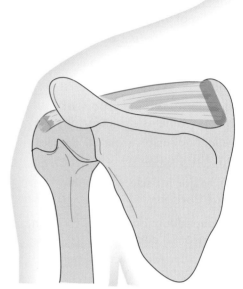

Figure 10-12.   The supraspinatus muscle (posterior view).

Teres Major Muscle

O	Axillary border of scapula near the inferior angle
I	Crest below lesser tubercle inferior to the latissimus dorsi muscle attachment
A	Shoulder extension, adduction, and medial rotation
N	Lower subscapular nerve (C5, C6, C7)

The **supraspinatus muscle** (Fig. 10-12) lies above the spine of the scapula. It passes underneath the acromion process to attach on the greater tubercle of the humerus. The portion located in the supraspinous fossa is deep to the trapezius muscle above and to the deltoid muscle laterally. Early kinesiology studies suggested that the supraspinatus muscle was most effective in only initiating shoulder abduction. However, electromyography studies have since shown that it is active throughout abduction. In addition to its joint movement function, the supraspinatus muscle is very important in stabilizing the head of the humerus against the glenoid fossa.

Supraspinatus Muscle

O	Supraspinous fossa of the scapula
I	Greater tubercle of the humerus
A	Shoulder abduction
N	Suprascapular nerve (C5, C6)

The **infraspinatus muscle** (Fig. 10-13) lies below the spine of the scapula. Most of the muscle is superficial; however, the trapezius and deltoid muscles cover portions of it. The distal attachment of the infraspinatus muscle is just inferior to the attachment of the supraspinatus muscle on the greater tubercle of the humerus. Although some authors refer to the infraspinatus muscle's ability to extend the shoulder joint, its more horizontal line of pull must be recognized. Therefore, its extension action is assistive at best.

Infraspinatus Muscle

O	Infraspinous fossa of scapula
I	Greater tubercle of humerus
A	Shoulder lateral rotation, horizontal abduction
N	Suprascapular nerve (C5, C6)

The **teres minor muscle** (see Fig. 10-13) is closely related to the infraspinatus muscle in both anatomical location and function. Both muscles are mostly superficial, with portions covered by the trapezius and the deltoid muscles. Both the teres major and teres minor muscles attach on the axillary border of the scapula and run obliquely up and outward to attach on the humerus. The teres minor muscle

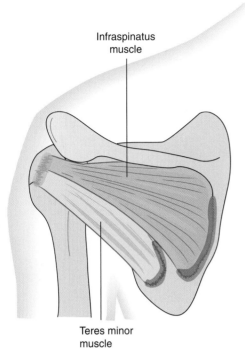

Figure 10-13. The infraspinatus and teres minor muscles (posterior view).

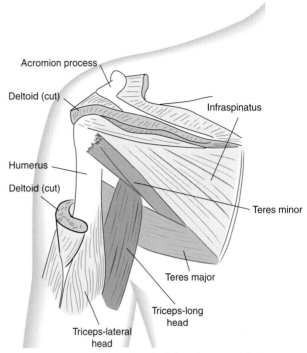

Figure 10-14. The long head of the triceps muscle separates the teres major and teres minor muscles at the axilla (posterior view).

attaches posteriorly on the greater tubercle of the humerus inferior to the infraspinatus, whereas the teres major muscle passes through the axilla to attach anteriorly below the lesser tubercle of the humerus. They are separated by the long head of the triceps muscle passing between them in the axilla (Fig. 10-14).

Teres Minor Muscle

O	Axillary border of scapula
I	Greater tubercle of humerus
A	Shoulder lateral rotation, horizontal abduction
N	Axillary nerve (C5, C6)

If you observe the distal attachments of the supraspinatus, infraspinatus, and teres minor muscles on the greater tubercle of the humerus, you will notice that they are essentially in a line (Fig. 10-15). For this reason, they are collectively referred to as the *SIT muscles,* taking the first letter from each muscle. These three muscles plus the subscapularis are referred to as the *rotator cuff,* or *SITS muscles.*

The **subscapularis** muscle (Fig. 10-16) gets its name from its location, which can be slightly misleading. In Latin, *sub* means "under." The subscapularis muscle is located deep on the "underside" of the scapula, lying next to the rib cage. This underside is actually the anterior, or

costal, surface of the scapula. From this attachment on the anterior surface, the subscapularis muscle runs laterally to cross the shoulder joint anteriorly and attach on the lesser tubercle of the humerus. This distal attachment blends into a common tendinous sheath with the other rotator cuff muscles to cover the humeral head and hold the head against the glenoid fossa. Because the subscapularis has a horizontal line of pull and attaches anteriorly on the humerus, it is a prime mover in medial rotation and assists in adduction of the shoulder.

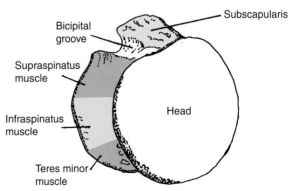

Figure 10-15. This superior view of the proximal end of the left humerus shows the attachments of the rotator cuff muscles.

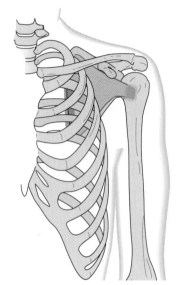

Figure 10-16. The subscapularis muscle (anterior view).

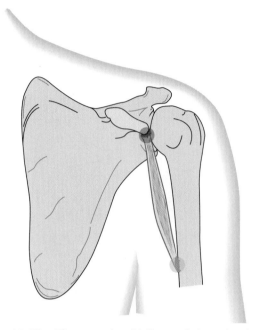

Figure 10-17. The coracobrachialis muscle (anterior view).

Subscapularis Muscle

O	Subscapular fossa of the scapula
I	Lesser tubercle of the humerus
A	Shoulder medial rotation
N	Upper and lower subscapular nerve (C5, C6)

The **coracobrachialis muscle** (Fig. 10-17) derives its name from its attachments on the coracoid process of the scapula and on the humerus, or arm (in Latin, *brachium*). It has an almost vertical line of pull quite close to the joint axis. Therefore, most of its force is directed back into the joint, stabilizing the head against the glenoid fossa. Some authors refer to this muscle's ability to flex and adduct the shoulder. However, because its vertical line of pull is so close to the joint axes, these actions are assistive at best.

Coracobrachialis Muscle

O	Coracoid process of the scapula
I	Medial surface of the humerus near the midpoint
A	Stabilizes the shoulder joint
N	Musculocutaneous nerve (C6, C7)

The biceps and triceps muscles are two-joint muscles that cross both the shoulder and the elbow. Their actions at the shoulder joint are assistive at best. Because their main functions are at the elbow, they will be discussed in Chapter 11.

Anatomical Relationships

The relationship between the shoulder girdle and shoulder joint muscles is logical. Shoulder girdle muscles attach to the scapula and trunk to move or stabilize the scapula. Shoulder joint muscles attach mostly to the scapula and humerus to move the arm. These muscles are superficial to muscles of the shoulder girdle. This arrangement allows both sets of muscles to function without getting in each other's way.

The deltoid forms a superficial cap over the anterior, lateral, and posterior sides of the shoulder (see Fig. 10-8). Anteriorly, the pectoralis major covers most of the superficial chest wall, while the biceps brachii (Fig. 10-18) and triceps brachii encompass most of the anterior and posterior arm, respectively.

Several shoulder muscles can be seen posteriorly if the trapezius muscle is removed (Fig. 10-19). The supraspinatus lies deep to the trapezius above the scapular spine. In descending order, the infraspinatus, teres minor, and teres major lie below the scapular spine. The latissimus dorsi covers the lumbar and lower thoracic region of the back.

Viewed anteriorly, the coracobrachialis lies deep to the pectoralis major and anterior deltoid and lies medial to the short head of the biceps (see Fig. 10-18). The subscapularis is truly a deep muscle. With the pectoralis major and deltoid muscles removed (Fig. 10-18, right side) and with the arm slightly abducted, the subscapularis can be seen as it passes between the rib cage and

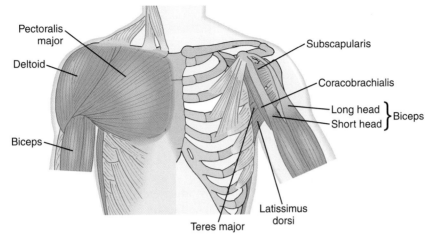

Figure 10-18.   Anterior shoulder muscles. Right side shows the superficial layer. Left side has that layer removed.

the scapula, and it runs horizontally through the axilla to the proximal end of the anterior humerus.

Glenohumeral Movement

The movement of the humeral head on the glenoid fossa must be given some additional attention. Notice that the articular surface of the humeral head is greater than that of the glenoid fossa (Fig. 10-20). If the humeral head simply rotated in the glenoid fossa,

it would run out of articular surface before much abduction occurred. Also, the vertical pull of the deltoid muscle would pull the head up against the acromion process.

It is the arthrokinematic motions of glide, spin, and roll (see Chapter 4 for a detailed description of these terms) that keep the head of the humerus articulating with the glenoid fossa. As abduction occurs, the humeral head rolls across the glenoid fossa. At the same time, the head glides inferiorly, keeping the

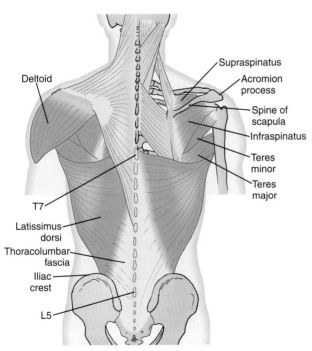

Figure 10-19.   Posterior shoulder muscles. Left side shows the superficial layer. Right side has that layer removed.

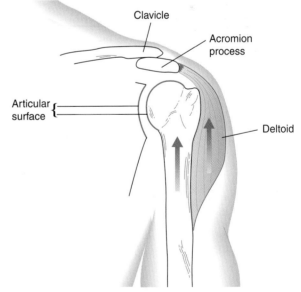

Figure 10-20.   The articular surfaces of the glenohumeral joint and the vertical pull of the deltoid muscle (anterior view). If the deltoid muscle acted alone, it would pull the humeral head upward and impinge it under the coracoacromial arch.

head of the humerus articulating with the glenoid fossa. This is accomplished by the rotator cuff muscles (Fig. 10-21). In addition to abducting the shoulder joint, the supraspinatus muscle pulls the humeral head into the glenoid fossa. The other rotator cuff muscles (subscapularis, infraspinatus, and teres minor) pull the head in and downward against the glenoid fossa. The glenoid labrum serves to slightly deepen the glenoid fossa, making the joint surfaces more congruent.

Another feature of shoulder abduction is that complete range of motion can be accomplished only if the shoulder joint is also laterally rotated. Try this on yourself. Start with your arm at your side (shoulder adduction) and in medial rotation; abduct your shoulder, keeping your thumb pointed down. This is referred to as the "empty can" position. Notice how much motion you can comfortably achieve.

Next, repeat the motion with your shoulder in a neutral position between medial and lateral rotation (fundamental position) and with your thumb pointed forward. Notice how much motion you can comfortably accomplish. Finally, repeat the motion with your shoulder in a laterally rotated position, keeping your thumb pointed up in the hitchhiking position. This is referred to as the "full can" position. It is this laterally rotated position that should allow the most comfortable shoulder motion, because the greater tubercle is being rotated from under the acromion process, allowing full abduction. The greater tubercle in the medially rotated or neutral position runs into the acromion process overhead.

Summary of Muscle Action

Table 10-1 summarizes the prime mover actions of the shoulder joint muscles.

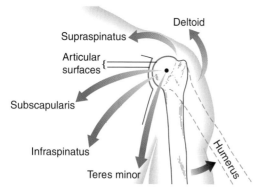

Figure 10-21. Force couple of the deltoid and rotator cuff muscles (SITS) rotating the humeral head in the glenoid fossa during shoulder abduction.

Table 10-1	Prime Mover Muscles of the Shoulder Joint
Action	**Muscles**
Flexion	Anterior deltoid, pectoralis major (clavicular)*
Extension	Posterior deltoid, latissimus dorsi, teres major, pectoralis major (sternal)†
Hyperextension	Latissimus dorsi, posterior deltoid
Abduction	Deltoid, supraspinatus
Adduction	Pectoralis major, teres major, latissimus dorsi
Horizontal abduction	Posterior deltoid, infraspinatus, teres minor
Horizontal adduction	Pectoralis major, anterior deltoid
Lateral rotation	Infraspinatus, teres minor, posterior deltoid
Medial rotation	Latissimus dorsi, teres major, subscapularis, pectoralis major, anterior deltoid

*To approximately 60 degrees.
†To approximately 120 degrees.

Summary of Muscle Innervation

Muscles of the shoulder joint receive innervation from various branches high on the brachial plexus (see Fig. 6-21). Tables 10-2 and 10-3 summarize the muscle innervation and the segmental innervation of the shoulder joint, respectively. There is some discrepancy among various sources regarding the spinal cord level of innervation.

Common Shoulder Pathologies

Acromioclavicular separation is the term commonly used to describe the various amounts of ligament injury at the acromioclavicular joint. In a *first-degree sprain,* the acromioclavicular ligament (see Fig. 9-7) is stretched. In a *second-degree sprain,* the acromioclavicular ligament is ruptured and the coracoclavicular ligament (see Fig. 9-7) is stretched. In a *third-degree sprain,* both the acromioclavicular and coracoclavicular ligaments are ruptured.

Clavicular fractures account for the most frequently broken bone in children. They usually result from a fall on the lateral aspect of the shoulder or on the outstretched hand. The clavicle usually breaks in its midportion. A **humeral neck fracture** is another injury

Table 10-2	Innervation of the Muscles of the Shoulder Joint		
Muscle	**Nerve**	**Plexus Portion**	**Segment**
Subscapularis	Upper and lower subscapular	Posterior cord	C5, C6
Teres major	Lower subscapular	Posterior cord	C5, C6
Pectoralis major	Lateral pectoral	Lateral cord	C5, C6, C7
	Medial pectoral	Medial cord	C8, T1
Latissimus dorsi	Thoracodorsal	Posterior cord	C6, C7, C8
Supraspinatus	Suprascapular	Superior trunk	C5, C6
Infraspinatus	Suprascapular	Superior trunk	C5, C6
Deltoid	Axillary		C5, C6
Teres minor	Axillary		C5, C6
Coracobrachialis	Musculocutaneous		C6, C7
Biceps	Musculocutaneous		C5, C6
Triceps	Radial		C7, C8

caused by a fall on the outstretched hand. It is common in the elderly and is usually an impacted fracture. **Midhumeral fractures** are often caused by a direct blow or a twisting force. Spiral fractures in this region increase the risk of a **radial nerve injury,** as the nerve passes next to the bone. **Pathological fractures** of the humerus may be caused by benign tumors or metastatic carcinoma from primary sites such as the lung, breast, kidney, and prostate.

One of the most common joint dislocations involves the shoulder, and most of those are **anterior shoulder dislocations.** A forced shoulder abduction and lateral rotation tends to be the dislocating motion causing the humeral head to slide anteriorly out of the glenoid fossa. **Glenohumeral subluxation** is commonly seen in individuals who have hemiplegia, usually from a cerebrovascular accident (stroke). Paralysis of the shoulder muscles leaves them no longer able to hold the head of the humerus in the glenoid fossa. This paralysis combined with the pull of gravity and the weight of the arm over time causes this partial dislocation.

Impingement syndrome is an overuse condition that involves compression between the acromial arch, humeral head, and soft tissue structures such as the coracoacromial ligament, rotator cuff muscles, long head of the biceps, and subacromial bursa. A type of impingement known as *swimmer's shoulder* is common with swimmers specializing in freestyle, butterfly, and backstroke. **Adhesive capsulitis** refers to the inflammation and fibrosis of the shoulder joint capsule, which leads to pain and loss of shoulder range of motion. It is also known as *frozen shoulder*. A **torn rotator cuff** involves the distal tendinous insertion of the supraspinatus, infraspinatus, teres minor, and

Table 10-3	Segmental Innervation of Shoulder Joint					
Spinal Cord Level	**C4**	**C5**	**C6**	**C7**	**C8**	**T1**
Supraspinatus		X	X			
Infraspinatus		X	X			
Teres minor		X	X			
Subscapularis		X	X			
Teres major		X	X			
Deltoid		X	X			
Biceps		X	X			
Pectoralis major		X	X	X	X	X
Coracobrachialis			X	X		
Latissimus dorsi			X	X	X	
Triceps				X	X	

subscapularis on the greater/lesser tubercle area of the humerus. Tears can be the result of acute trauma or gradual degeneration.

Chronic inflammation of the supraspinatus tendon can lead to an accumulation of mineral deposits and can result in **calcific tendonitis,** which may be asymptomatic or quite painful. **Bicipital tendonitis** usually involves the long head of the biceps proximally as it crosses the humeral head, changes direction, and descends into the bicipital groove. The biceps long head tendon commonly *ruptures* during repetitive or forceful overhead positions. Irritation as it slides in the groove can lead to **subluxing of the biceps tendon** (long head). Overloading the muscle in an abducted and laterally rotated position tends to be the force subluxing the tendon out of the bicipital groove.

Points to Remember

- The shoulder is a triaxial ball-and-socket joint.
- The close-packed position is abduction and lateral rotation.
- Concave joint surfaces move in the same direction as the joint motion.
- Convex joint surfaces move in the opposite direction as the joint motion.
- A force couple has muscles pulling in different directions to achieve the same motion.

Review Questions

General Anatomy Questions

1. There are four sets of motions that occur at the shoulder joint. Which motions occur
   a. in the frontal plane around the sagittal axis?
   b. in the transverse plane around the vertical axis?
   c. in the sagittal plane around the frontal axis?

2. Describe circumduction and the shoulder joint motions involved.

3. Which fossa is located on the anterior surface of the scapula?

4. The spine of the scapula divides the posterior surface into which two fossas?

5. What landmarks can be used to determine if a model of an unattached bone is a right or left humerus?

6. What are the SITS muscles, and why are they called "rotator cuff muscles"?

7. Name the shoulder joint muscles attaching on the anterior surface of the scapula.

8. Name the shoulder joint muscles attaching on the posterior surface of the scapula.

9. Which shoulder joint muscles do not attach on the scapula?

10. Regarding the pectoralis major:
    a. Which portion of it is effective in shoulder flexion?
    b. What part of the range is it more effective?
    c. Why?

Functional Activity Questions

Identify the shoulder joint motions and the accompanying shoulder girdle motions in the following actions.

1. Putting your billfold in your left back pocket with your left hand
   a. Shoulder joint motion _____
   b. Shoulder girdle motion _____

2. Reaching up to get hold of your seat belt (driver's side with left hand)
   a. Shoulder joint motion _____
   b. Shoulder girdle motion _____

3. Fastening your seat belt with your left hand
   a. Shoulder joint motion _____
   b. Shoulder girdle motion _____

4. Placing a book on the upper bookshelf
   a. Shoulder joint motion _____
   b. Shoulder girdle motion _____

5. Tucking and holding a book under your arm
   a. Shoulder joint motion _____
   b. Shoulder girdle motion _____

Review Questions—cont'd

Clinical Exercise Questions

1. Lie prone on a table with your arm over the edge and with your shoulder flexed 90 degrees, elbow extended, and a weight in your hand (Fig. 10-22A). Lift the weight away from the table in a sideward motion (Fig. 10-22B).
   a. What is the shoulder joint motion?
   b. What type of contraction (isometric, concentric, eccentric) is occurring?
   c. What muscles are prime movers in this shoulder joint motion?

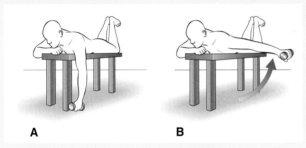

A   **B**

Figure 10-22.   **(A)** Starting position. **(B)** Ending position.

2. Repeat the exercise in Question 1, except flex the elbow to 90 degrees as you lift the weight up.
   a. Does flexing the elbow shorten the force arm?
   b. Does flexing the elbow shorten the resistance arm?
   c. Why is this exercise easier than the one in Question 1?

3. Stand with your arm adducted at the side of your body, elbow flexed to 90 degrees, and hold a loop of elastic tubing whose other end is anchored in front of you at the same level as your hand. In a sawing motion (back and forth motion like you are sawing wood), pull back on the tubing.
   a. What is the shoulder joint motion?
   b. What type of contraction (isometric, concentric, eccentric) is occurring?
   c. What muscles are prime movers in this shoulder joint motion?

4. Return to the starting position of the exercise in Question 3.
   a. What is the shoulder joint motion?
   b. What type of contraction (isometric, concentric, eccentric) is occurring?
   c. What muscles are prime movers in this shoulder joint motion?

5. Stand and hold a cane or weight bar in both hands.
   a. With your hands approximately 12 inches apart and elbows extended, raise the bar. What shoulder motion is occurring?
   b. With your arms as far apart as possible and elbows extended, raise the bar. What predominant shoulder motion is occurring?
   c. In what plane is the motion in part (b) occurring? (Hint: It is not sagittal, frontal, or transverse.)

6. Lie on your right side with your left elbow flexed to 90 degrees and holding a weight in your hand. Keep your left elbow resting on the left side of your body.

   First part: roll the weight up toward the ceiling.
   a. What is the shoulder joint motion?
   b. What type of contraction (isometric, concentric, eccentric) is occurring?
   c. What muscles are prime movers in this shoulder joint motion?

   Second part: hold for the count of five.
   a. What is the shoulder joint motion?
   b. What type of contraction (isometric, concentric, eccentric) is occurring?
   c. What muscles are prime movers in this shoulder joint motion?

   Third part: slowly return to the starting position.
   a. What is the shoulder joint motion?
   b. What type of contraction (isometric, concentric, eccentric) is occurring?
   c. What muscles are prime movers in this shoulder joint motion?

(continued on next page)

Review Questions—cont'd

7. The ability of this gymnast (Fig. 10-23) to perform this iron cross maneuver may be limited by the strength of which group of shoulder joint muscles?

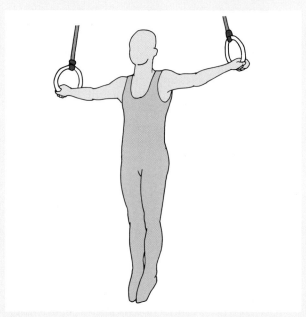

Figure 10-23.   Iron cross.

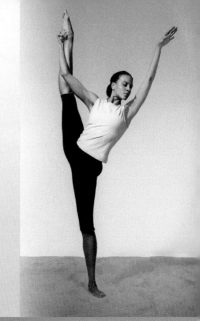

CHAPTER 11
Elbow Joint

Joint Structure and Motions

Bones and Landmarks

Ligaments and Other Structures

Muscles of the Elbow and Forearm

Anatomical Relationships

Summary of Muscle Action

Summary of Muscle Innervation

Common Elbow Pathologies

Points to Remember

Review Questions

General Anatomy Questions

Functional Activity Questions

Clinical Exercise Questions

Joint Structure and Motions

The elbow complex includes three bones, three ligaments, two joints, and one capsule. The articulation of the humerus with the ulna and radius is commonly called the **elbow joint** (Fig. 11-1). On the humerus, the trochlea articulates with the trochlear notch of the ulna and the capitulum articulates with the head of the radius.

The elbow is a uniaxial hinge joint that allows only **flexion** and **extension** (Fig. 11-2). Measured from the 0-degree position of extension, the joint has approximately 145 degrees of flexion.

Unlike the shoulder joint, the elbow has no active hyperextension. This motion is blocked by the olecranon process of the ulna fitting into the olecranon fossa of the humerus. Some individuals may be able to hyperextend a few degrees, but this is due to a laxity of ligaments rather than bony structure.

The articulation between the radius and ulna is known as the **radioulnar joint** (Fig. 11-3). They articulate with each other at both ends. At the proximal end,

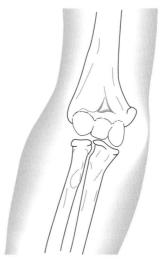

Figure 11-1. The right elbow joint (anterior view).

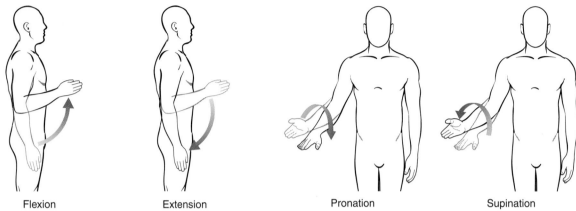

Flexion   Extension

Figure 11-2.   Elbow motions.

Pronation   Supination

Figure 11-4.   Forearm motions.

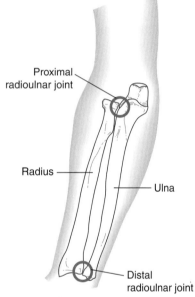

Proximal radioulnar joint

Radius

Ulna

Distal radioulnar joint

Figure 11-3.   The radioulnar joints (anterior view).

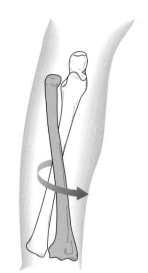

Figure 11-5.   The radius moves around the ulna (anterior view).

the head of the radius pivots within the radial notch of the ulna, forming the **superior** or **proximal radioulnar joint.** Due to the shape of the radius, the distal end of the radius rotates around the distal end of the ulna, forming the **inferior** or **distal radioulnar joint.** Functionally, they are considered one joint. The radioulnar joint is a uniaxial pivot joint, allowing only **pronation** and **supination** of the forearm (Fig. 11-4). Measured from the neutral or midposition, there are approximately 90 degrees of supination and 80 degrees of pronation.

When pronation and supination occur, the radius moves around the ulna (Fig. 11-5). The ulna does not rotate, as it is locked in place by its bony shape at the proximal end. You can confirm this on your own elbow. With your elbow flexed, place the fingers of your opposite hand on either side of the olecranon process and then pronate and supinate your forearm. Note that the

olecranon process does not move. If you put your fingers on the shaft of the ulna, you again will notice that the ulna does not move. Remember this when figuring out muscle action. The radius moves and the ulna does not. Therefore, a muscle must attach on the radius to be able to pronate or supinate the forearm.

In the anatomical position, the longitudinal axes of the humerus and forearm form an angle called the **carrying angle** (Fig. 11-6). This angle tends to be greater in women than in men. Normal carrying angle measures approximately 5 degrees in males and between 10 and 15 degrees in females. This angle occurs because the distal end of the humerus is not level. The medial side (trochlea) is lower than the lateral side (capitulum). Therefore, as the ulna and radius rotate around the trochlea and capitulum of the humerus, they do not rotate in a straight line like a typical hinge joint, in

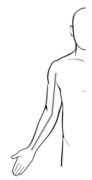

Figure 11-6.   The carrying angle (anterior view).

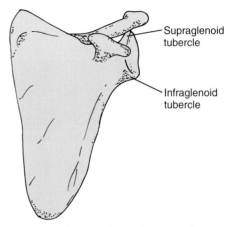

Figure 11-7.   Attachments for the biceps and triceps muscles (anterior view).

which the long axis of the lower segment is in line with the long axis of the upper segment. The effect of this carrying angle can be seen if a line is drawn along the long axis of the humerus and extended down the forearm. You will notice that during elbow extension, the hand is on the outside of that imaginary line. When the elbow is flexed, the hand moves to the inside of the imaginary line. This angle is quite functional in getting your hand to your mouth.

There are two distinctly different end feels at the elbow joint. With flexion, the end feel is soft because the muscle bulk of the arm and forearm compresses together and limits further motion. This is called soft tissue approximation. The end feel for extension is just the opposite. It is described as hard due to bone-on-bone contact as the olecranon process of the ulna moves into the olecranon fossa of the humerus, limiting further motion. This is called a bony end feel.

The end feels at the forearm are not quite as distinct. In supination, the end feel is firm because of muscle and ligament tension. This is called soft tissue stretch. Pronation end feel is hard (bony) due to contact between the radius and ulna. This bony end feel is more subtle than that felt during elbow extension.

The distal end of the humerus has two convex areas: the trochlea articulating with the ulna and the capitulum articulating with the radius. The concave trochlear notch is at the proximal end of the ulna, and the concave radial head is at the proximal end of the radius. With open-chain activities, the concave radial and ulnar joint surfaces slide on the humerus in the same direction as the motion of the forearm.

Bones and Landmarks

Some bony landmarks of the scapula were covered in Chapters 9 and 10, but those important to elbow function are as follows (Fig. 11-7):

Infraglenoid Tubercle
The raised portion on the inferior lip of the glenoid fossa that provides attachment of the long head of the triceps muscle

Supraglenoid Tubercle
Raised portion on the superior lip of the glenoid fossa that provides attachment for the long head of the biceps muscle

Coracoid Process
Projection on the anterior surface that provides attachment for the short head of the biceps muscle (described in Chapter 9)

The distal end of the **humerus** (Fig. 11-8) provides the bony landmarks important to elbow function:

Trochlea
Located on the medial side of the distal end; articulates with the ulna

Capitulum
On the lateral side next to the trochlea; articulates with head of radius

Medial Epicondyle
Located on the medial side of the distal end above the trochlea; larger and more prominent than the lateral epicondyle. It provides attachment for the pronator teres muscle.

Lateral Epicondyle
Located on the lateral side of the distal end above the capitulum; provides attachment for the anconeus and supinator muscles

Lateral Supracondylar Ridge
Located above the lateral epicondyle; provides attachment for the brachioradialis muscle

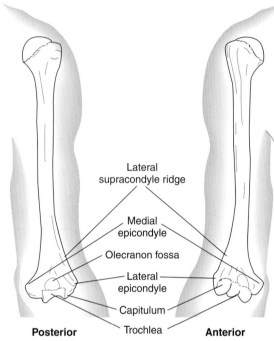

Figure 11-8.   The right humerus.

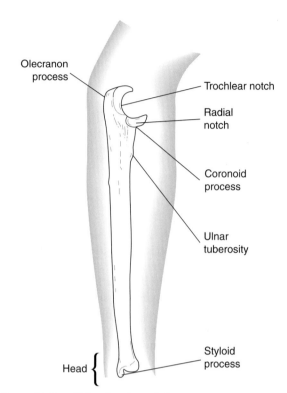

Figure 11-9.   Right ulna, lateral view.

Olecranon Fossa

Located on the posterior surface between the medial and lateral epicondyles; articulates with the olecranon process of the ulna

The **ulna** is the medial bone of the forearm lying parallel to the radius. The bony landmarks important to elbow function are as follows (Fig. 11-9):

Olecranon Process

Located at the proximal end of the ulna, on the posterior surface; forms the prominent point of the elbow and provides attachment for the triceps muscle

Trochlear Notch

Also called the *semilunar notch*; articulates with the trochlea of the humerus; makes up the anterior surface at the proximal end

Coronoid Process

Located just below the trochlear notch; with the ulnar tuberosity, provides attachment for the brachialis muscle

Radial Notch

Located at the proximal end on the lateral side just distal to the trochlear notch; articulation point for the head of the radius

Ulnar Tuberosity

Located below the coronoid process; provides an attachment for the brachialis muscle

Styloid Process

At the distal end on the posterior medial surface

Head

At the distal end on the lateral surface; the ulnar notch of the radius pivots around it during pronation and supination.

The **radius,** located lateral to the ulna, provides many important bony landmarks for elbow function (Fig. 11-10):

Head

Proximal end; has a cylinder shape with a depression in the superior surface where it articulates with the capitulum of the humerus

Radial Tuberosity

Located on the medial side near the proximal end; provides attachment for the biceps muscle

Styloid Process

Located on the posterior lateral side of the radius at the distal end; provides attachment for the brachioradialis muscle

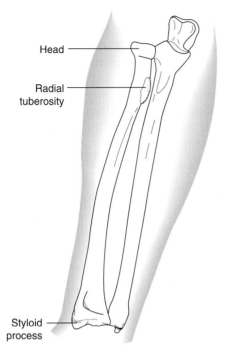

Figure 11-10.   Right radius, anterior view.

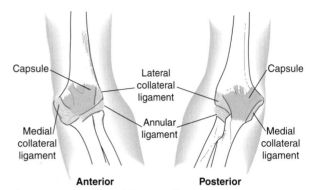

Figure 11-11.   Elbow joint capsule and ligaments.

Ligaments and Other Structures

The three ligaments of the elbow are the medial and lateral collateral ligaments and the annular ligament (Fig. 11-11). The **medial collateral ligament** is triangular and spans the medial side of the elbow. It attaches on the medial epicondyle of the humerus and runs obliquely to the medial sides of the coronoid process and olecranon process of the ulna. The **lateral collateral ligament** is also triangular. It attaches proximally on the lateral epicondyle of the humerus and distally on the annular ligament and the lateral side of the ulna. These two ligaments provide a great deal of medial and lateral stability to the elbow. The **annular ligament** attaches anteriorly and posteriorly to the radial notch of the ulna, encompassing the head of the radius and holding it against the ulna.

The **joint capsule** attaches around the distal end of the humerus and encompasses the trochlea and capitulum, and the fossas located above them. It attaches around the proximal end of the ulna, under the radial notch and coronoid process, and around the trochlear notch. It attaches around the radius just under the head. The capsule is strengthened anteriorly and somewhat posteriorly by the annular ligament. The collateral ligaments reinforce the capsule on the sides of the joint.

In addition to the annular ligament, the radioulnar articulations are held together by the **interosseous membrane** (Fig. 11-12). This broad, flat membrane is located between the radius and the ulna for most of their length. The interosseous membrane keeps the two bones from separating and provides more surface area for attachment of the forearm and wrist muscles.

The cubital fossa is a shallow, somewhat triangular depression on the anterior elbow. It is bordered laterally by the brachioradialis, medially by the pronator teres, and superiorly by an imaginary line between the medial and lateral epicondyles. This line corresponds closely to the skin crease in the bend of the elbow. The floor is formed by the brachialis and supinator muscles. From lateral to medial, the main vertical structures within the fossa are the biceps tendon, the brachial artery, and the median nerve. The radial nerve lies between the biceps tendon and the brachioradialis muscles but is not usually considered to be within the fossa. The brachial

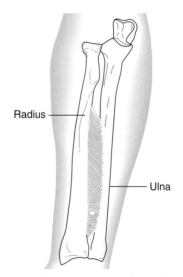

Figure 11-12.   The interosseous membrane (anterior view).

artery divides into the radial (superficial) and ulnar (deeper) arteries near the inferior apex of the fossa. Superficial to the fossa, and not considered part of it, are the three superficial veins: median cubital, cephalic, and basilic veins. The brachial pulse can be palpated in the cubital fossa, and during blood pressure measurements, the stethoscope is placed over the brachial artery in this location.

Muscles of the Elbow and Forearm

The muscles of the elbow and forearm are as follows:

Brachialis
Brachioradialis
Biceps
Supinator
Triceps
Anconeus
Pronator teres
Pronator quadratus

The **brachialis muscle** (Fig. 11-13) gets its name from its location (Latin for "arm"). It attaches to the distal half of the humerus on the anterior surface and spans the elbow joint anteriorly to attach on the coronoid process and ulnar tuberosity of the ulna. It lies deep to the biceps muscle. Because the brachialis muscle has no attachment on the radius, it has no role in pronation or supination. However, this muscle is a very strong elbow flexor, regardless of the forearm's position, and is therefore sometimes called the "workhorse of the elbow joint."

Brachialis Muscle

O	Distal half of humerus, anterior surface
I	Coronoid process and ulnar tuberosity of the ulna
A	Elbow flexion
N	Musculocutaneous nerve (C5, C6)

The **biceps brachii muscle** has two heads and is located on the arm (Fig. 11-14). This muscle is commonly referred to simply as the *biceps*. Both heads attach on the scapula. The **long head** arises from the supraglenoid tubercle, runs over the head of the humerus and out the joint capsule to descend through the intertubercular (bicipital) groove, and joins with the **short head** that comes from the coracoid process.

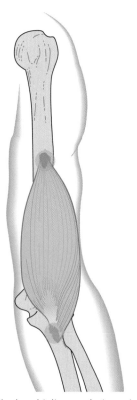

Figure 11-13. The brachialis muscle (anterior view).

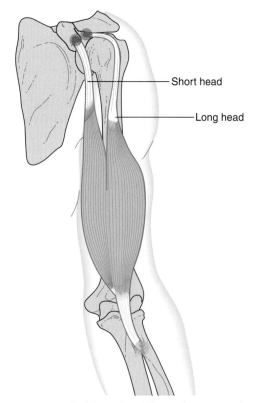

Short head

Long head

Figure 11-14. The biceps brachii muscle, commonly referred to as the *biceps,* has two heads (anterior view).

Because tendons of both heads cross the shoulder joint anteriorly, the biceps assists in shoulder flexion. However, its main function is at the elbow. After joining, the two heads form a common muscle belly that covers the anterior surface of the arm. The biceps muscle tendon crosses the elbow joint to attach on the radial tuberosity. It is the superficial muscle of the anterior arm. Because the biceps brachii muscle spans the elbow joint anteriorly, it is a good elbow flexor, especially in the midrange. Because it attaches obliquely on the radius, it contributes to supination of the forearm.

To understand the supination component of the biceps muscle, think of it as a corkscrew. The tendon crosses the elbow joint anteriorly to attach medially on the radial tuberosity. When the forearm is in pronation, the radial tuberosity rotates further medially toward the posterior side. In effect, the tendon of the biceps muscle wraps partially around the radius in the pronated position. During supination, the biceps muscle contracts and essentially "unwraps" or "untwists" the forearm (Fig. 11-15). It is most effective in supination when the elbow is in approximately 90 degrees of flexion, and it loses its effectiveness as the elbow is extended. This is because the muscle's moment arm is greatest at 90 degrees; therefore, its angular force is also greatest. As the elbow is extended, the moment arm decreases, as does angular force, and the stabilizing force increases. (See Chapter 8 for a discussion of torque.)

Biceps Brachii Muscle

O	Long head: supraglenoid tubercle of scapula
	Short head: coracoid process of scapula
I	Radial tuberosity of radius
A	Elbow flexion, forearm supination
N	Musculocutaneous nerve (C5, C6)

The **brachioradialis muscle** gets its name from its two attachments: one on the humerus (brachii) and the other on the radius (Fig. 11-16). Proximally, it is attached on the supracondylar ridge, which is slightly above the lateral epicondyle of the humerus. It crosses the elbow anteriorly and laterally to attach distally near the styloid process of the radius. It is a superficial muscle and easy to identify. Place your hand in your lap in a neutral position between supination and pronation and then give resistance to elbow flexion. The brachioradialis muscle should be quite prominent on the top of your forearm near the elbow. Because of its more lateral attachment, it is most effective as an elbow flexor when the forearm is in a neutral position. This is because its line of pull is vertical with essentially no diagonal component and goes through the axis for pronation and supination. Therefore, the brachioradialis muscle has no real effect in pronation or supination, even though it has an attachment on the radius.

Brachioradialis Muscle

O	Lateral supracondylar ridge on the humerus
I	Styloid process of the radius
A	Elbow flexion
N	Radial nerve (C5, C6)

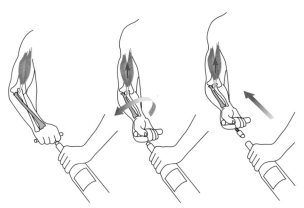

Figure 11-15. Supination action of biceps (anterior view). The action of the biceps as a forearm supinator and elbow flexor is used when pulling a cork out of a bottle with a corkscrew. First, it unscrews the cork (supination); then it pulls on the cork (flexion).

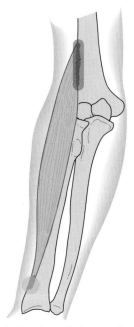

Figure 11-16. The brachioradialis muscle (anterior view).

The **triceps brachii muscle,** commonly called the **triceps,** derives its name from its three heads. This muscle is located posteriorly and makes up the entire muscle mass of the posterior arm (Fig. 11-17). The **long head** comes from the inferior rim of the glenoid fossa of the scapula and descends between the teres minor and teres major muscles to join the other two heads. The **lateral head** is attached laterally on the posterior surface of the humerus below the greater tubercle. The **medial head** lies deep to the long and lateral heads and is attached below the lateral head to most of the posterior surface. The three heads come together to form the muscle belly. The triceps muscle tendon crosses the elbow posteriorly to attach to the olecranon process of the ulna. Because it spans the elbow quite vertically, it is very effective in elbow extension. Because it has no attachment on the radius, it can play no role in pronation or supination.

Triceps Muscle

O	Long head: infraglenoid tubercle of scapula
	Lateral head: inferior to greater tubercle on posterior humerus
	Medial head: posterior surface of humerus
I	Olecranon process of ulna
A	Elbow extension
N	Radial nerve (C7, C8)

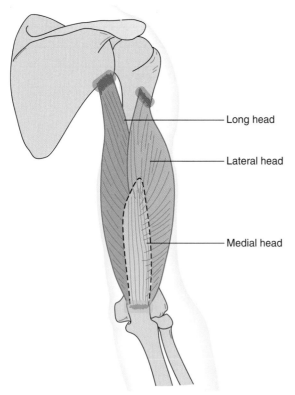

Figure 11-17.   The triceps brachii muscle, commonly referred to as the *triceps,* has three heads (posterior view). The dotted line indicates the portion of the muscle that lies deep.

The **anconeus muscle** is a very small muscle that attaches next to the much larger triceps muscle (Fig. 11-18). It attaches proximally to the posterior surface of the lateral epicondyle and then spans the elbow posteriorly to attach laterally and inferior to the olecranon process. It is a small muscle in comparison to the triceps and therefore does not play any significant role in elbow extension. This muscle lies on top of the annular ligament and attaches to part of it. When it contracts, the anconeus pulls on the ligament and keeps it from being pinched in the olecranon fossa during elbow extension.

Anconeus Muscle

O	Lateral epicondyle of humerus
I	Lateral and inferior to olecranon process of ulna
A	Not a prime mover in any joint action; assists in elbow extension
N	Radial nerve (C7, C8)

The **pronator teres muscle** (Fig. 11-19) gets its name partially from its action (pronation) and partially from its long shape (*teres,* Latin for "long"). It is a superficial muscle as it crosses the elbow, but it is covered by the brachioradialis muscle at its distal attachment. Proximally, it attaches on the medial epicondyle of the

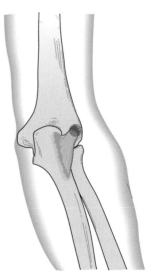

Figure 11-18.   The anconeus muscle (posterior view).

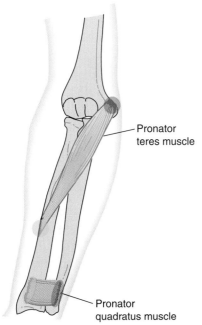

Figure 11-19.   The pronator muscles (anterior view).

humerus and the medial aspect of the coronoid process of the ulna. It crosses the anterior surface of the elbow, running diagonally to attach distally on the lateral surface of the radius at about the midpoint. Because it crosses the elbow anteriorly, it has the ability to flex the elbow. This muscle's role is only as an assisting mover because of its smaller size and diagonal line of pull.

Pronator Teres Muscle

O	Medial epicondyle of humerus and coronoid process of ulna
I	Lateral aspect of radius at its midpoint
A	Forearm pronation, assistive in elbow flexion
N	Median nerve (C6, C7)

The **pronator quadratus muscle** (see Fig. 11-19) also gets its name from its action (pronation) and partially from its shape (quadratus). It is a small, flat, quadrilateral muscle located deep on the anterior surface of the distal forearm; therefore, cannot be palpated. It attaches from the distal one-fourth of the ulna to the distal one-fourth of the radius. It has a horizontal line of pull, and works with the pronator teres muscle to pronate the forearm.

Pronator Quadratus Muscle

O	Distal one-fourth of ulna
I	Distal one-fourth of radius

A	Forearm pronation
N	Median nerve (C8, T1)

The **supinator muscle** (Fig. 11-20) is a deep muscle that wraps around the elbow joint laterally from the posterior surface to the anterior surface. It attaches posteriorly to the lateral epicondyle and adjacent surface of the ulna. It crosses the elbow joint laterally to wrap around the proximal end of the radius to attach distally on the proximal anterior surface of the radius. It combines with the biceps muscle as a prime mover in forearm supination (Fig. 11-21).

Supinator Muscle

O	Lateral epicondyle of humerus and adjacent ulna
I	Anterior surface of the proximal radius
A	Forearm supination
N	Radial nerve (C6)

Anatomical Relationships

The muscle bellies of the biceps, brachialis, and triceps are proximal to the joint, while the muscle bellies of the brachioradialis, pronator teres, pronator quadratus, and supinator are at or distal to the elbow. Figure 11-22 shows the anterior muscles. You can feel the biceps if you put your hand on the anterior surface of your arm. Lying directly underneath the biceps is the brachialis. The dotted lines in Figure 11-22 indicate that the brachialis lies beneath the biceps except at the distal humerus, where it can be palpated on either side of the biceps tendon. The brachioradialis is the most superficial muscle on the

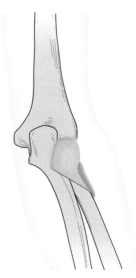

Figure 11-20.   The supinator muscle (posterior view).

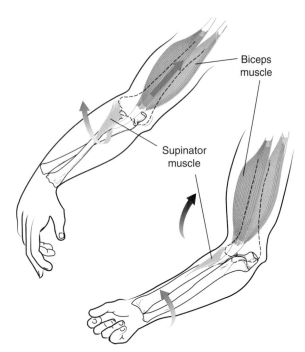

Figure 11-21.   The supinator and biceps muscles combine in a force couple action to move the radius around the ulna from a pronated forearm to a supinated forearm (anterior view).

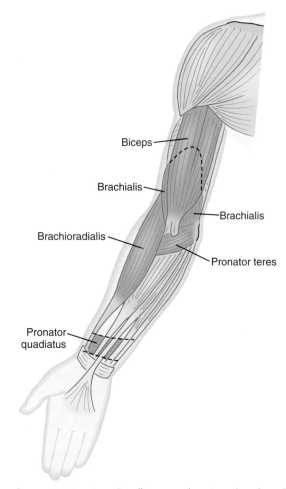

Figure 11-22.   Anterior elbow muscles. Note that dotted lines indicate the brachialis muscle lying underneath the biceps.

lateral side of the forearm. The pronator teres is also superficial, but it has its proximal attachment on the medial side, along with the wrist flexors and palmaris longus. The pronator quadratus is located deep to several wrist and hand tendons at the distal end of the anterior forearm.

Figure 11-23 shows the posterior muscles. The triceps makes up the entire posterior arm. The long and lateral heads are superficial and the medial head is deep. The medial head is almost the same shape as the triceps distal tendon and lies deep to it (as indicated by the dotted lines in Fig. 11-23). The anconeus is a very small muscle located superficially on the posterior elbow, just distal to the triceps insertion. The supinator lies deep to the wrist extensors and the brachioradialis near their origin (Fig. 11-24).

Summary of Muscle Action

Table 11-1 summarizes the muscle action of the prime movers of the elbow and forearm.

Summary of Muscle Innervation

Terminal nerves of the brachial plexus innervate all muscles of the elbow. The musculocutaneous nerve innervates muscles of the anterior arm involved with elbow flexion. The radial nerve travels through the axilla and around the middle portion of the humerus to innervate the posterior surface of the arm, forearm, and hand. It is responsible for all elbow extension. The median nerve descends the arm anteriorly, sending branches to the pronator muscles. Table 11-2 on page 158 summarizes the innervation of elbow joint musculature. Table 11-3 on page 158 summarizes the segmental innervation. Please note that there is some discrepancy among various sources regarding the spinal cord level of innervation.

Common Elbow Pathologies

Lateral epicondylitis, also known as **tennis elbow,** is a very common overuse condition that affects the common extensor tendon where it inserts into the

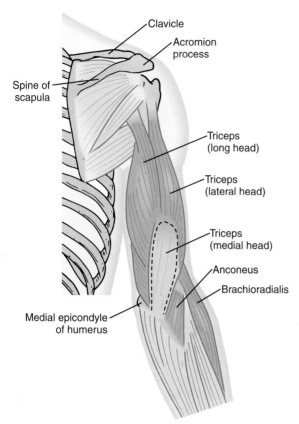

Figure 11-23. Posterior elbow muscles.

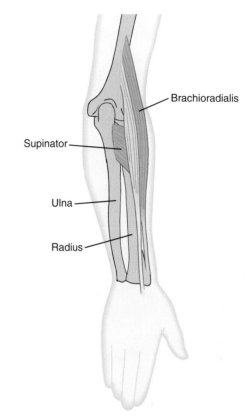

Figure 11-24. Supinator, a deep muscle, in relation to surrounding muscles. Note that most of the extensor muscles of the wrist and hand that lie over the supinator have not been included.

lateral epicondyle of the humerus. The extensor carpi radialis brevis is particularly affected. It is common in racquet sports and other repetitive wrist extension activities. **Medial epicondylitis,** also know as **golfer's elbow,** is an inflammation of the common flexor tendon that inserts into the medial epicondyle. It is an overuse condition that results in tenderness over the medial epicondyle and pain on resisted wrist flexion.

Little League elbow is an overuse injury of the medial epicondyle, usually caused by a repetitive throwing motion. It is seen in young baseball players who have not reached skeletal maturity. The throwing motion places a valgus stress on the elbow, causing lateral compression and medial distraction on the joint. **Pulled elbow,** or **nursemaid's elbow** is seen in young children under the age of 5 years who have experienced a sudden strong traction force on the arm. This often occurs when an adult suddenly pulls on the child's arm, or the child falls away from an adult while being held by the arm. This force causes the radial head to sublux out from under the annular ligament.

Elbow dislocation is caused when a great deal of force is applied to an elbow that is in a slightly flexed position. This causes the ulna to slide posterior to the distal end of the humerus. **Supracondylar fractures** are among the most common fractures in children and are caused by falling on the outstretched hand. The distal end of the humerus fractures just above the

Table 11-1	Prime Movers of the Elbow and Forearm	
Action	**Muscle**
Elbow flexion	Biceps
	Brachialis
	Brachioradialis
Elbow extension	Triceps
Forearm pronation	Pronator teres
	Pronator quadratus
Forearm supination	Biceps
	Supinator

Table 11-2	Innervation of the Muscles of the Elbow Joint	
Muscle	Nerve	Spinal Segment
Brachialis	Musculocutaneous	C5, C6
Biceps	Musculocutaneous	C5, C6
Brachioradialis	Radial	C5, C6
Triceps	Radial	C6, C7
Anconeus	Radial	C7, C8
Pronator teres	Median	C6, C7
Pronator quadratus	Median	C8, T1
Supinator	Radial	C6

Table 11-3 Segmental Innervation of the Elbow Joint					
Spinal Cord Level	C5	C6	C7	C8	T1
Biceps	X	X			
Brachialis	X	X			
Brachioradialis	X	X			
Supinator		X			
Pronator teres		X	X		
Triceps			X	X	
Anconeus			X	X	
Pronator quadratus				X	X

condyles. The great danger of this fracture as well as the elbow dislocation is the potential damage to the brachial artery because of the close proximity. This can lead to **Volkmann's ischemic contracture,** a rare but potentially devastating ischemic necrosis of the forearm muscles.

Points to Remember

- Synovial joint shapes can be irregular (plane), hinge, pivot, condyloid, saddle, and ball-and-socket.
- Synovial joints can have zero to three axes.
- When a muscle has contracted (shortened) over all its joints as far as it can, it has become actively insufficient.
- When a muscle has elongated (stretched) over all of its joints as far as possible, it has become passively insufficient.
- An activity can be an open- or closed-kinetic-chain movement, depending on whether the distal segment is fixed.
- The concave-convex rule has the convex joint surface moving in a direction opposite to the movement of the body segment and the concave joint surfacing moving in the same direction as the body segment.

Review Questions

General Anatomy Questions

1. In terms of the elbow and forearm joints, identify the following:
   a. Name of bones involved:
      Forearm _____
      Elbow _____
   b. Number of axes:
      Forearm _____
      Elbow _____
   c. Shape of joint:
      Forearm _____
      Elbow _____
   d. Joint motion allowed:
      Forearm _____
      Elbow _____

2. If you were handed an unattached model of an ulna, how could you orient landmarks to determine on which side of the body it belonged?

3. Name the ligament that stabilizes
   a. the lateral side of the elbow.
   b. the medial side of the elbow.
   c. the radius and allows it to rotate.

4. Which muscles of the elbow and/or forearm are two-joint muscles?

5. To which bone must a muscle attach to do forearm supination or pronation?

6. Which elbow or forearm muscles do not attach to the humerus?

7. Which muscles connect the scapula to the ulna and/or radius?

8. Which muscles connect the humerus and ulna?

9. The only part of the triceps that crosses the shoulder joint is _____.

10. What positions would you put the upper extremity in to achieve
    a. active insufficiency of the biceps?
    b. passive insufficiency of the biceps?

11. In a closed-chain activity, does the humeral joint surface move in the same or opposite direction as the forearm?

12. a. If you put your hand on the anterior surface of your arm, you would be touching what muscle?
    b. Placing your hand on the posterior surface is over what muscle?
    c. Touching the lateral forearm is touching what muscle?

Functional Activity Questions

Identify the elbow and forearm motion in each of the following activities:

1. Place a dinner plate in an upper kitchen cabinet.
   a. Elbow _____
   b. Forearm _____

2. Put a piece of chocolate in your mouth.
   a. Elbow _____
   b. Forearm _____

3. When answering the telephone, reach for the receiver (Fig. 11-25A).
   a. Elbow _____
   b. Forearm _____

4. Next, put the receiver to your ear (Fig. 11-25B).
   a. Elbow _____
   b. Forearm _____

5. With a hammer in your hand, pound on a nail that has been set in the wall.
   a. Elbow _____
   b. Forearm _____

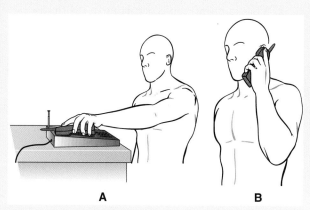

Figure 11-25. Elbow and forearm motion when answering the telephone. **(A)** Starting position. **(B)** Ending position.

(continued on next page)

Review Questions—cont'd

Clinical Exercise Questions

1. In a sitting position, place your right forearm on the table palm down with your elbow flexed as necessary (Fig. 11-26A). Using your left hand, push against the radial side of the right forearm just proximal to the wrist until the right palm is facing up (Fig. 11-26B). The right forearm remains relaxed.
   a. What joint motion is occurring in the right forearm?
   b. What muscles are being stretched?

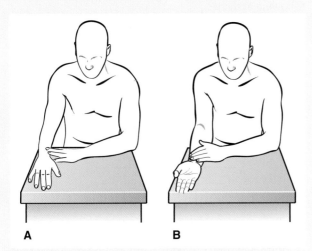

Figure 11-26.   Self-stretch at the forearm. **(A)** Starting position. **(B)** Ending position.

2. Sit in a chair that has armrests and place your hands on them. Do a chair push-up, lifting your buttocks off the seat.
   a. What joint motion is occurring in the right elbow?
   b. What type of contraction (isometric, concentric, or eccentric) is occurring?
   c. What muscles are being strengthened?
   d. Is this an open- or closed-kinetic-chain activity?

3. Stand with your right arm extended straight up toward the ceiling. Using your left hand, push your right hand down behind your head (Fig. 11-27). Allow your elbow to bend.
   a. What joint motion is occurring in the right elbow?
   b. What muscles are being stretched?

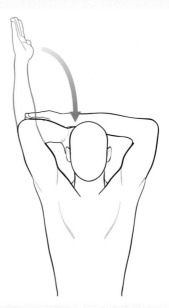

Figure 11-27.   Self-stretch at the elbow.

4. In a sitting position, place your hands and forearms on the table. Push on the table as if you are trying to hold it down.
   a. What joint motion is occurring in the right elbow?
   b. What type of contraction (isometric, concentric, or eccentric) is occurring?
   c. What muscles are being strengthened?

5. Stand with your right hand next to your right shoulder, and hold a small weight. Move your hand to anatomical position.
   a. What joint motion is occurring in the right elbow?
   b. What type of contraction (isometric, concentric, or eccentric) is occurring?
   c. What muscles are being strengthened?
   d. Is this an open- or closed-kinetic-chain activity?

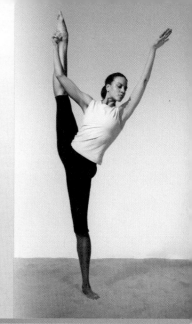

CHAPTER 12

Wrist Joint

Joint Structure

Joint Motions

Bones and Landmarks

Ligaments and Other Structures

Muscles of the Wrist

Anatomical Relationships

Summary of Muscle Action

Summary of Muscle Innervation

Points to Remember

Review Questions

General Anatomy Questions

Functional Activity Questions

Clinical Exercise Questions

Joint Structure

The wrist joint is perhaps one of the most complex joints of the body. It is actually made up of two joints: the radiocarpal joint and the midcarpal joint. The **radiocarpal joint** (Fig. 12-1) consists of the distal end of the radius and the radioulnar disk proximally and the scaphoid, lunate, and triquetrum distally. Because an articular disk is located between the ulna and the proximal row of carpals, the ulna is not considered part of this joint. The pisiform, located in the proximal row of carpal bones, does not articulate with the disk because it is more anterior to the triquetrum. Therefore, it is not considered part of this joint, either.

As a synovial joint, the radiocarpal joint is classified as a **condyloid joint,** with the concave distal end of the radius and the articular disk articulating with the convex scaphoid, lunate, and triquetrum. The convex-shaped proximal row of carpal bones moves in a direction that is opposite to the hand. Therefore, during wrist flexion, the carpals glide posteriorly on the radius and articular disk. During wrist extension, they glide anteriorly. With radial deviation, they glide in an ulnar direction, and in ulnar deviation, they glide in the opposite direction.

The radiocarpal joint is also classified as a biaxial joint, allowing flexion and extension, and radial deviation and ulnar deviation. The combination of all four of these motions is called *circumduction*. There is no rotation at the wrist.

The **midcarpal,** or **intercarpal, joints** (see Fig. 12-1) are located between the two rows of carpal bones and contribute to wrist motion. Their shape is **irregular,** and they are classified as **plane joints.** They are nonaxial joints that allow gliding motions, which collectively contribute to radiocarpal joint motion.

The **carpometacarpal (CMC) joints** appear between the distal row of carpal bones and the proximal end of the metacarpal bones (see Fig. 12-1). Because

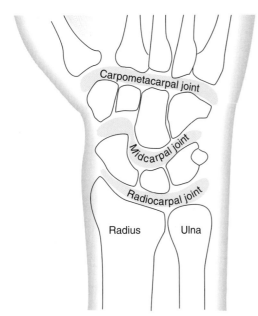

Figure 12-1.   The joints of the left wrist (anterior view).

they have a more direct function in the movement of the hand, they will be discussed in more detail in Chapter 13.

Joint Motions

When discussing wrist motion, several terms are frequently used. *Wrist flexion* and *palmar flexion* are synonymous, as are *extension, hyperextension,* and *dorsiflexion.* Approximately midway between flexion and extension, putting the hand in a straight line with the forearm, is *neutral position.* This is the position of the wrist joint in anatomical position. *Extension* is the return from *flexion.* Movement beyond the neutral position is *hyperextension.* However, the most commonly used terms are **flexion, neutral,** and **extension,** and they will be used here. Nevertheless, you should be familiar with these other terms, which are summarized in Table 12-1.

Flexion and extension occur in the sagittal plane around the frontal axis. There are approximately 90 degrees of flexion and 70 degrees of extension. **Radial** and **ulnar deviation** occur in the frontal plane around the sagittal axis. There are approximately 25 degrees of radial deviation and 35 degrees of ulnar deviation. Figure 12-2 illustrates these motions.

Due to tension of ligaments and the joint capsule, the end feel for all wrist motions, except radial deviation, is soft tissue stretch. The end feel for radial deviation is bony, due to bony contact between the radial styloid process and the scaphoid (carpal) bone.

Bones and Landmarks

The carpal bones consist of two rows of four bones each (Fig. 12-3). Starting on the thumb side of the proximal row are the **scaphoid, lunate, triquetrum,** and **pisiform.** In the distal row, lateral to medial, are the **trapezium, trapezoid, capitate,** and **hamate.** These are short bones arranged in an arch, with the concavity on the anterior (palmar surface) side and the convexity on the posterior side. This arched arrangement contributes greatly to the thumb's ability to oppose.

The bony landmarks for the wrist are as follows:

Styloid Processes
Distal projection on the lateral side of the radius (see Fig. 12-3) and distal medial posterior side of the ulna (see Fig. 11-9), providing attachment for the collateral ligaments

Hook of the Hamate
Projection on the anterior surface of the hamate, providing attachment for the transverse carpal ligament

Medial Epicondyle
Located on the distal medial side of the humerus; attachment for the common flexor tendon (see Fig. 11-8)

Table 12-1	Comparison of Wrist Joint Terminology*	
Preferred Terminology	**Alternate Terminology**	**Motion or Position**
Flexion	Flexion, palmar flexion	Anterior from anatomical position
Neutral	Extension, neutral	Anatomical position
Extension	Hyperextension, dorsiflexion	Posterior from anatomical position
Radial deviation	Abduction	Lateral from anatomical position
Ulnar deviation	Adduction	Medial from anatomical position

*__Bold print__ indicates which terms are used in this book.

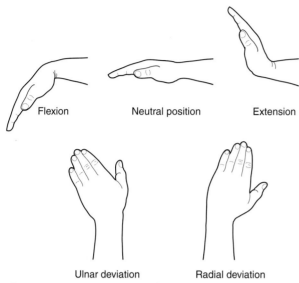

Figure 12-2.   Joint motions of the wrist.

Lateral Epicondyle
Located on the distal lateral side of the humerus; attachment for the common extensor tendon (see Fig. 11-8)

Supracondylar Ridge
Located just proximal to the lateral epicondyle; attachment for the extensor carpi radialis longus muscle (see Fig. 11-8)

Ligaments and Other Structures

There are basically four ligaments of the radiocarpal joint that provide the major support of the wrist. In addition, there are numerous smaller ligaments supporting the intercarpal joints. The **radial collateral ligament** attaches to the styloid process of the radius and to the scaphoid and trapezium bones. The **ulnar collateral ligament** attaches to the styloid process of the ulna and to the pisiform and triquetrum. These ligaments provide lateral and medial support, respectively, to the wrist joint. They are illustrated in Figures 12-3, 12-4, and 12-5.

The **palmar radiocarpal ligament** is a thick, tough ligament that limits wrist extension. It is a broad band that attaches from the anterior surface of the distal radius and ulna to the anterior surface of the proximal carpal bones, and to the capitate bone in the distal row (see Fig. 12-4). It is perhaps more important to wrist function than its counterpart, the dorsal radiocarpal ligament, because most activities of the hand occur with the wrist extended, as opposed to being flexed. Therefore, the palmar radiocarpal ligament is also more apt to be stretched

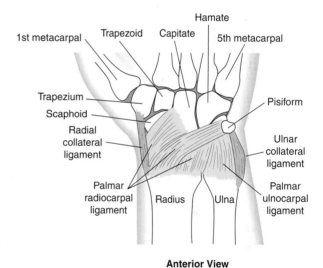

Anterior View

Figure 12-4.   Palmar radiocarpal ligament (left hand).

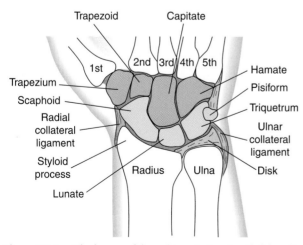

Figure 12-3.   The bones of the wrist, anterior view (left hand).

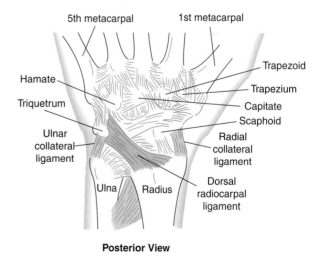

Posterior View

Figure 12-5.   Dorsal radiocarpal ligament (left hand).

or sprained. It should be noted that some sources separate the radiocarpal ligament from the ulnocarpal ligament, and some do not. Functionally, they essentially act as one.

The **dorsal radiocarpal ligament** attaches from the posterior surface of the distal radius to the same surface of the scaphoid, lunate, and triquetrum (see Fig. 12-5). This ligament limits the amount of flexion allowed at the wrist. Because forces causing excessive flexion are not as great as those causing excessive extension, this ligament is not as strong as the palmar radiocarpal ligament.

A **joint capsule,** which encloses the radiocarpal joint, is reinforced by the radial and ulnar collateral ligaments and by the palmar and dorsal radiocarpal ligaments. The **articular disk** (see Fig. 12-3) is located on the distal end of the ulna and articulates with the triquetrum and lunate bones. It acts as a shock absorber and as filler between the distal ulna and its adjacent carpal bones—the triquetrum and lunate. The disk fills the gap created, because the ulna and its styloid process do not extend as far distally as the radius and its styloid process.

The **palmar fascia** is a relatively thick, triangular fascia located superficially in the palm of the hand (Fig. 12-6). It is also called the *palmar aponeurosis.* It covers the tendons of the extrinsic muscles and provides some protection to the structures in the palm. The palmar fascia serves as the distal attachment of the palmaris longus, which blends into this fascia, as does the flexor retinaculum.

Muscles of the Wrist

The muscles spanning and having a primary function at the wrist will be discussed here; the muscles that cross the wrist but have a more significant function at the thumb or fingers will be discussed in Chapter 13. The following are the muscles to be discussed in this section:

Anterior	Posterior
Flexor carpi ulnaris	Extensor carpi radialis longus
Flexor carpi radialis	Extensor carpi radialis brevis
Palmaris longus	Extensor carpi ulnaris

Some general statements can be made about the proximal muscle attachments of the wrist muscles. First, the flexors attach on the medial epicondyle, and the extensors attach on the lateral epicondyle. Second, the distal attachment for all the wrist muscles is a metacarpal, except for the palmaris longus muscle. Third, the names of the muscles tell generally what their action is (flexor, extensor), what they act on (*carpi* means "wrist"), and on what side of the wrist the distal attachment is located (*radialis* means "radial"; *ulnaris* means "ulnar"). Their names will also describe whether the muscle functions in ulnar or radial deviation.

The **flexor carpi ulnaris muscle** is a superficial muscle running along the ulnar, slightly anterior, side of the forearm (Fig. 12-7). Its proximal attachment is

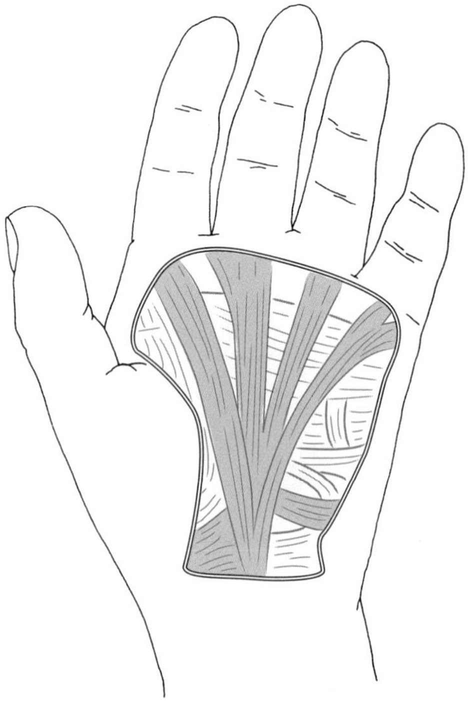

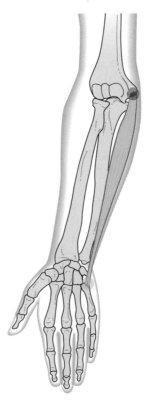

Figure 12-6.   Palmar fascia (anterior view).

Figure 12-7.   The flexor carpi ulnaris muscle (anterior view).

mostly on the medial epicondyle of the humerus, and its distal attachment is the base of the fifth metacarpal and pisiform bone. It is the only wrist muscle attaching to a carpal bone. It is a prime mover in wrist flexion and ulnar deviation.

Flexor Carpi Ulnaris Muscle

O	Medial epicondyle of humerus
I	Pisiform and base of fifth metacarpal
A	Wrist flexion, ulnar deviation
N	Ulnar nerve (C8, T1)

The **flexor carpi radialis muscle** is also a relatively superficial muscle running from the medial epicondyle diagonally across the anterior forearm to attach laterally at the base of the second and third metacarpals (Fig. 12-8). It is a prime mover in wrist flexion and radial deviation.

Flexor Carpi Radialis Muscle

O	Medial epicondyle of the humerus
I	Base of second and third metacarpals
A	Wrist flexion, radial deviation
N	Median nerve (C6, C7)

The **palmaris longus muscle** is also a superficial muscle running down the anterior surface of the forearm from the common flexor attachment of the medial epicondyle. It attaches in the midline to the palmar fascia (Fig. 12-9). It is easily identified in the midline at the base of the wrist, especially against slight resistance to wrist flexion. This muscle is rather unique because it has only one bony attachment, which is at the proximal end. This muscle is missing in approximately 21% of individuals, either unilaterally or bilaterally (Moore, 1985, p 698). Because the palmaris longus muscle is quite small, its absence does not result in any real loss of strength. Although it is in an ideal position to flex the wrist, it is assistive at best because of its size.

Palmaris Longus Muscle

O	Medial epicondyle of humerus
I	Palmar fascia
A	Assistive in wrist flexion
N	Median nerve (C6, C7)

On the posterior side of the wrist is the **extensor carpi radialis longus muscle.** This muscle is mostly superficial (Fig. 12-10). It attaches proximally just above the lateral epicondyle on the lateral supracondylar ridge. It then runs down the lateral

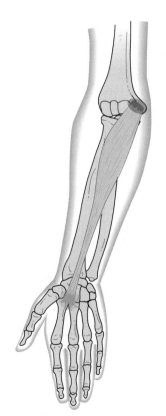

Figure 12-8.   The flexor carpi radialis muscle (anterior view).

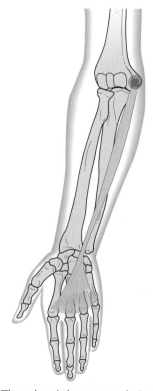

Figure 12-9.   The palmaris longus muscle (anterior view).

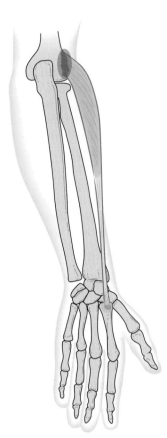

Figure 12-10. The extensor carpi radialis longus muscle (posterior view).

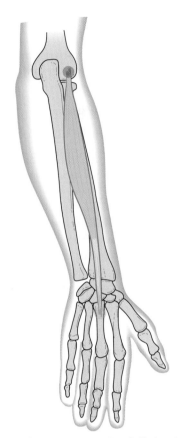

Figure 12-11. The extensor carpi radialis brevis muscle (posterior view).

posterior side of the forearm, under two tendons that go to the thumb, and then under the extensor retinaculum (see Fig. 12-15) to attach at the base of the second metacarpal. It is a prime mover in wrist extension and radial deviation. It assists in elbow extension.

Extensor Carpi Radialis Longus Muscle

O	Supracondylar ridge of humerus
I	Base of second metacarpal
A	Wrist extension, radial deviation
N	Radial nerve (C6, C7)

Because the extensor carpi radialis muscle also has *longus* in its name, this implies that there is a "brevis." The **extensor carpi radialis brevis muscle** lies next to the extensor carpi radialis longus muscle (Fig. 12-11). It arises from the common extensor tendon on the lateral epicondyle. Like the "longus," it passes under two tendons that go to the thumb and then under the extensor retinaculum. Its distal attachment is at the base of the third metacarpal. Because its attachment is close to the axis of motion for radial and ulnar deviation, it is only assistive in radial deviation. However, it is a prime mover in wrist extension. It also assists in elbow extension.

Extensor Carpi Radialis Brevis Muscle

O	Lateral epicondyle of humerus
I	Base of third metacarpal
A	Wrist extension
N	Radial nerve (C6, C7)

The **extensor carpi ulnaris muscle** is also a superficial muscle arising from the common extensor tendon on the lateral epicondyle (Fig. 12-12). It runs down the medial side of the posterior forearm to attach at the base of the fifth metacarpal. It is a prime mover in wrist extension and ulnar deviation, and assists in elbow extension.

Extensor Carpi Ulnaris Muscle

O	Lateral epicondyle of humerus
I	Base of fifth metacarpal
A	Wrist extension, ulnar deviation
N	Radial nerve (C6, C7, C8)

Anatomical Relationships

For the most part, the wrist flexors are relatively superficial, are located on the anterior surface of the

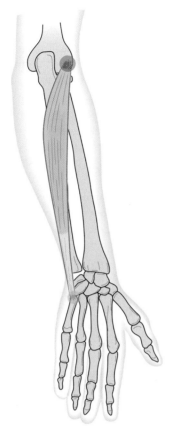

Figure 12-12.   The extensor carpi ulnaris muscle (posterior view).

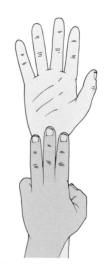

Figure 12-13.   Tendon position of anterior wrist muscles.

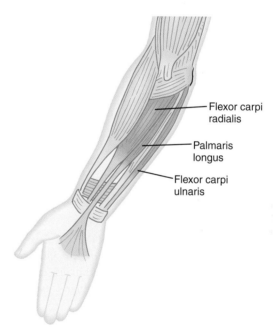

Flexor carpi radialis

Palmaris longus

Flexor carpi ulnaris

Figure 12-14.   Anterior wrist muscles in relation to muscles of hand and thumb.

forearm, and originate on the medial epicondyle. As shown in Figure 12-13, if you take the index, middle, and ring fingers of your left hand and place them at your right wrist (anterior surface), this represents the location and order of the flexor carpi radialis (index finger), the palmaris longus (middle finger), and the flexor carpi ulnaris (ring finger). These attachments also line up with the second, third, and fifth fingers, respectively. Figure 12-14 shows the three superficial wrist flexors. The brachioradialis is also superficial, but it is an elbow muscle that does not cross the wrist. Beneath the wrist flexors are the flexors of the thumb and hand, which will be described in Chapter 13.

The muscles of the wrist extensor group are also relatively superficial but are on the posterior surface of the forearm (Fig. 12-15). Their common origin is mostly the lateral epicondyle. Just distal to that landmark, they parallel each other. The extensor carpi radialis longus is most lateral, followed by the extensor carpi radialis brevis. The extensor digitorum and extensor digiti minimi (both hand muscles) lie in the midline. Medial to them and on the ulnar side is the extensor carpi ulnaris. Note

that all wrist, hand, and thumb tendons are contained by the **extensor retinaculum** (see Fig. 12-15).

Summary of Muscle Action

Table 12-2 summarizes the muscle action of the prime movers of the wrist.

Summary of Muscle Innervation

Innervation of the wrist muscles is quite straight forward. The radial nerve innervates the posterior

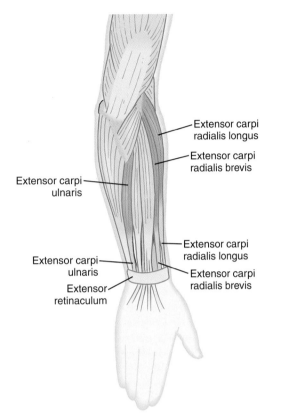

Extensor carpi radialis longus

Extensor carpi radialis brevis

Extensor carpi ulnaris

Extensor carpi radialis longus

Extensor carpi ulnaris

Extensor carpi radialis brevis

Extensor retinaculum

Figure 12-15.   Posterior wrist muscles in relation to muscles of hand and thumb.

muscles. The median nerve innervates the anterior muscles on the thumb side, and the ulnar nerve innervates muscles on the ulnar side. Tables 12-3 and 12-4 summarize the innervation of the muscles of the wrist. There is some variation among sources regarding segmental innervation.

Points to Remember

- An isometric contraction has relatively no joint motion.
- The muscle attachments move closer together with a concentric contraction.
- An eccentric contraction is a deceleration activity.
- A mnemonic to help remember the order of the wrist bones: "Sam Likes To Push The Toy Car Hard" = scaphoid, lunate, triquetrum, pisiform, trapezium, trapezoid, capitates, and hamate.
- When using a longer lever arm, less force is needed.
- Working against gravity requires more work than working with gravity or with gravity eliminated.

Table 12-2	Muscle Action of the Wrist
Action	**Muscles (Prime Movers)**
Flexion	Flexor carpi radialis, flexor carpi ulnaris
Extension	Extensor carpi radialis longus and brevis, extensor carpi ulnaris
Radial deviation	Flexor carpi radialis, extensor carpi radialis longus
Ulnar deviation	Flexor carpi ulnaris, extensor carpi ulnaris

Table 12-3	Innervation of the Muscles of the Wrist	
Muscle	**Nerve**	**Spinal Segment**
Extensor carpi radialis longus	Radial	C6, C7
Extensor carpi radialis brevis	Radial	C6, C7
Extensor carpi ulnaris	Radial	C6, C7, C8
Flexor carpi radialis	Median	C6, C7
Palmaris longus	Median	C6, C7
Flexor carpi ulnaris	Ulnar	C8, T1

Table 12-4	Segmental Innervation of the Wrist Joint			
Spinal Cord Level	**C6**	**C7**	**C8**	**T1**
Extensor carpi radialis longus	X	X		
Extensor carpi radialis brevis	X	X		
Extensor carpi ulnaris	X	X	X	
Palmaris longus	X	X		
Flexor carpi radialis	X	X		
Flexor carpi ulnaris			X	X

Review Questions

General Anatomy Questions

1. Name the bones of the wrist joint, starting laterally on the proximal row and going medially. Use the same order for the distal row.

2. Which wrist motions occur in
   a. the sagittal plane around the frontal axis?
   b. the frontal plane around the sagittal axis?
   c. the transverse plane around the vertical axis?

3. Describe the wrist joints:
   a. Number of axes
      Radiocarpal _____
      Intercarpal _____
   b. Shape of joint
      Radiocarpal _____
      Intercarpal _____
   c. Joint motion allowed
      Radiocarpal _____
      Intercarpal _____

4. Which muscles attach on the medial epicondyle of the humerus?

5. Which muscles attach on or close to the lateral epicondyle of the humerus?

6. If you were shown a drawing of only a wrist joint, what landmarks could tell you if the drawing were a posterior or anterior view?

7. Which muscles cross the wrist on the radial side?

8. Which muscles cross the wrist on the ulnar side?

9. Which muscle, if present, is very easy to identify but has little functional importance?

10. Starting on the anterior surface of the ulnar side and moving in the direction of the radial side, name the wrist muscles that cross the wrist. Go completely around the wrist.

11. Why is the ulna not considered part of the wrist joint?

12. Generally speaking, you use wrist muscles when hammering. However, when extra force is needed, you may use elbow or even shoulder muscles. Why does that create greater force?

13. When hammering overhead, why are your wrist ulnar deviators working harder than when hammering at waist level?

14. The wrist motions have what types of end feels?

15. What is the name of the bony landmark just proximal to the lateral epicondyle?

Functional Activity Questions

Many, but not all, functional activities have the wrist in a neutral or slightly extended position. Often an isometric contraction is required to maintain that position. In the following activities, identify the wrist joint position and the muscle group contracting isometrically.

1. Holding a cup of coffee
   a. Wrist position _____
   b. Wrist muscle group _____

2. Typing on a conventional computer keyboard
   a. Wrist position _____
   b. Wrist muscle group _____

3. Pushing down on a stapler
   a. Wrist position _____
   b. Wrist muscle group _____

4. Brushing long hair with a comb (with right hand brushing on left side; Fig. 12-16)
   a. Wrist position _____
   b. Wrist muscle group _____

(continued on next page)

Review Questions—cont'd

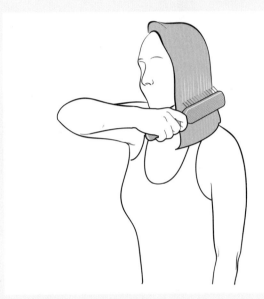

Figure 12-16.　Brushing hair.

5. Holding a box from the bottom (Fig. 12-17)
   a. Wrist position _____
   b. Wrist muscle group _____

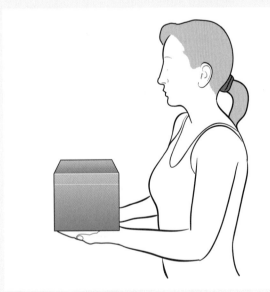

Figure 12-17.　Holding a box.

Clinical Exercise Questions

Remember that elastic tubing loses its recoil quickly and is not as effective in the end range of an eccentric contraction. There may be more effective ways to perform eccentric contractions than examples given here. You should be able to recognize an eccentric contraction regardless of an exercise's effectiveness.

1. Sit with your forearm resting on your thigh, palm up, and holding a weight in your hand. Bend your wrist up.
   a. What joint motion is occurring in the wrist?
   b. What type of contraction (isometric, concentric, or eccentric) is occurring?
   c. What muscles are being strengthened?

2. Slowly lower the weight to the starting position described in the exercise in Question 1.
   a. What joint motion is occurring in the wrist?
   b. What type of contraction (isometric, concentric, or eccentric) is occurring?
   c. What muscles are being strengthened?

3. Standing with your arm at your side, elbow flexed, palm down, hold on to a loop of elastic tubing that has the other end anchored under your foot. Curl your wrist up.
   a. What joint motion is occurring in the wrist?
   b. What type of contraction (isometric, concentric, or eccentric) is occurring?
   c. What muscles are being strengthened?
   d. What muscle group is also acting at the elbow?
   e. What type of contraction is occurring at the elbow?

4. Slowly lower your wrist to the starting position described in the exercise in Question 3.
   a. What joint motion is occurring in the wrist?
   b. What type of contraction (isometric, concentric, or eccentric) is occurring?
   c. What muscles are being strengthened?

5. Standing with your arm at your side, elbow flexed, forearm in a neutral position, hold on to a loop of elastic tubing that has the other end anchored above your head to some stationary object. Bend your wrist down.
   a. What joint motion is occurring in the wrist?
   b. What type of contraction (isometric, concentric, or eccentric) is occurring?
   c. What muscles are being strengthened?

6. Slowly return to the starting position described in the exercise in Question 5.
   a. What joint motion is occurring in the wrist?
   b. What type of contraction (isometric, concentric, or eccentric) is occurring?
   c. Explain why it is this type of contraction.
   d. What muscles are being strengthened?

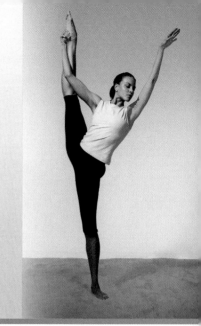

CHAPTER **13**

Hand

Joints and Motions of the Thumb

Joints and Motions of the Fingers

Bones and Landmarks

Ligaments and Other Structures

Muscles of the Thumb and Fingers

Extrinsic Muscles

Intrinsic Muscles

Anatomical Relationships

Common Wrist and Hand Pathologies

Summary of Muscle Actions

Summary of Muscle Innervation

Hand Function

Grasps

Points to Remember

Review Questions

General Anatomy Questions

Functional Activity Questions

Clinical Exercise Questions

The hand is the distal end of the upper extremity. It is made up of the thumb and finger metacarpals and phalanges. The hand is the key point of function for the upper extremity. We use our hands to accomplish an inexhaustible number of activities, ranging from very simple to quite complex tasks. The main purpose of the upper extremity's other joints is to place the hand in various positions to accomplish these tasks. Not only is the hand extremely useful and versatile, but it is also quite complex. This chapter will deal only with the hand's more basic structures and functions.

Joints and Motions of the Thumb

The first digit, the thumb, has three joints: the carpometacarpal (CMC) joint, the metacarpophalangeal (MCP) joint, and the interphalangeal (IP) joint (Fig. 13-1). The **CMC joint** is made up of the trapezium bone, which articulates with the base of the first metacarpal (Fig. 13-2). It is a saddle joint, and both joint surfaces are concave and convex. The shape and relationship of these joint surfaces can be compared to two Pringles potato chips stacked one on top of the other. The shape of the inferior surface of the top chip is similar to the shape of the first metacarpal; the shape of the superior surface of the bottom chip is similar to the trapezium bone. Each surface is concave in one direction and convex in the other. Sometimes the CMC joint is described as a modified ball-and-socket joint, implying that it has motion in all three planes. If you look at your thumb in anatomical position, you will notice that the pad is perpendicular to the palm. When you oppose your thumb, the pad is now facing, or parallel to, the palm. Clearly, rotation has occurred. However, if you try to rotate the thumb without any other joint movement, you will find it impossible to do so. The rotation at the CMC joint is a passive, not voluntary, motion, which occurs as a result of the joint's shape. This type of motion is commonly referred to as an

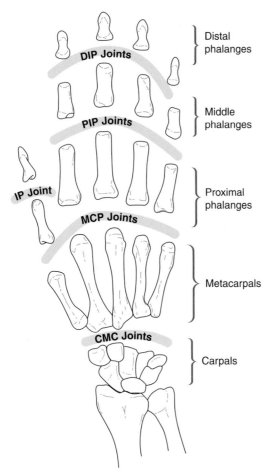

Figure 13-1. Joints and bones of the fingers and thumb (anterior view). Note that each finger has a DIP and PIP joint, whereas the thumb has only an IP joint.

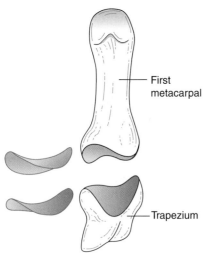

Figure 13-2. The saddle shape of the carpometacarpal (CMC) joint of the thumb can be compared to the shape of two Pringles potato chips.

accessory movement (a movement that accompanies the active movement and is essential to normal motion).

The CMC joint of the thumb allows more mobility than the CMC joints of the other four fingers, yet it also provides as much stability. This is unusual. It allows flexion and extension, abduction and adduction, and opposition and reposition (Fig. 13-3). Thumb motions differ from the usual way we name joint motions. **Flexion** and **extension** occur in a plane *parallel* to the palm. **Abduction** and **adduction** occur in a plane *perpendicular* to the palm. In other words, with the forearm supinated and the palm facing up, the thumb moving side to side across the palm is flexion and extension. The thumb moving up toward the ceiling, away from the palm, is abduction, and its return is adduction. **Opposition** is a combination of flexion and abduction, with "built-in" accessory motion of rotation; **reposition**

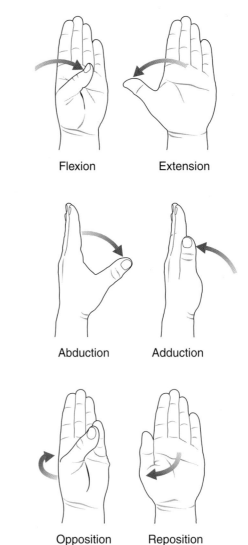

Figure 13-3. Motions of the CMC joint of the thumb

is the return to anatomical position. It is because of this accessory rotation that the CMC joint is usually considered a "modified" biaxial joint.

Although the CMC joint of the thumb is quite mobile, the MCP and IP joints are not. The MCP joint is a hinge joint that allows only flexion and extension and is therefore a uniaxial joint. The IP joint, the only phalangeal joint, also allows only flexion and extension.

Joints and Motions of the Fingers

The second, third, fourth, and fifth digits, commonly known as the *index, middle, ring,* and *little fingers,* respectively, have four joints each. These joints are the CMC joint, MCP joint, proximal interphalangeal (PIP) joint, and distal interphalangeal (DIP) joint (see Fig. 13-1).

The **carpometacarpal joints** are classified as nonaxial plane (irregular) synovial joints that provide more stability than mobility. The trapezium articulates with the base of the first metacarpal, as described previously in the discussion of the thumb joint. The trapezoid articulates with the second metacarpal, the capitate with the third metacarpal, and the hamate with the fourth and fifth metacarpals (Fig. 13-4). The fifth CMC joint is the most mobile of the fingers and allows for a small amount of **fifth finger opposition.** It does not allow as much opposition as the thumb (the first CMC

joint). The fourth CMC joint is slightly mobile, but the second and third CMC joints are not.

This can be demonstrated by looking at your knuckles with your forearm supinated and your elbow flexed. Note that with a relaxed fist, the MCP joints are essentially in a straight line. When you make a tight fist, the fifth MCP joint moves a great deal and the fourth MCP joint moves to a lesser extent, while the second and third MCP joints remain stationary. This MCP movement actually is initiated at the CMC joints.

The **metacarpophalangeal joints (MCP)** of the fingers are biaxial condyloid joints. The convex, rounded heads of the metacarpals articulate with the base of the proximal phalanges, which have a concave shape (see Fig. 13-1 and Fig. 4-1). These are commonly referred to as the "knuckles." The motions allowed at these joints are flexion, extension, and hyperextension, plus abduction and adduction (Fig. 13-5). The middle finger is the point of reference for abduction and adduction. **Abduction** occurs when the second, fourth, and fifth fingers move away from the middle (third) finger and also when the middle finger moves in either direction. **Adduction** is the return from abduction and occurs with the second, fourth, and fifth fingers. There is no adduction of the middle finger, only abduction occurring in either direction.

There are two **interphalangeal joints** in the fingers. The PIP joint is between the proximal and middle

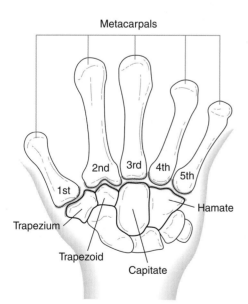

Figure 13-4. The carpometacarpal (CMC) joints of the thumb and fingers (posterior view). Note that the trapezium articulates with the first metacarpal, the trapezoid with the second metacarpal, the capitate with the third metacarpal, and the hamate with the fourth and fifth metacarpals.

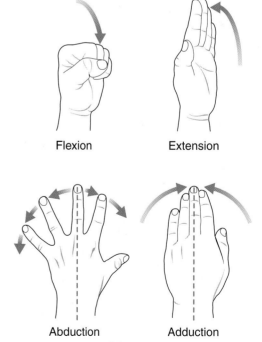

Figure 13-5. Motions of the metacarpophalangeal (MCP) joints and fingers.

phalanges, and the DIP joint is between the middle and distal phalanges. They are uniaxial hinge joints and allow only flexion and extension.

Bones and Landmarks

Although the thumb and fingers have essentially the same bony structure, there is one major difference. The thumb has two phalanges, whereas the fingers each have three. This feature makes the thumb shorter, allowing opposition to be more functional.

Therefore, the hand, made up of the thumb and four fingers, has five metacarpals, five proximal phalanges, and five distal phalanges, but only four middle phalanges (see Fig. 13-1). There are no significant landmarks on these bones other than the bone ends. The proximal end of the metacarpals and phalanges is called the *base,* and the distal end is called the *head.* There is one indistinct landmark on the forearm, which is sometimes referred to when describing muscle attachments:

Oblique Line
Located on the anterior surface of the radius from below the tuberosity, running diagonally to approximately midradius

Ligaments and Other Structures

Although there are numerous structures in the hand, only a few of those more commonly referred to will be described here. The **flexor retinaculum** ligament is a fibrous band that spans the anterior surface of the wrist in a mediolateral (horizontal) direction (Fig. 13-6). Its main function is to hold these tendons close to the wrist, thus preventing the tendons from pulling away from the wrist (bow-stringing) when the wrist flexes. It also prevents the two sides of the carpal bones from spreading apart or separating. In construction, this horizontal structure is called a "tie beam." The flexor retinaculum is made up of two parts that formerly were known as the *palmar carpal ligament* and the *transverse carpal ligament.* Currently, they are grouped together as the *flexor retinaculum.* Because of their clinical significance, these two parts will be described individually.

The **palmar carpal ligament** is more proximal and superficial than the transverse carpal ligament. Its distal fibers do blend with the transverse carpal ligament. The palmar carpal ligament attaches to the styloid processes of the radius and ulna and crosses over the flexor muscles.

The **transverse carpal ligament** lies deeper and more distal. It attaches to the pisiform and hook of the

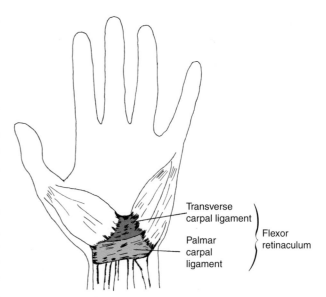

Figure 13-6.   The flexor retinaculum is made up of the palmar and transverse carpal ligaments (anterior view).

hamate on the medial side and to the scaphoid and trapezium bones laterally. It arches over the carpal bones, forming a tunnel through which the median nerve and nine extrinsic flexor tendons of the fingers and thumb (four tendons each of the flexor digitorum superficialis and flexor digitorum profundus, and one tendon for the flexor pollicis longus) pass. Figure 13-7 shows the bony floor of the carpal bones and the fibrous ceiling of the transverse carpal ligament. Together they form the tunnel through which the tendons and nerve pass. The figure also shows the area of the hand innervated by the median nerve.

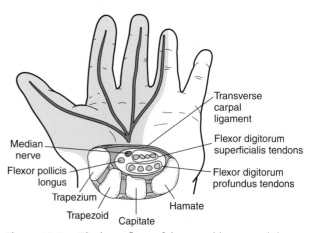

Figure 13-7.   The bony floor of the carpal bones and the fibrous ceiling of the transverse carpal ligament form the carpal tunnel (anterior superior view). The median nerve and several tendons pass through this tunnel. Note the area of the hand innervated by this nerve.

The **extensor retinaculum ligament** is a fibrous band traversing the posterior side of the wrist in a horizontal mediolateral direction (Fig. 13-8). It attaches medially to the styloid process of the ulna and to the triquetrum, pisiform, and lateral side of the radius. It holds the extensor tendons close to the wrist, especially during wrist extension.

The **extensor expansion ligament,** also called the *extensor hood* (Fig. 13-9), is a small, triangular, flat aponeurosis covering the dorsum and sides of the proximal phalanx of the fingers. The extensor digitorum tendon blends into the expansion. It is wider at its base over the MCP joint, actually wrapping over the sides somewhat. As it approaches the PIP joint, it is joined by tendons of the lumbricales and interossei muscles. It narrows toward its distal end at the base of the distal phalanx. The extensor digitorum, lumbricales, and interossei muscles form an attachment to the middle or distal phalanx by way of this expansion. The **extensor hood** area, formed by the extensor expansion proximally, covers the head of the metacarpal and keeps the extensor tendon in the midline.

When the hand is relaxed, the palm assumes a cupped position. This palmar concavity is due to the arrangement of the bony skeleton reinforced by ligaments. There are three arches that are responsible for this shape (Fig. 13-10). The **proximal carpal arch** is formed by the proximal end of the metacarpals (base)

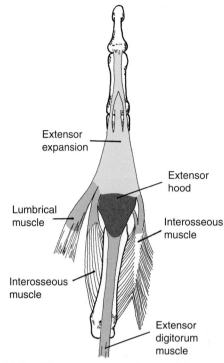

Figure 13-9.   The extensor expansion provides an attachment on the middle and/or distal phalanx for several muscles (posterior view).

and carpal bones and is maintained by the flexor retinaculum (see Fig. 13-6). The shallower **distal carpal arch** is made up of the metacarpal heads. The **longitudinal arch** begins at the wrist and runs the length of the metacarpal and phalanges for each digit. It is perpendicular to the other two arches. These arches contribute to the function of the various grasps described at the end of this chapter.

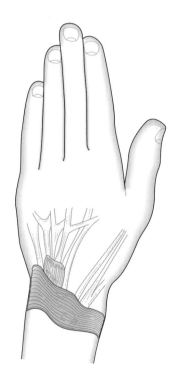

Figure 13-8.   Extensor retinaculum (posterior view).

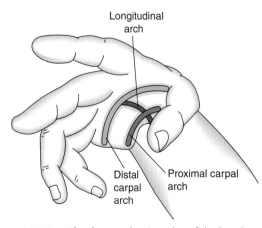

Figure 13-10.   The three arches in palm of the hand.

Muscles of the Thumb and Fingers

Extrinsic Muscles

In addition to the wrist muscles previously described, there are several other muscles that span the wrist and cross the joints in the hand. These muscles are called **extrinsic muscles** of the hand, because their proximal attachment is above, or proximal to, the wrist joint. They have an assistive role in wrist function, but their primary function is at the thumb or finger. Their names give much information about function and location. For example, it is rather easy to distinguish the muscles having a function on the thumb because *pollicis* means "thumb" in Latin. The extrinsic muscles are as follows:

Anterior	Posterior
Flexor digitorum superficialis	Abductor pollicis longus
Flexor digitorum profundus	Extensor pollicis brevis
Flexor pollicis longus	Extensor pollicis longus
	Extensor digitorum
	Extensor indicis
	Extensor digiti minimi

The **flexor digitorum superficialis** muscle lies deep to the wrist flexors and palmaris longus muscle (Fig. 13-11). Its broad proximal attachment is part of the common flexor tendon on the medial epicondyle of the humerus. It also has an attachment on the coronoid process of the ulna and the oblique line of the radius. It divides into four tendons and crosses the wrist (Fig. 13-12). Its distal attachment splits into two parts and attaches on each side of the middle phalanx of each finger. Its action is to flex the MCP and PIP joints of the second through fifth fingers.

Flexor Digitorum Superficialis Muscle

O	Common flexor tendon on the medial epicondyle, coronoid process, and radius
I	Sides of the middle phalanx of the four fingers
A	Flexes the MCP and PIP joints of the fingers
N	Median nerve (C7, C8, T1)

The **flexor digitorum profundus muscle** lies deep to the flexor digitorum superficialis muscle; these two muscles traverse the forearm and hand together (Fig. 13-13). The profundus muscle has its proximal attachment on the ulna on the anterior and medial surfaces, from the

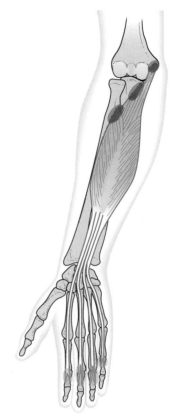

Figure 13-11.   Flexor digitorum superficialis muscle (anterior view).

coronoid process to approximately three-fourths of the way down the ulna. It runs beneath the flexor digitorum superficialis muscle until the superficialis tendon splits into two parts at its distal attachment. The profundus muscle passes through this split and continues distally to attach at the base of the distal phalanx of the second through fifth fingers (see Fig. 13-12). Its action is to flex the MCP, PIP, and DIP joints of the second through fifth fingers.

Flexor Digitorum Profundus Muscle

O	Upper three-fourths of the ulna
I	Distal phalanx of the four fingers
A	Flexes all three joints of the fingers (MCP, PIP, and DIP)
N	Median and ulnar nerves (C8, T1)

The **flexor pollicis longus muscle** is a deep muscle that has its proximal attachment on the anterior surface of the radius and interosseous membrane and its distal attachment at the base of the thumb's distal phalanx (Fig. 13-14). It is a prime mover in flexion of the CMC, MCP, and IP joints of the thumb.

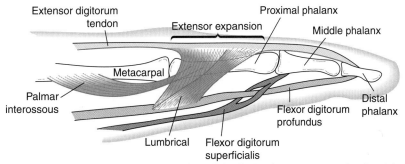

Figure 13-12.   Side view of a digit showing tendon relationship of the flexor digitorum superficialis with the flexor digitorum profundus, and the two flexor tendons with the extensor digitorum tendon.

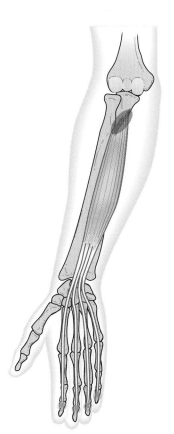

Figure 13-13.   Flexor digitorum profundus muscle (anterior view).

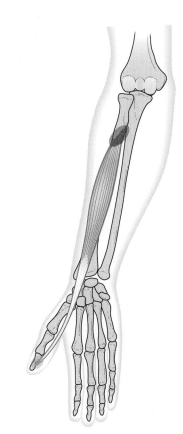

Figure 13-14.   Flexor pollicis longus muscle (anterior view).

Flexor Pollicis Longus Muscle

O	Radius, anterior surface
I	Distal phalanx of thumb
A	Flexes all three joints of the thumb (CMC, MCP, IP)
N	Median nerve (C8, T1)

The **abductor pollicis longus muscle** is located deep on the posterior forearm (Fig. 13-15). It attaches to the radius just distal to the supinator, the interosseous membrane, and the middle portion of the ulna. It becomes superficial just proximal to crossing the wrist and attaches to the base of the first metacarpal on the radial side. It effectively abducts the thumb at the CMC joint even though it is attached only to the metacarpal, because the distal joints (MCP and IP) allow only flexion and extension. Therefore, the thumb moves as one unit in the direction of abduction and

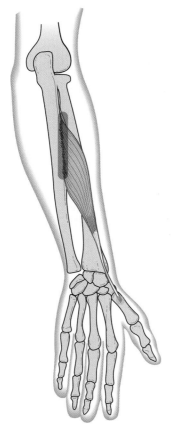

Figure 13-15. Abductor pollicis longus muscle (posterior view).

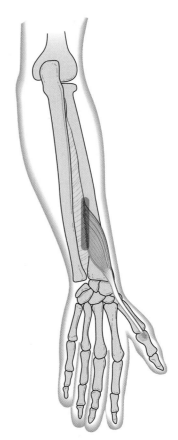

Figure 13-16. Extensor pollicis brevis muscle (posterior view).

adduction. Similarly, adducting the metacarpal also adducts the entire thumb. Therefore, in this text, when referring to thumb abduction, adduction, opposition, and reposition, it is implied that the action occurs at the CMC joint.

Abductor Pollicis Longus Muscle

O	Posterior radius, interosseous membrane, middle ulna
I	Base of the first metacarpal
A	Abducts thumb (CMC)
N	Radial nerve (C6, C7)

The **extensor pollicis brevis muscle** is also located deep on the posterior forearm and spans the wrist just medial to the abductor pollicis longus muscle. Its proximal attachment is on the posterior radius near the distal end and just below the abductor pollicis longus muscle. Its distal attachment is on the posterior surface at the base of the thumb's proximal phalanx (Fig. 13-16). It functions to extend the CMC and MCP joints of the thumb.

Extensor Pollicis Brevis Muscle

O	Posterior distal radius
I	Base of the proximal phalanx of thumb
A	Extends CMC and MCP joints of thumb
N	Radial nerve (C6, C7)

The **extensor pollicis longus muscle** is located near the two previously mentioned muscles, deep on the posterior forearm. Its proximal attachment is on the middle third of the ulna and interosseous membrane (Fig. 13-17). Like the other two muscles, it becomes superficial just before crossing the wrist. Its distal attachment is at the base of the thumb's distal phalanx, on the posterior side. It functions to extend the CMC, MCP, and IP joints of the thumb.

Extensor Pollicis Longus Muscle

O	Middle posterior ulna and interosseous membrane
I	Base of distal phalanx of thumb

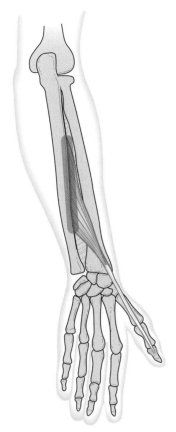

Figure 13-17. Extensor pollicis longus muscle (posterior view).

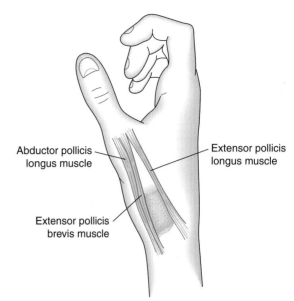

Abductor pollicis longus muscle

Extensor pollicis longus muscle

Extensor pollicis brevis muscle

Figure 13-18. The borders of the anatomical snuffbox are defined by the tendon of the extensor pollicis longus muscle on one side and the tendons of the abductor pollicis longus and brevis muscles on the other side (side view).

A	Extends all three joints of the thumb (CMC, MCP, and IP)
N	Radial nerve (C6, C7, C8)

If you extend your thumb, you will notice that a depression is formed between what appears to be two tendons. Actually, there are three tendons. The abductor pollicis longus and extensor pollicis brevis muscles form the lateral border, and the extensor pollicis longus muscle forms the medial border. This depression is called the **anatomical snuffbox** (Fig. 13-18).

The **extensor digitorum muscle** is a superficial muscle on the posterior forearm and hand (Fig. 13-19). It attaches proximally to the lateral epicondyle of the humerus as part of the common extensor tendon. It passes under the extensor retinaculum to attach distally on the distal phalanx of the second through fifth fingers via the extensor expansion (see Fig. 13-12). In the area of the metacarpals are interconnecting bands joining the four extensor digitorum tendons. These interconnecting bands limit independent finger extension. The extensor digitorum muscle is the only common extensor muscle of the fingers. It extends the MCP,

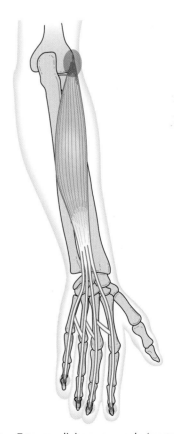

Figure 13-19. Extensor digitorum muscle (posterior view).

PIP, and DIP joints of the second, third, fourth, and fifth fingers.

Extensor Digitorum Muscle

O	Lateral epicondyle of the humerus
I	Base of distal phalanx of the second through fifth fingers
A	Extends all three joints of the fingers (MCP, PIP, and DIP)
N	Radial nerve (C6, C7, C8)

The **extensor indicis muscle** is a deep muscle that has its proximal attachment on the posterior surface of the distal ulna (Fig. 13-20). It crosses the wrist under the extensor retinaculum medial to the extensor digitorum muscle and attaches into the extensor expansion, with the extensor digitorum muscle. It extends the MCP, PIP, and DIP joints of the index finger.

Extensor Indicis Muscle

O	Distal ulna
I	Base of distal phalanx of the second finger
A	Extends all three joints of the second finger (MCP, PIP, and DIP)
N	Radial nerve (C6, C7, C8)

The **extensor digiti minimi muscle** is a long, narrow muscle (Fig. 13-21) that is deep to the extensor digitorum and extensor carpi ulnaris muscles near its proximal attachment. It becomes superficial before crossing the wrist. It comes off the common extensor tendon on the lateral epicondyle of the humerus, crosses the wrist under the extensor retinaculum, and attaches to the base of the distal phalanx of the fifth finger via the extensor expansion. It is a prime mover in extending the MCP, PIP, and DIP joints of the fifth finger.

Extensor Digiti Minimi Muscle

O	Lateral epicondyle of humerus
I	Base of distal phalanx of fifth finger
A	Extends all three joints of fifth finger (MCP, PIP, and DIP)
N	Radial nerve (C6, C7, C8)

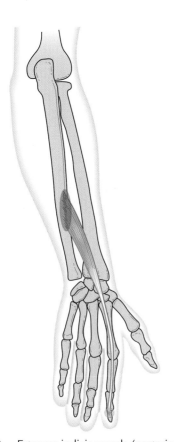

Figure 13-20. Extensor indicis muscle (posterior view).

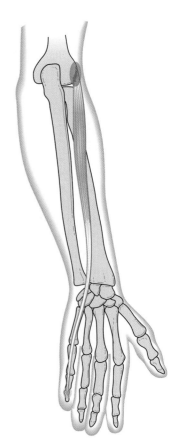

Figure 13-21. Extensor digiti minimi muscle (posterior view).

In review, the extrinsic muscles have their proximal attachment above the wrist and their distal attachment on the hand. Because they cross the wrist, they could have a function there; however, any wrist function is usually assistive at best. The prime function of the extrinsic muscles is in moving the fingers or thumb.

Intrinsic Muscles

Intrinsic muscles have their proximal attachment at, or distal to, the carpal bones and have a function on the thumb or fingers. These muscles are responsible for the hand's fine motor control and precision movement. The intrinsic muscles can be further divided into the thenar, hypothenar, and deep palm muscles. The **thenar muscles** are those that function to move the thumb. They form the thenar eminence, or ball of the thumb. The **deep palm muscles** are located deep in the palm of the hand between the thenar and hypothenar muscles. They perform some of the more intricate motions that usually involve multiple muscles. These muscles are the adductor pollicis, the interossei (of which there are four dorsal and four palmar), and the lumbricales (of which there are also four muscles). The **hypothenar muscles,** forming the hypothenar eminence, act primarily on the little finger. Table 13-1 summarizes the three groups of intrinsic muscles.

In the thenar group, the **flexor pollicis brevis muscle** is a relatively superficial muscle. It attaches proximally to the trapezium and the flexor retinaculum, and distally to the base of the proximal phalanx of the thumb (Fig. 13-22). Its primary actions are to flex the CMC and MCP joints of the thumb.

Flexor Pollicis Brevis Muscle

O	Trapezium and flexor retinaculum
I	Proximal phalanx of the thumb
A	Flexes the CMC and MCP joints of thumb
N	Median nerve (C6, C7)

The **abductor pollicis brevis muscle** lies just lateral to the flexor pollicis brevis muscle. It attaches proximally to the flexor retinaculum, scaphoid, and trapezium, and

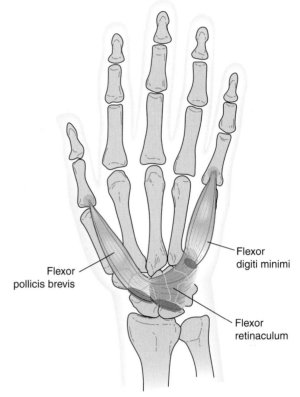

Flexor pollicis brevis

Flexor digiti minimi

Flexor retinaculum

Figure 13-22.   The flexor pollicis brevis and flexor digiti minimi muscles (anterior view).

distally to the base of the thumb's proximal phalanx (Fig. 13-23). It acts to abduct the CMC joint of the thumb.

Abductor Pollicis Brevis Muscle

O	Scaphoid, trapezium, and flexor retinaculum
I	Proximal phalanx of the thumb
A	Abducts the thumb (CMC joint)
N	Median nerve (C6, C7)

The **opponens pollicis muscle** lies deep to the abductor pollicis brevis muscle. It attaches proximally to the trapezium and flexor retinaculum and distally to the entire lateral surface of the first metacarpal (Fig. 13-24). Its primary function is to oppose the thumb. Remember, this action occurs at the CMC joint.

Table 13-1	Intrinsic Muscles of the Hand	
Thenar	**Deep Palm**	**Hypothenar**
Flexor pollicis brevis	Adductor pollicis	Flexor digiti minimi
Abductor pollicis brevis	Interossei	Abductor digiti minimi
Opponens pollicis	Lumbricales	Opponens digiti minimi

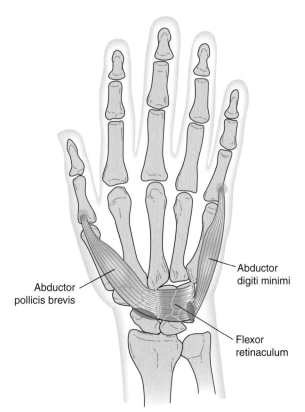

Figure 13-23. The abductor pollicis brevis and abductor digiti minimi muscles (anterior view).

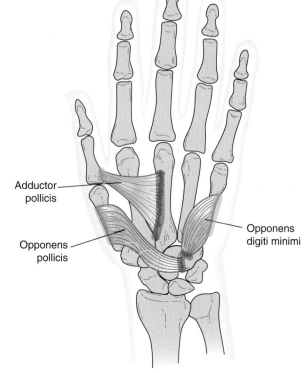

Figure 13-24. The opponens pollicis, adductor pollicis, and opponens digiti minimi muscles (anterior view).

Opponens Pollicis Muscle

O	Trapezium and flexor retinaculum
I	First metacarpal
A	Opposes the thumb (CMC joint)
N	Median nerve (C6, C7)

Thumb opposition is perhaps the most important function of the hand. Because it is a combination of flexion, abduction, and rotation of the thumb, other muscles such as the flexor pollicis brevis and abductor pollicis muscles assist in this function.

The muscles located in the area between the thenar and hypothenar muscle groups are often called the **deep palm group,** or the *intermediate group.* The adductor pollicis muscle is sometimes placed in this group, because it is located deep within the palm. Other sources place it with the thenar group because of its action on the thumb. It is placed here in the deep palm group for perhaps no other reason than to discuss the intrinsic muscles in groups of three!

The **adductor pollicis muscle** is a thumb muscle, although it is not usually considered part of the thenar group. This is probably because it is located deep and

does not make up the muscle bulk of the thenar eminence. It has its proximal attachments on the capitate, the base of the second metacarpal, and the palmar surface of the third metacarpal. Its distal attachment is at the base of the proximal phalanx of the thumb (see Fig. 13-24). As its name implies, its function is to adduct the thumb (at the CMC joint).

Adductor Pollicis Muscle

O	Capitate, base of the second metacarpal, palmar surface of the third metacarpal
I	Base of proximal phalanx of thumb
A	Adducts thumb (CMC joint)
N	Ulnar nerve (C8, T1)

There are two sets of interossei muscles: dorsal and palmar. There are four **dorsal interossei** muscles. They each attach proximally to two adjacent metacarpals and distally to the base of the proximal phalanx (Fig. 13-25). Table 13-2 summarizes the attachments and actions of each of the dorsal interossei muscles. Their action is to abduct the second, third, and fourth fingers at the MCP joint. Remember that the third finger abducts in both on, the middle finger. Distally, they attach to the base of the proximal phalanx of the same finger as the proximal attachment (Fig. 13-26). These attachments are summarized in Table 13-3. Like the dorsal interossei muscles, the palmar interossei muscles are innervated by the ulnar nerve.

Palmar Interossei Muscles

O	1st, 2nd, 4th, and 5th metacarpals
I	Base of respective proximal phalanx
A	Adduct fingers at MCP joint
N	Ulnar nerve (C8, T1)

As mentioned, the middle finger is the point of reference for abduction and adduction. Movement away from the middle finger is abduction, and movement toward it is adduction. Note that the middle finger

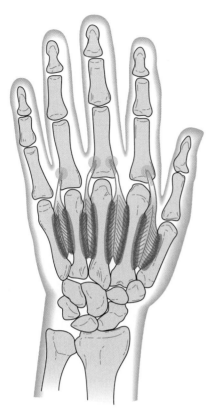

Figure 13-25.   Dorsal interossei muscles. Note that the middle finger has two attachments (posterior view).

directions. The fifth finger is abducted by the abductor digiti minimi. The ulnar nerve innervates all dorsal interossei muscles.

Dorsal Interossei

O	Adjacent metacarpals
I	Base of proximal phalanx
A	Abduct fingers at MCP joint
N	Ulnar nerve (C8, T1)

Like the dorsal interossei muscles, there are four **palmar interossei** muscles. They attach proximally to the palmar surface of the first, second, fourth, and fifth metacarpals. They do not attach to, or have a function

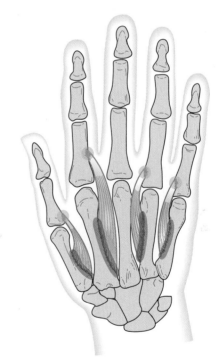

Figure 13-26.   Palmar interossei muscles (anterior view). Note that the middle finger has no attachments.

Table 13-2	Dorsal Interossei Muscles of the Hand		
Muscle	Proximal Attachment	Distal Attachment	Action
First	First and second metacarpals	Lateral side of index finger	Abduct index finger
Second	Second and third metacarpals	Lateral side of middle finger	Abduct middle finger laterally
Third	Third and fourth metacarpals	Medial side of middle finger	Abduct middle finger medially
Fourth	Fourth and fifth metacarpals	Medial side of ring finger	Abduct ring finger

Table 13-3	Palmar Interossei Muscles		
Muscles	Proximal Attachment	Distal Attachment	Action
First	First metacarpal	Medial side of thumb	Adduct thumb
Second	Second metacarpal	Medial side of index finger	Adduct index finger
Third	Fourth metacarpal	Lateral side of ring finger	Adduct ring finger
Fourth	Fifth metacarpal	Lateral side of little finger	Adduct little finger

abducts in two directions and therefore does not adduct.

The last muscle group to be discussed is rather unique. The **lumbricales,** of which there are four, have no bony attachment. They are located quite deep and attach only to tendons. Proximally, they attach to the tendon of the flexor digitorum profundus muscle, spanning the MCP joint anteriorly (Fig. 13-27). This allows them to flex the MCP joint. They then pass posteriorly at the proximal phalange to attach to the tendinous expansion of the extensor digitorum muscle (Fig. 13-28). This allows them to extend the PIP and DIP joint. Therefore, their action is to flex the MCP

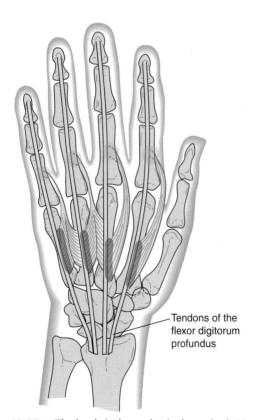

Tendons of the flexor digitorum profundus

Figure 13-27. The lumbrical muscles (palmar view). Note that the distal attachment on the tendons of the extensor digitorum cannot be seen in this view.

joint and extend the PIP and DIP joints of the second through fifth fingers. This combined motion is referred to as the "tabletop position." Incidentally, the plural of lumbrical can be spelled with an "s" or "es".

Lumbrical Muscles

O	Tendon of the flexor digitorum profundus muscle
I	Tendon of the extensor digitorum muscle
A	Flex the MCP joint while extending the PIP and DIP joints
N	First and second lumbricales: medial nerve
	Third and fourth lumbricales: ulnar nerve (C6, C7, C8)

The counterpart to the thenar muscle group is the hypothenar group. The **flexor digiti minimi muscle** serves the same function on the little finger as the flexor pollicis brevis does on the thumb. It is attached proximally to the hook of the hamate and the flexor retinaculum, and distally to the base of the little finger's proximal phalanx (see Fig. 13-22). It flexes the MCP joint of that finger. Remember, although most thumb motion occurs at the CMC joint, most finger motion occurs at the MCP joint.

Flexor Digiti Minimi Muscle

O	Hamate and flexor retinaculum
I	Base of proximal phalanx of the fifth finger
A	Flexes CMC and MCP joints of the fifth finger
N	Ulnar nerve (C8, T1)

The **abductor digiti minimi muscle** lies superficially just medial to the flexor digiti minimi muscle on the ulnar border of the hypothenar eminence. It attaches proximally to the pisiform and to the tendon of the flexor carpi ulnaris muscle and distally to the base of the proximal phalanx of the fifth finger (see Fig. 13-23). It abducts the MCP joint of that finger.

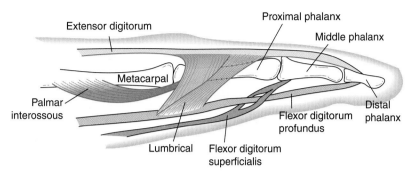

Figure 13-28. The lumbrical muscles (side view).

Abductor Digiti Minimi Muscle

O	Pisiform and tendon of flexor carpi ulnaris
I	Proximal phalanx of fifth finger
A	Abducts the MCP joint of the fifth finger
N	Ulnar nerve (C8, T1)

The **opponens digiti minimi muscle** lies deep to the other hypothenar muscles. Its proximal attachments, the hook of the hamate and the flexor retinaculum, are similar to the proximal attachments of the flexor digiti minimi muscle. Distally, it attaches to the ulnar border of the fifth metacarpal (see Fig. 13-24). Its primary action is in opposition of the fifth finger. This occurs at the CMC joint.

Opponens Digiti Minimi Muscle

O	Hamate and flexor retinaculum
I	Fifth metacarpal
A	Opposes the fifth finger (CMC joint)
N	Ulnar nerve (C8, T1)

Anatomical Relationships

Describing the muscles of the hand in relationship to each other is a rather involved process. It is difficult to separate wrist and hand extrinsic muscles. One must consider not only anterior and posterior groups, but also extrinsic and intrinsic muscles. We will start with the extrinsic muscles spanning the wrist anteriorly. The palmaris longus is the most superficial muscle, but it has no significant function. The tendons of the flexor digitorum superficialis are deep to it. The flexor digitorum profundus tendons are deep to both, essentially forming the third layer of extrinsic muscle tendons in the palm. The other extrinsic muscle on the anterior surface is the flexor pollicis longus, which crosses the wrist to attach on the thumb.

In Figure 13-29, remove the palmaris longus and look at the palm. On the fifth finger side and heading toward the thumb, you will see three intrinsic muscles that move the little finger: the opponens digiti minimi, the adductor digiti minimi, and the flexor digiti minimi. In the middle of the palm are the tendons of the flexor digitorum profundus (attaching on the distal phalanx of each finger), beneath the tendons of the flexor digitorum superficialis (attaching to either side of the middle phalanx of each finger). Each muscle has tendons going to the second, third, fourth, and fifth fingers. The flexor digitorum profundus gives rise to the proximal attachments of the lumbricales. Moving toward the thumb side, you will see the muscles that move the thumb—the adductor pollicis, flexor pollicis brevis, abductor pollicis brevis, and opponens pollicis—and the

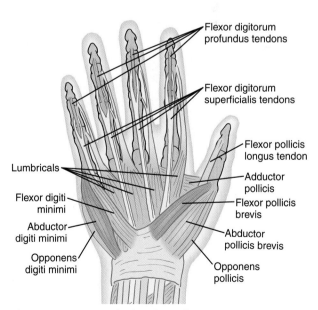

Figure 13-29. Anterior hand muscles.

tendon of the flexor pollicis longus. Remove the tendons of the flexor digitorum superficialis and profundus, and you can see the deepest layer, the palmar interossei.

On the lateral and posterior side of the thumb, the extrinsic muscles are, in order of appearance, the abductor pollicis longus, the extensor pollicis brevis, and the extensor pollicis longus, which together make up the anatomical snuffbox (see Figs. 13-18 and 13-20). Next, and most superficial in the middle of the posterior forearm, are the extensor digitorum and extensor digiti minimi muscles (Fig. 13-30). Deep to the extensor digitorum above the wrist is the extensor indicis. The only intrinsic muscle on the posterior side is the dorsal interossei. Deep to the extensor digitorum tendons below the wrist is the dorsal interossei.

Common Wrist and Hand Pathologies

Wrist and hand pathologies have been included together, since many tendons involved cross the wrist and attach in the hand. A **Colles' fracture** is a common injury of elderly people, resulting from a fall on the outstretched

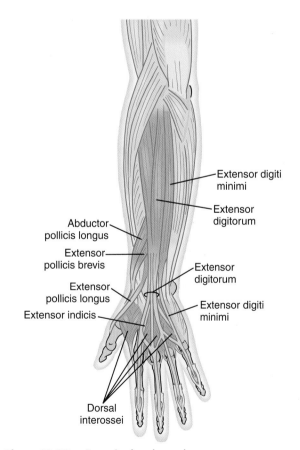

Extensor digiti minimi

Extensor digitorum

Abductor pollicis longus

Extensor pollicis brevis

Extensor pollicis longus

Extensor indicis

Extensor digitorum

Extensor digiti minimi

Dorsal interossei

Figure 13-30.   Posterior hand muscles.

hand. This transverse fracture of the distal radius includes a posterior displacement of the distal fragment. In **Smith's fracture,** the distal fragment is displaced anteriorly (reverse Colles') and is caused by a fall on the back of the hand. A **"greenstick" fracture** refers to an incomplete fracture, usually of the radius and more proximal than a Colles' fracture. It is more common in children than adults. This fracture is similar to the breaking of a young or new tree limb. If you try to break the limb, you will find that it does not break completely in half like an older, more brittle limb. A **ganglion cyst** is a benign tumor mass commonly seen as a bump on the dorsal surface of the wrist.

Carpal tunnel syndrome is an extremely common condition caused by compression of the median nerve within the carpal tunnel. Symptoms include numbness and tingling in the hand, which often begins at night. Patients often complain of tingling, pain, and weakness in the hand, particularly in the thumb, index, and middle fingers. Tapping over the carpal tunnel often produces symptoms. Some fibers of the transverse carpal ligament are often surgically cut to relieve the symptoms. **De Quervain's disease** is caused by an inflammation and thickening of the sheath containing the extensor pollicis brevis and abductor pollicis longus, resulting in pain on the radial side of the wrist. Because it is an inflammation of tendons and their surrounding sheaths, it is called a **tenosynovitis.** Making a fist with your thumb inside and then moving the wrist into ulnar deviation can elicit pain in those tendons and is considered a positive test. Care should be exercised in doing this test because it often causes some discomfort in a normal wrist.

Dupuytren's contracture occurs when the palmar aponeurosis undergoes a nodular thickening. It is most common in the area of the palm in line with the ring and little fingers. Often those fingers will develop flexion contractures. **Stenosing tenosynovitis,** commonly known as **trigger finger,** is a problem with the sliding mechanism of a tendon in its sheath. When a nodule or swelling of the sheath lining or the tendon develops, the tendon can no longer slide in and out smoothly. It may pass into the sheath when the finger flexes, but it becomes stuck as the finger attempts to extend. The \finger can become locked in that position, and it must be manually extended. The flexor tendons of the middle and ring fingers are most commonly involved. **Skier's thumb,** a common hand injury among athletes, involves an acute tear of the ulnar collateral ligament of the thumb. **Gamekeeper's thumb** is an old term referring to a stretching injury of this ligament developed over time by English gamekeepers as they twisted the necks of small game.

Swan neck deformity is characterized by flexion of the MCP joint, (hyper)extension of the PIP joint, and flexion of the DIP joint. With a **boutonnière deformity,** the deformity is in the opposite direction—extension of the MCP joint, flexion of the PIP joint, and extension of the DIP joint. **Ulnar drift** results in ulnar deviation of the fingers at the MCP joints. **Mallet finger** is caused by disruption of the extensor mechanism of the DIP joint, either because the tendon was severed or because the portion of bone where the tendon attached has avulsed from the distal phalanx. In either case, the distal phalanx remains in a flexed position and cannot be extended. The scaphoid is the most frequently injured carpal bone. A **scaphoid fracture** usually results from a fall on the outstretched hand of a younger person. Because of a poor vascular supply, it has a high incidence of avascular necrosis. **Kienböck's disease** refers to the necrosis of the lunate, which may develop after trauma.

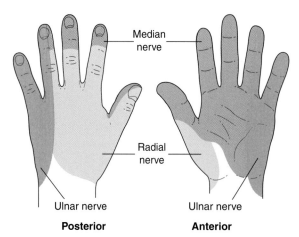

Figure 13-31. Sensory innervation of the hand. Motor innervation follows a similar pattern.

Summary of Muscle Actions

The actions of the prime movers of the hand are summarized in Table 13-4.

Summary of Muscle Innervation

Innervation of the hand is almost as straightforward as innervation of the wrist (Fig. 13-31). However, a few exceptions must be discussed. Similar to the wrist,

muscles on the posterior surface of the hand are innervated mostly by the radial nerve. Anteriorly, muscles on the thumb side are supplied primarily by the median nerve, and muscles on the little finger side are supplied primarily by the ulnar nerve.

The adductor pollicis muscle appears to be the exception; it is innervated by the ulnar nerve rather than the median nerve like all the other thumb (pollicis) muscles. However, remember that the adductor

Table 13-4	Prime Movers of the Hand	
Action	Joint	Muscle
Thumb		
Flexion	CMC, MCP	Flexor pollicis brevis
	IP (MCP, CMC)	Flexor pollicis longus
Extension	CMC, MCP	Extensor pollicis brevis
	IP (MCP, CMC)	Extensor pollicis longus
Abduction	CMC	Abductor pollicis brevis, abductor pollicis longus
Adduction	CMC	Adductor pollicis
Opposition	CMC	Opponens pollicis
Reposition	CMC	Adductor pollicis, extensor pollicis longus, extensor pollicis brevis
Action	Joint	Muscle
Finger		
Flexion	MCP	Lumbricales, flexor digitorum superficialis, flexor digitorum profundus
	PIP	Flexor digitorum superficialis, flexor digitorum profundus
	DIP	Flexor digitorum profundus
Extension	MCP	Extensor digitorum, extensor indicis, extensor digiti minimi
	PIP and DIP	Lumbricales, extensor digitorum, extensor digiti minimi, extensor indicis
Abduction	MCP	Dorsal interossei, abductor digiti minimi
Adduction	MCP	Palmar interossei
Opposition (fifth)	CMC	Opponens digiti minimi

Table 13-5	Innervation of the Muscles of the Hand	
Muscle	Nerve	Spinal Segment
Extensor digitorum	Radial	C6, C7, C8
Extensor indicis	Radial	C6, C7, C8
Extensor digiti minimi	Radial	C6, C7, C8
Extensor pollicis longus	Radial	C6, C7, C8
Extensor pollicis brevis	Radial	C6, C7
Abductor pollicis longus	Radial	C6, C7
Flexor digitorum superficialis	Median	C7, C8, T1
Flexor digitorum profundus	Median	C8, T1
	Ulnar	C8, T1
Flexor pollicis longus	Median	C8, T1
Flexor pollicis brevis	Median	C6, C7
Abductor pollicis brevis	Median	C6, C7
Opponens pollicis	Median	C6, C7
Lumbricales 1 and 2	Median	C6, C7
Lumbricales 3 and 4	Ulnar	C8
Flexor digiti minimi	Ulnar	C8, T1
Abductor digiti minimi	Ulnar	C8, T1
Opponens digiti minimi	Ulnar	C8, T1
Adductor pollicis	Ulnar	C8, T1
Dorsal and palmar interossei	Ulnar	C8, T1

pollicis muscle attaches in the middle of the palm to the third metacarpal (see Fig. 13-24). It is here that the ulnar nerve changes direction and runs toward the thumb. As it does, it sends branches to the adductor pollicis and dorsal and palmar interossei muscles (see Fig. 6-27). The flexor digitorum profundus muscle receives its innervation from both the median and ulnar nerve, as do the lumbricales. This is not surprising, because the lumbricales have their proximal attachment on the tendons of the flexor digitorum

Table 13-6	Segmental Innervation of the Hand			
Spinal Cord Level	C6	C7	C8	T1
Extensor digitorum	X	X	X	
Extensor indicis	X	X	X	
Extensor digiti minimi	X	X	X	
Extensor pollicis longus	X	X	X	
Extensor pollicis brevis	X	X		
Abductor pollicis longus	X	X		
Abductor pollicis brevis	X	X		
Flexor pollicis brevis	X	X		
Opponens pollicis	X	X		
Flexor digitorum superficialis		X	X	X
Flexor digitorum profundus			X	X
Flexor pollicis longus			X	X
Lumbricales	X	X	X	
Flexor digiti minimi			X	X
Abductor digiti minimi			X	X
Opponens digiti minimi			X	X
Adductor pollicis			X	X
Dorsal and palmar interossei			X	X

profundus muscle. Table 13-5 further summarizes hand muscle innervation. This table shows that injury to the lower cervical vertebrae will affect all hand function. Table 13-6 summarizes the segmental innervation. Note that there is some discrepancy among various sources regarding the spinal cord level of innervation.

Hand Function

The human hand performs many functions. The primary function is grasp, or *prehension*. This means that the hand is designed to hold or manipulate objects. There are also many nonprehensile hand functions such as expressing emotions; scratching; using a fist as a club; and using the open palm, as in pushing down on an armrest to assist in standing. Because no manipulative movement occurs with these types of activities, no further description of nonprehensile function will be made here.

With prehension (grasping or holding an object), the manner in which the hand is used depends on the size, shape, and weight of the object, how that object will be used, and the involvement of the proximal segments of the upper extremity. Generally speaking, the shoulder girdle and shoulder joint position the hand in space. The elbow allows the hand to move closer or farther away from the body, especially the face. The wrist provides stability while the hand is manipulating objects and is important in the tenodesis action described in Chapter 5. Although much attention tends to focus on the grasping aspect of hand function, release is equally important. Release is the role of the MP, PIP, and DIP extensors. Without the ability to release, the hand's grasp function is greatly diminished.

Of paramount importance to hand function is sensation. Without intact sensation, an individual must compensate with visual clues to find items, know what is being held, and how hard the object is being grasped. For example, if you were presented with a laundry bag full of clothes and told to find the small box of soap, you could feel around inside the bag until locating the soap. However, if your hand's sensation were not intact, you would have to empty the bag and visually search for the box. A person with an upper extremity amputation who uses a prosthetic device is a good example of having hand function without sensation. That person would need visual feedback to find the soap and to know if the terminal device had grasped it. Hand sensation is provided by the radial, ulnar, and median nerves. Figure 13-31 shows the pattern of sensory distribution. This distribution varies somewhat among authors.

There is an optimal wrist and hand position for the hand to be most effective in terms of strength and precision. This position is called the **functional position of the hand.** In this position, the wrist is in a slightly extended position, the MCP and PIP joints of the fingers are slightly flexed, and the thumb is in opposition. Figure 13-32 illustrates this position. Maintenance of the thenar web is vital to thumb opposition.

Grasps

There are basically two types of prehension: power grips and precision grips. The activity dictates which grip is needed. A **power grip** is used when an object must be held forcefully while being moved about by more proximal joint muscles (holding a hammer or doorknob; Fig. 13-33). Often a power grip involves an isometric contraction with no movement occurring between the hand and the object being held.

A **precision grip,** often referred to as *precision prehension,* is used when an object must be manipulated in a finer type movement, such as holding a pen or threading a needle (Fig. 13-34).

Power Grips

A power grip usually involves a significant amount of force and is considered the most powerful grip. The

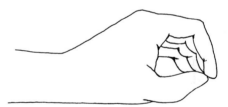

Figure 13-32.   Functional position of the wrist and hand. The wrist is in slight extension, the MCP and PIP joints are in some degree of flexion, and the thumb is in opposition.

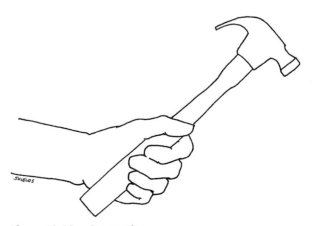

Figure 13-33.   Power grip.

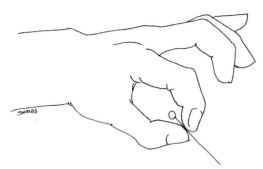

Figure 13-34.   Precision grip.

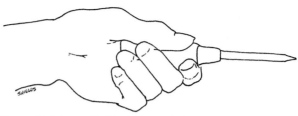

Figure 13-36.   Cylindrical grip variation.

fingers tend to flex around the object in one direction and the thumb wraps around in the opposite direction, providing a counterforce to keep the object in contact with the palm or fingers. Once the object is firmly set in the hand, it can be moved about in space by more proximal joint musculature. The long finger flexors (extrinsics) grip the object, and the long finger extensors (also extrinsics) assist in holding the wrist in a neutral or slightly extended position. When the thumb is involved, it tends to be in an adducted position.

The three commonly described power grips are cylindrical, spherical, and hook. The **cylindrical grip** (Fig. 13-35) has all the fingers flexed around the object, which usually lies at a right angle to the forearm. The thumb is wrapped around the object in the opposite direction, often overlapping the fingers. Examples of a cylindrical grip would be holding a hammer, a racquet, or a wheelbarrow handle.

A variation of the cylindrical grip has the fingers flexed around a handle in a graded fashion (Fig. 13-36). The fifth finger joints are flexed the most, and the second finger joints are only partly flexed. The thumb lies

parallel and against the handle, and the wrist is in slight ulnar deviation. The advantage of this grip over a cylindrical grip is that it allows a forceful but more controlled use of the tool. Examples of this type of grip would involve holding a golf club or a screwdriver.

A **spherical grip** has all the fingers and thumb abducted around an object, and, unlike the cylindrical grip, the fingers are more spread apart. The palm of the hand is often not involved (Fig. 13-37). Activities involving a spherical grip include holding an apple or a doorknob or picking up a glass by its top.

The **hook grip** involves the second through fifth fingers flexed around an object in a hooklike manner (Fig. 13-38). The MCP joints are extended, and the PIP and DIP joints are in some degree of flexion. The thumb is usually not involved. Therefore, this is the only power grip possible if a person has a median nerve injury and loses the ability to oppose the thumb.

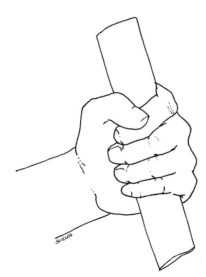

Figure 13-35.   Cylindrical grip.

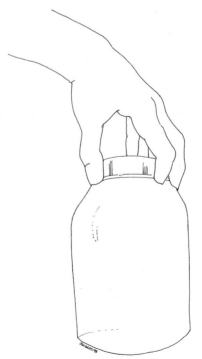

Figure 13-37.   Spherical grip.

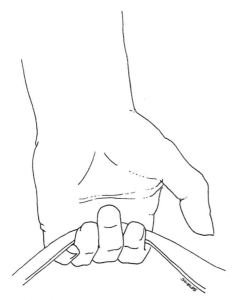

Figure 13-38.   Hook grip.

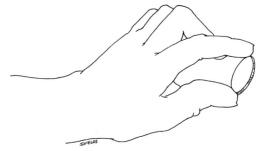

Figure 13-39.   Pinch grip.

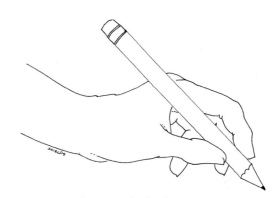

Figure 13-40.   Three-jaw chuck grip.

Examples of a hook grip are seen when holding on to a handle, such as on a suitcase, a wagon, or a bucket.

Precision Grips

Precision grips tend to hold the object between the tips of the fingers and the thumb. The intrinsic muscles are involved along with the extrinsics. The thumb tends to be abducted or opposed. These grips provide more fine movement and accuracy. The object is usually small, even fragile. The palm does not tend to be involved, and the proximal joints do not tend to move. There are four commonly recognized types of precision grip.

With the **pad-to-pad grip,** the MCP and PIP joints of the finger(s) are flexed, the thumb is abducted and opposed, and the distal joints of both are extended, bringing the pads of the finger(s) and thumb together. When it involves the thumb and one finger, usually the index finger, it is called a **pinch grip** (Fig. 13-39). It may also involve the thumb and two fingers, usually the index and middle fingers. This is called a **three-jaw chuck.** If you observe how a power drill holds the drill bit in place, you will see the similarity to this grip (Fig. 13-40). There are three "jaws" pinching in on the drill bit; the entire holding mechanism is called a *chuck.* Holding a pen or pencil would be an example of this grip. This is by far the most common precision grip.

Similar to the pad-to-pad grip, the **tip-to-tip grip** involves bringing the tip of the thumb up against the tip of another digit, usually the index finger, to pick up a small object such as a coin or a pin (see Fig. 13-34). It is also called **pincer grip.** This type of grip becomes difficult, if not impossible, with very long fingernails.

The **pad-to-side grip,** also called *lateral prehension,* has the pad of the extended thumb pressing an object against the radial side of the index finger (Fig. 13-41). This is a strong grip, but it allows less fine movements than the other two types. The terminal device of upper extremity prostheses adapts this type of grip. Also, because this grip does not require an opposed thumb, a person who has lost opposition but has retained thumb adduction can grasp and hold small objects.

The **side-to-side grip,** somewhat similar to pad-to-side grip, requires adduction of two fingers, usually the index or middle fingers (Fig. 13-42). It is a weak grip and does not permit much precision. It is perhaps most frequently used to hold a cigarette. It is also used to

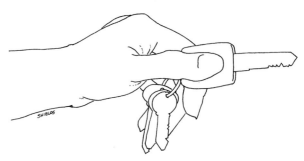

Figure 13-41.   Pad-to-side grip.

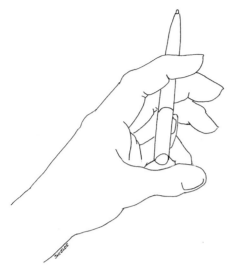

Figure 13-42.   Side-to-side grip.

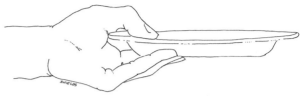

Figure 13-43.   Lumbrical grip.

hold an object, like a pencil, between two fingers while using another pencil or pen. Because the thumb is not involved, this grip could be used in the absence of the thumb.

The **lumbrical grip,** sometimes referred to as the **plate grip,** has the MCP flexed and the PIP and DIP joints extended. The thumb opposes the fingers holding an object horizontal (Fig. 13-43). This grip is usually used when something needs to be kept horizontal such as a plate or a tray. It is called a lumbrical grip because the action of the lumbrical muscles is to flex the MCP joints while extending the IP joints.

Points to Remember

- Isometric contractions are used to stabilize or hold a body part in position.
- Cylindrical, spherical, and hook grips are used for power hand movements.
- Pad-to-pad, pinch, three-jaw chuck, tip-to-tip, pad-to-side, side-to-side, and lumbrical grips are used for precision hand movements.
- A convex joint surface moves in the opposite direction of the body segment's movement.
- A concave joint surface moves in the same direction as the body segment's movement.
- In anatomical position, the sagittal plane divides the body into right and left parts. The frontal plane divides the body into front and back parts. The transverse plane divides the body into top and bottom parts.

Review Questions

General Anatomy Questions

1. Which finger and thumb motions occur in
   a. the frontal plane around the sagittal axis?
   b. the sagittal plane around the frontal axis?
   c. the transverse plane around the vertical axis?

2. Compare the thumb and fingers:
   a. Number of bones
      Thumb _____
      Finger _____
   b. Number of joints
      Thumb _____
      Finger _____
   c. Names of the joints
      Thumb _____
      Finger _____

3. Thumb opposition is a combination of what motions?

4. Which of the thumb opposition motions is an accessory motion?

5. What is the purpose of the retinaculum?

6. What structures make up the carpal tunnel? Which tendons and nerve run through the carpal tunnel?

7. What is an extrinsic muscle? List the extrinsic muscles of the hand.

Review Questions—cont'd

8. What is an intrinsic muscle? List the intrinsic muscles of the hand.

9. Explain the difference between thenar muscles and hypothenar muscles, and give an example of each.

10. What is the "anatomical snuffbox"? Which muscles act as the borders of this area?

11. What hand muscle does not have a bony attachment? To what two tendons does it attach?

12. a. What is the shape of the proximal end of the proximal phalange of the fingers?

    b. What is the shape of the distal end of the finger metacarpals?

    c. Is the joint surface of the proximal phalange moving in the same or opposite direction as the finger in MCP flexion/extension?

Functional Activity Questions

For Questions 1–9, identify the type of power or precision grip used in the following activities:

1. Holding the handle of a skillet

2. Pulling a little red wagon

3. Turning pages of a book

4. Fastening a snap or button

5. Carrying a coffee mug by its handle

6. Holding a hand of playing cards

7. Holding an apple

8. Holding on to a barbell

9. Picking up a CD

10. Analyze the following activity in terms of the entire upper extremity action. Hold an infant with your hands on either side of the infant's trunk so that you are looking eye-to-eye (Fig. 13-44).

    a. A combination of what two types of grasp is used?

    b. The wrist is being held in a neutral position by isometric contractions occurring in two different planes. What are the two muscle groups involved?

    c. Name the wrist muscle prime movers of these two muscles groups.

    d. The forearm is in midposition between pronation and supination. What muscle group is holding the elbow in position isometrically?

    e. Name the elbow prime movers of this muscle group.

    f. The shoulder joint is being held in position by isometric contractions occurring in two different planes. What are the two muscle groups involved?

    g. Name the shoulder prime movers of these two muscle groups.

    h. What shoulder girdle positions occur with the shoulder joint positions?

    i. Name the shoulder girdle prime movers.

Clinical Exercise Questions

Identify the joint motion and prime movers involved in the following exercises:

1. Keeping the fingers straight, spread them wide apart; bring them together.

2. With your forearm supinated and the thumb next to the radial side of the index finger, raise it straight up from the palm.

3. Touch the tip of your thumb to the tip of the little finger.

4. Keep the fingers straight and bend at the knuckles.

5. Starting with the thumb next to the radial side of the index finger, move it across the palm toward the little finger.

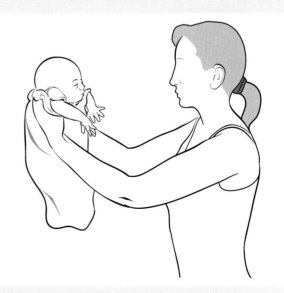

Figure 13-44.   Activity analysis: holding a baby.

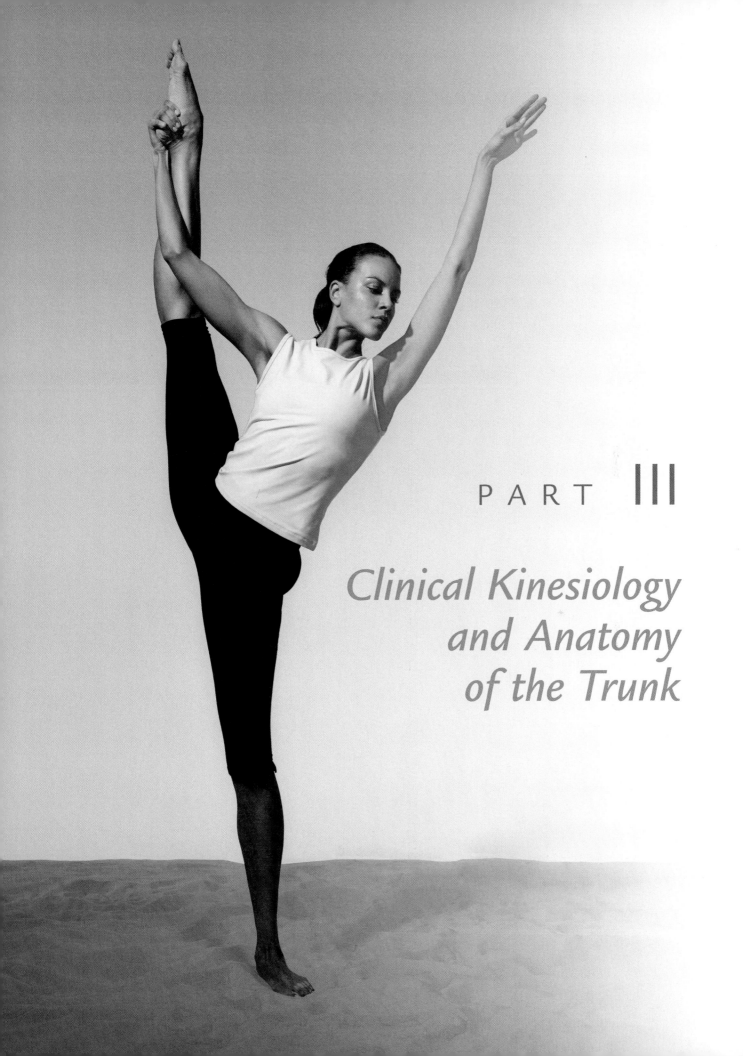

PART III

Clinical Kinesiology
and Anatomy
of the Trunk

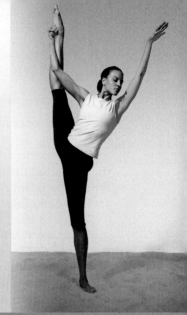

CHAPTER 14
Temporomandibular Joint

Joint Structure and Motions

Bones and Landmarks

Ligaments and Other Structures

Mechanics of Movement

Muscles of the TMJ

Anatomical Relationships

Summary of Muscle Action

Summary of Muscle Innervation

Points to Remember

Review Questions

General Anatomy Questions

Functional Activity Questions

Clinical Exercise Questions

Joint Structure and Motions

The temporomandibular joint, often referred to as the TMJ, is one of the most frequently used joints in the body. It is used during chewing, swallowing, yawning, talking, and any other activity involving jaw motion. The TMJ is located anterior to the ear and at the posterior superior end of the jaw (Fig. 14-1). It is made up of the articular fossa of the temporal bone superiorly, articulating with the condyle of the mandible inferiorly. The TMJ is a synovial joint and is best described as having a hingelike shape. Because it also allows some gliding motion, it is not a pure hinge joint.

The TMJ consists of two bones, a disk that divides the joint into two joint spaces, a joint capsule, four ligaments, and four main muscles that create five motions. As shown in Figure 14-2, the joint motions are

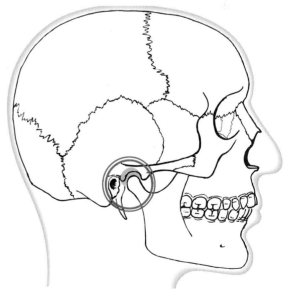

Figure 14-1. The temporomandibular joint (TMJ) is highlighted within the circle (lateral view).

depression (opening the mouth); **mandibular elevation** (closing the mouth); **lateral deviation** (side-to-side jaw movement); **protrusion,** or *protraction* (moving the jaw forward); and **retrusion,** or *retraction* (moving the jaw posteriorly). Retrusion is basically the return to anatomical position from a protruded position.

When the mandible is at rest, the condyle of the mandible is seated in the mandibular fossa of the temporal bone. The normal resting position of the mandible is lips closed and teeth several millimeters apart. This position is maintained by low levels of activity of the temporalis muscles. The mouth should open far enough for you to be able to put two to three fingers between the front upper and lower teeth.

Bones and Landmarks

The skull has two parts: the bones of the large cranium cavity, which encase the brain, and the bones of the face (Fig. 14-3). The TMJ is made up of the mandible, a facial bone articulating with the temporal bone, which is a cranial bone. Surrounding bones provide an area for muscle and ligament attachment. The following is a description of the bones and landmarks significant to the TMJ.

The **mandible,** or **mandibular bone** (Figs. 14-4 and 14-5), is shaped somewhat like a horseshoe and articulates with the temporal bone on each side of the face. It consists of a body and two upwardly projecting rami. Although the mandible is considered one bone, each lateral end articulates with a temporal bone, forming two identical joints on either side of the face. The mandible makes up the inferior part of the face and is often referred to as the *jaw* or *lower jaw.* Its significant landmarks are as follows:

Angle
Located between the body and the ramus, it is the joining point of the two landmarks. It is often referred to as the *angle of the ramus.*

Body
The horizontal portion of the mandible; the superior surface of the body holds the lower teeth.

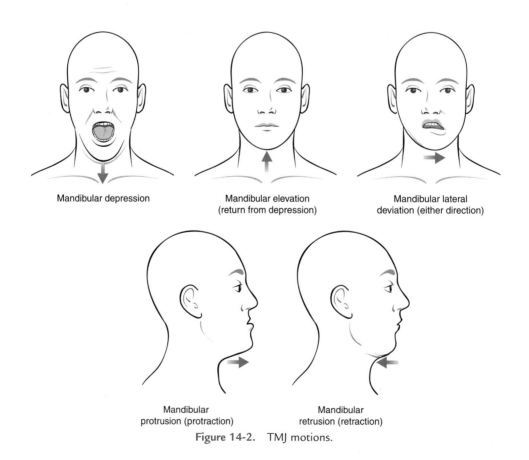

Mandibular depression

Mandibular elevation
(return from depression)

Mandibular lateral
deviation (either direction)

Mandibular
protrusion (protraction)

Mandibular
retrusion (retraction)

Figure 14-2.   TMJ motions.

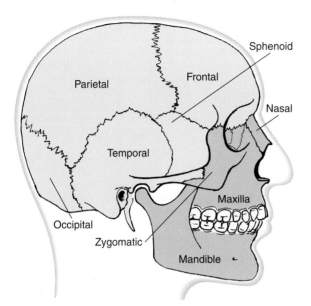

Figure 14-3.   Bones of the skull (lateral view).

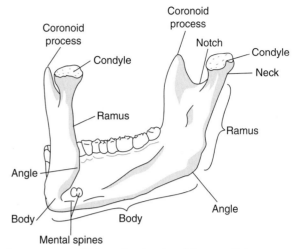

Figure 14-5.   The bony landmarks of the mandible. Posterior and slightly lateral view.

Condyle
Also called the *condylar process*. It is the posterior projection on the ramus, and it articulates with the temporal bone.

Coronoid Process
Located anterior to the condyle on the ramus. It serves as an attachment for the masseter muscle.

Mental Spine
Located on the interior side (inside) of the mandible near the midline. It serves as an attachment for the geniohyoid muscle.

Neck
Located just inferior to the condyle.

Notch
Located between the condyle and coronoid process on the ramus.

Ramus
The vertical portion of the mandible from the angle to the condyle.

The **temporal bone** is located on the side of the skull posterior to the zygomatic bone, inferior to the parietal bone, posterior to the greater wing of the sphenoid, and anterior to the occipital bone (see Fig. 14-3). The articular portion of the temporal bone consists of the concave articular (mandibular) fossa in the middle, with the convex articular tubercle located anteriorly and the convex postglenoid tubercle located posteriorly (Fig. 14-6). Its main landmarks consist of:

Articular Tubercle
Makes up the anterior portion of the articulating surface of the temporal bone. When the mandible is depressed, the condyle of the mandible rests under this landmark.

Articular Fossa
Also called the *mandibular fossa*, it lies anterior to the external auditory meatus and articulates with the condyle of the mandible.

Postglenoid Tubercle
Makes up the posterior wall of the fossa and is located just anterior to the external auditory meatus.

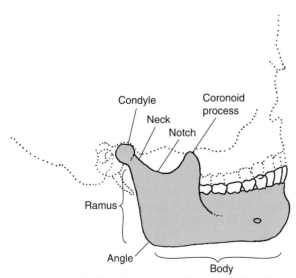

Figure 14-4.   The bony landmarks of the mandible (right lateral view).

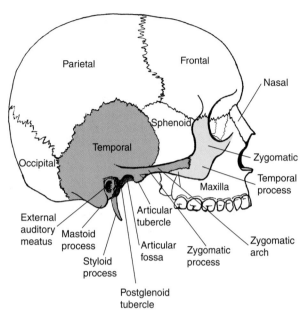

Figure 14-6. The bony landmarks of the temporal and zygomatic bones. Right lateral view of skull with mandible removed.

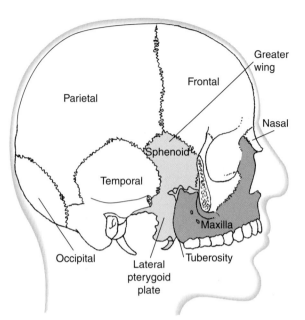

Figure 14-7. Sphenoid and maxillary bones. Right lateral view with zygomatic arch removed.

Styloid Process

A slender projection positioned down and forward from the temporal bone on the inferior, slightly interior, surface. It serves as attachment for various muscles and ligaments.

Mastoid Process

Bony prominence posterior and inferior to the ear to which the digastric muscle attaches.

External Auditory Meatus

The external opening for the ear, located posterior to the TMJ.

Zygomatic Process

Makes up the posterior portion of the zygomatic arch. It serves as the attachment for the masseter.

The **sphenoid bone** is located at the lateral base of the skull anterior to the temporal bone. It resembles a bat with extended wings (Fig. 14-7). Because of its location, the sphenoid bone connects with six other cranial bones and two facial bones. Only the following external surface features are relevant to TMJ function:

Greater Wing

A large bony process located medially to the zygomatic bone and arch, and anteriorly to the rest of the temporal bone. As part of the temporal fossa, it provides attachment for the temporalis and lateral pterygoid muscles.

Lateral Pterygoid Plate

Lies deep to the zygomatic arch. It serves as an attachment for the lateral and medial pterygoid muscles.

Spine

Lies deep to the articular fossa of the temporal bone and provides attachment for the sphenomandibular ligament.

The **zygomatic bone** forms the prominence of the cheek and contributes the lateral wall and floor of the eye orbit (see Fig. 14-6). The frontal, maxilla, sphenoid, and temporal bones border it. The zygomatic bone, along with the zygomatic process of the temporal bone, forms the zygomatic arch, to which the masseter attaches. Only the following features are relevant to TMJ function:

Temporal Process

Lies posterior and inferior and joins with the zygomatic process of the temporal bone to form the zygomatic arch.

The following are made up of combinations of skull bones:

Temporal Fossa (Fig. 14-8)

Bony floor formed by the zygomatic, frontal, parietal, sphenoid, and temporal bones. It contains the attachment of the temporalis muscle.

Zygomatic Arch (see Fig 14-6)

Formed by two bones: the zygomatic process of the temporal bone posteriorly and the temporal process of the zygomatic bone anteriorly.

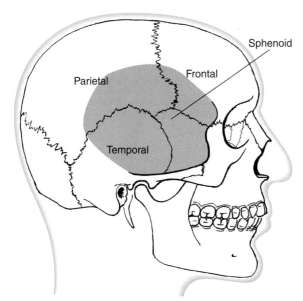

Figure 14-8. Temporal fossa includes portions of the temporal, parietal, frontal, and sphenoid bones (lateral view).

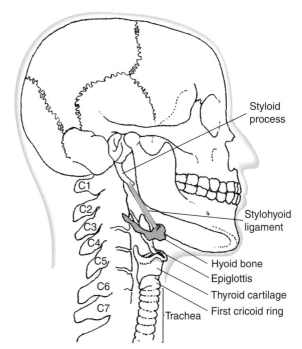

Figure 14-9. The hyoid bone is suspended from the styloid process of the temporal bone by the stylohyoid ligament (right side view).

The **maxilla** or **maxillary bone** is commonly called the *upper jaw.* It is located in the upper part of the face and houses the upper teeth. It connects with the nasal bone superiorly and with the zygomatic bone laterally (see Fig. 14-7). Its main landmark is:

Tuberosity
A rounded projection located on the inferior posterior angle. It serves as attachment for the medial pterygoid.

The **hyoid bone** is a horseshoe-shaped bone lying just superior to the thyroid cartilage at about the level of C3. It has no bony articulation but is suspended from the styloid processes of the temporal bones by the stylohyoid ligaments (Fig. 14-9). Its main function is to provide attachment for the tongue muscles. However, it also provides attachment for the suprahyoid and infrahyoid muscles that assist in mandibular depression.

The **thyroid cartilage** is the largest of the nine cartilages of the larynx. It is commonly called the "Adam's apple" and tends to be more prominent in males. It lies just inferior to the hyoid bone at about the level of C3 to C4 (see Fig. 14-9). It provides attachment for the infrahyoid muscles.

Ligaments and Other Structures

The **lateral ligament** is also known as the **temporomandibular ligament.** Anteriorly, it attaches on the neck of the mandibular condyle and disk, and then runs superiorly to the articular tubercle of the temporal bone (Fig. 14-10). It limits downward, posterior, and lateral motions of the mandible.

The **sphenomandibular ligament** attaches to the spine of the sphenoid bone and runs to the middle of the ramus on the internal surface of the mandible (see Figs. 14-10 and 14-11). It suspends the mandible and limits excessive anterior motion.

The **stylomandibular ligament** runs from the styloid process of the temporal bone to the posterior inferior border of the mandible's ramus (see Figs. 14-10 and 14-11). It lies between the masseter and medial pterygoid muscles and plays a role in limiting excessive anterior motion.

The **stylohyoid ligament** attaches from the styloid process of the temporal bone to the hyoid bone (see Fig. 14-9). Its function is to hold the hyoid bone in place.

The **joint capsule** envelops the TMJ by attaching superiorly to the articular tubercle and borders of the fossa of the temporal bone. Inferiorly, it attaches to the neck of the condyle of the mandible (see Figs. 14-10 and 14-11).

The **articular disk** of the TMJ is similar to the articular disk of the sternoclavicular joint. It is connected circumferentially to the capsule and tendon of

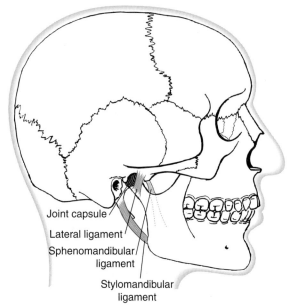

Figure 14-10. The ligaments that suspend and/or limit excessive motion of the mandible (right lateral view). Dotted lines show the sphenomandibular ligament (distal attachment on medial side).

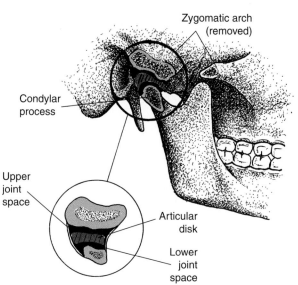

Figure 14-12. Lateral view of the right TMJ with zygomatic arch removed and condylar process cut. This shows the relationship of the mandibular condyle, disk, and articular fossa in a closed-jaw position. The articular disk divides the joint space into upper and lower spaces.

the lateral pterygoid (Fig. 14-12). It also divides the joint space into two separate compartments: a larger upper joint space and a smaller lower joint space. The superior surface is both concave and convex to accommodate the shape of the fossa. The concave inferior surface of the articular disk accommodates the convex surface of the condyle and allows the joint to remain congruent (compatible) throughout the motion. The disk's shape and attachments also allow it to rotate in an anterior/posterior direction on the condyle. Because the articular disk is more firmly attached to the mandible than the temporal bone, it allows the disk to move forward with the condyle of the mandible when the mouth opens. It returns posteriorly when the mouth closes.

Mechanics of Movement

Depression of the mandible (opening the jaw) involves two motions (Fig. 14-13). The first part is accomplished by anterior rotation of the mandibular condyle on the disk (see Fig. 14-3A). The second part of the motion involves sliding the disk and condyle forward and downward under the articular tubercle (see Fig. 14-3B). Elevation of the mandible (closing the jaw) is the reverse action. It involves sliding the disk and condyle posteriorly and superiorly, which rotates the condyle posteriorly on the disk. These movements occur in the sagittal plane.

Protrusion and retrusion involve anterior/posterior movement in the horizontal plane. There is no rotation. Forward and backward motion of all parts of the mandible is equal. The mandibular condyle and disk move as one unit against the articular fossa of the temporal bone.

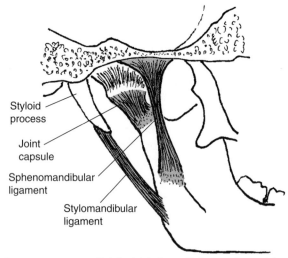

Figure 14-11. Medial (inside) view of left TMJ shows joint capsule and ligaments. Lateral ligament is not visible from this view.

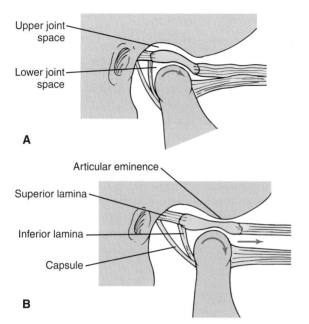

Figure 14-13. Joint motion during mandibular depression (mouth opening). **(A)** The condyle first rotates in the mandibular fossa, and **(B)** the condyle then glides downward and forward over the articular tubercle.

Lateral movement also occurs in the horizontal plane. It involves one condyle rotating in the articular fossa while the other condyle glides forward. To move the mandible toward the left, the left condyle will spin and the right condyle will glide forward (Fig. 14-14). This rotation occurs around a vertical axis.

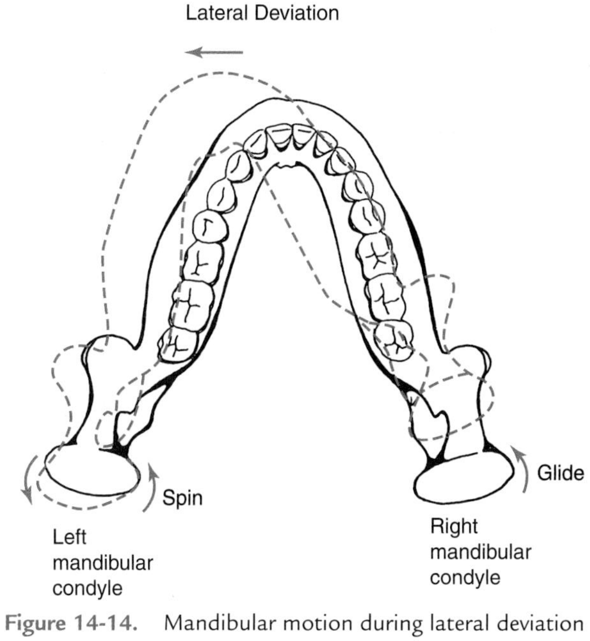

Lateral Deviation

Figure 14-14. Mandibular motion during lateral deviation to the left side (superior view).

Muscles of the TMJ

The TMJ is involved in activities such as talking, chewing, biting, swallowing, and yawning. Several muscles come into play, often synergistically. The muscles primarily involved are listed below. Unless stated otherwise, the action is considered to be bilateral and occurs at each joint (right and left) simultaneously.

Temporalis	Medial pterygoid
Masseter	Lateral pterygoid

Other muscles involved in TMJ movements are the following:

Suprahyoid muscles	Infrahyoid muscles
Mylohyoid	Sternohyoid
Geniohyoid	Sternothyroid
Stylohyoid	Thyrohyoid
Digastric	Omohyoid

The **temporalis** is a rather broad and fan-shaped muscle that lies in the temporal fossa (see Figs. 14-8 and 14-15). Because of its fan shape, the more anterior fibers run almost vertically, the middle fibers are at a diagonal, and the posterior fibers are nearly horizontal. From the temporal fossa, the fibers come together to form a tendon that passes deep to the zygomatic arch to insert on the coronoid process and anterior border of the ramus of the mandible. Its primary function is to elevate the mandible. Because of the horizontal direction of the posterior fibers, they also retract the jaw. In side-to-side movements, the temporalis contracts on one side, moving the mandible to the same side (ipsilaterally).

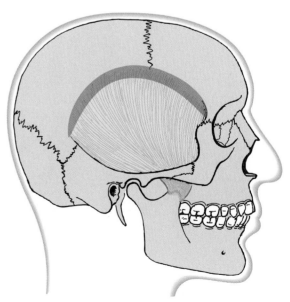

Figure 14-15. Temporalis muscle (lateral view).

Temporalis Muscle

O	Temporal fossa
I	Coronoid process and ramus of mandible
A	Bilaterally: elevation, retrusion (posterior fibers) Unilaterally: ipsilateral lateral deviation
N	Trigeminal nerve (cranial nerve V)

The powerful **masseter** is a thick, almost quadrilateral-shaped muscle that produces the fullness of the posterior part of the cheek between the mandibular angle and zygomatic arch (Fig. 14-16). It is made up of two parts: the larger, superficial part, and the smaller, deep portion. The superficial part arises from the zygomatic process of the maxilla and the inferior border of the zygomatic arch of the temporal bone. The deep part comes from the inferior and medial borders of the zygomatic arch. The two parts run inferiorly and posteriorly, coming together to attach on the angle of the ramus and coronoid process of the mandible. Both parts act as one muscle to elevate the mandible (close the jaw). Acting unilaterally, the masseter is an ipsilateral (same side) lateral deviator.

Masseter Muscle

O	Zygomatic arch of temporal bone and zygomatic process of maxilla
I	Angle of the ramus and coronoid process of mandible
A	Bilaterally: elevation Unilaterally: ipsilateral lateral deviation
N	Trigeminal nerve (cranial nerve V)

Although it is less powerful, the **medial pterygoid** is very similar to the masseter muscle. The medial pterygoid is located on the medial side (inside) of the mandibular ramus (Fig. 14-17), while the more superficial masseter is on the lateral side (outside). The medial pterygoid arises from the medial side of the lateral pterygoid plate of the sphenoid bone and the tuberosity of the maxilla. It runs inferiorly, laterally, and posteriorly to attach on the medial side of the ramus and angle of the mandible (Fig. 14-18). Its actions are mandibular elevation, protrusion, and contralateral (opposite side) lateral deviation.

Medial Pterygoid Muscle

O	Lateral pterygoid plate of the sphenoid bone and tuberosity of the maxilla
I	Ramus and angle of the mandible
A	Bilaterally: elevation, protrusion Unilaterally: contralateral lateral deviation
N	Trigeminal nerve (cranial nerve V)

The **lateral pterygoid** muscle is short, thick, and somewhat cone-shaped. It has two heads: superior and inferior. The superior part comes off the lateral surface of the greater wing of the sphenoid bone. The inferior,

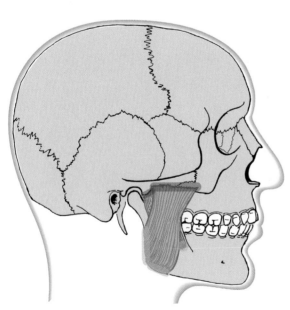

Figure 14-16.   Masseter muscle (lateral view).

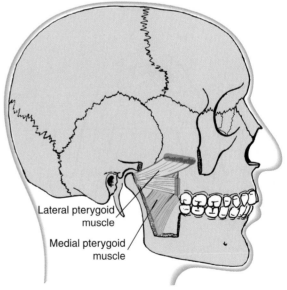

Lateral pterygoid muscle

Medial pterygoid muscle

Figure 14-17.   Lateral and medial pterygoid muscles (lateral view). The mandible and zygomatic arch are cut to show inside the mandible.

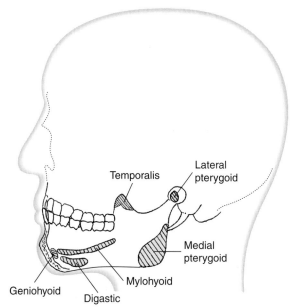

Figure 14-18. Medial (inside) view of mandible showing muscle attachments.

more horizontal part comes off the lateral surface of the lateral pterygoid plate. Both parts run nearly horizontal in a posterior and lateral direction. They attach on the neck of the mandibular condyle, the articular disk, and the capsule (see Figs. 14-17 and 14-18). This muscle depresses, protrudes, and laterally deviates the mandible to the opposite side (contralateral).

Lateral Pterygoid Muscle

O	Lateral pterygoid plate and greater wing of the sphenoid
I	Mandibular condyle and articular disk
A	Bilaterally: depression, protrusion Unilaterally: contralateral lateral deviation
N	Trigeminal nerve (cranial nerve V)

The **suprahyoid muscles,** as their name implies, are a group of muscles located above the hyoid bone. They connect the hyoid bone to the skull, primarily to the mandible. Individually, these muscles are known as the mylohyoid, geniohyoid, stylohyoid, and digastric muscles. Although their primary function is to elevate the hyoid, they can assist in mandibular depression when the infrahyoid muscles stabilize the hyoid bone. Therefore, these muscles will be described here in terms of their importance to the TMJ only.

The **mylohyoid** is a broad muscle that runs from the interior (inside) medial part of the mandible to the superior border of the hyoid bone (Figs. 14-18

through 14-20). The **geniohyoid** is a narrow muscle located superior to the mylohyoid (see Fig. 14-19). It attaches to the mental spine on the inside midline of the mandible and runs down to the hyoid. In Figure 14-20, the geniohyoid can be seen on the right side with the mylohyoid and digastric muscles reflected out of the way. In this view from under the mandible, the geniohyoid muscle is deep to the mylohyoid. The **digastric** muscle has two bellies connected in the middle by a tendon (Figs. 14-20 and 14-21). The anterior belly goes from the internal inferior surface of the mandible near the midline posteriorly and inferiorly, where it attaches to the tendinous inscription at the hyoid bone. The tendon is held in place by a fibrous sling attached to the hyoid bone. From this point, the posterior belly runs posterior and superior to attach to the mastoid process of the temporal bone. This pulleylike tendon is an example of how a muscle changes its line of pull. The **stylohyoid** is almost parallel to the digastric muscle. It attaches to the styloid process of the temporal bone and goes to the hyoid bone (see Fig. 14-20).

Mylohyoid Muscle

O	Interior medial mandible
I	Hyoid
A	Assists in depressing mandible
N	Branch of trigeminal nerve (cranial nerve V)

Geniohyoid Muscle

O	Mental spine of mandible
I	Hyoid
A	Assists in depressing mandible
N	Branch of C1 via hypoglossal nerve (cranial nerve XII)

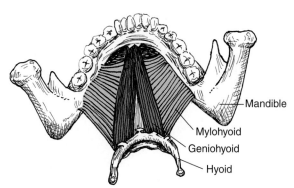

Figure 14-19. Muscles of the floor of the mouth. Posterior, superior view (looking down toward the front inside of the mandible).

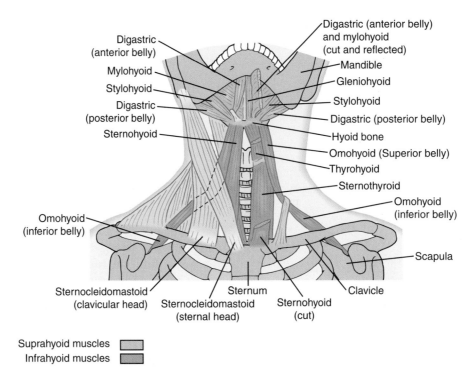

Figure 14-20.   The suprahyoid and infrahyoid muscles

Stylohyoid Muscle

O	Styloid process of temporal bone
I	Hyoid
A	Assists in depressing mandible
N	Branch of facial nerve (cranial nerve VII)

Digastric Muscle

O	Anterior: internal inferior mandible
	Posterior: mastoid process
I	Via pulleylike tendon to hyoid
A	Assists in depressing mandible
N	Branch of trigeminal nerve (cranial nerve V) and branch of facial nerve (cranial nerve VII)

As their name implies, the **infrahyoid muscles** are located below the hyoid bone and serve to depress it (see Fig. 14-20). Individually, these muscles are known as the sternohyoid, sternothyroid, thyrohyoid, and omohyoid muscles. They stabilize the hyoid bone, allowing the suprahyoid muscles to depress the mandible. These muscles will be described here in terms of their importance to the TMJ only.

The **sternohyoid** is a thin, narrow muscle that runs vertically next to the midline from the posterior aspect of the medial end of the clavicle, sternoclavicular ligament, and sternal manubrium. It is covered distally by the sternocleidomastoid muscle. Like all the infrahyoid muscles, the sternohyoid attaches to the inferior border of the hyoid bone. The **sternothyroid muscle** is shorter, wider, and lies deep to the sternohyoid, running vertically from the sternal manubrium and cartilage of the first rib to the thyroid cartilage. It indirectly pulls down on the hyoid bone by pulling down on the thyroid

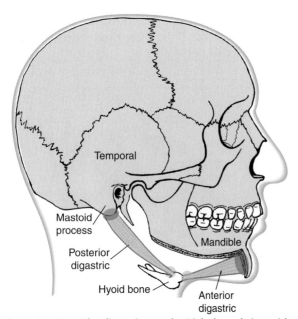

Figure 14-21.   The digastric muscle. Right lateral view with the mandible cut away to show anterior attachment.

cartilage, which, in turn, is connected to the hyoid bone via the thyrohyoid muscle. The **thyrohyoid** is a short, rectangular muscle that acts much like a continuation of the sternothyroid muscle. It runs vertically from the thyroid cartilage to the inferior border of the hyoid bone. The thyrohyoid serves to close the laryngeal opening, thus preventing food from entering the larynx during swallowing. In terms of the TMJ, it pulls down on the hyoid bone, stabilizing it so that the suprahyoid muscles can assist in depressing the jaw.

The **omohyoid** has two bellies connected by a tendon in between, much like the digastric muscle. The inferior belly comes off the superior border of the scapula and runs mostly horizontally. At the tendinous insertion, the muscle changes direction and the superior belly runs mostly vertically to the inferior border of the hyoid bone. The tendon is held in place by a fibrous sling attached to the clavicle that allows the muscle to make an almost right-angle turn. This is another example of an internal fixed pulley changing a muscle's line of pull. This muscle also stabilizes the hyoid bone by pulling down on it.

Sternohyoid Muscle

O	Medial end of clavicle, sternoclavicular ligament, and manubrium of sternum
I	Inferior border of hyoid bone
A	Stabilize hyoid bone
N	Branch of hypoglossal nerve (cranial nerve XII) communicating with C1 to C3

Sternothyroid Muscle

O	Manubrium of sternum and cartilage of the first rib
I	Thyroid cartilage
A	Stabilize hyoid bone
N	Branch of hypoglossal nerve (cranial nerve XII) communicating with C1 to C3

Thyrohyoid Muscle

O	Thyroid cartilage
I	Inferior border of hyoid bone
A	Stabilize hyoid bone
N	Branch of hypoglossal nerve (cranial nerve XII) communicating with C1

Omohyoid Muscle

O	Superior border of the scapula
I	Inferior border of hyoid bone
A	Stabilize hyoid bone
N	Branch of hypoglossal (cranial nerve XII) communicating with C1 to C3

Anatomical Relationships

There are four prime movers of the temporomandibular joint and many assistive movers. The temporalis and masseter are most superficial. The muscle belly of the temporalis lies above the zygomatic arch, and the belly of the masseter lies below (Fig. 14-22). Deep to these muscles at the level of the zygomatic arch and inside the mandible are the lateral and medial pterygoids. The medial pterygoid is deep to the lateral pterygoid (Fig. 14-23).

Also deep to the masseter and lying in a horizontal direction is the buccinator muscle. It is not considered a muscle of the TMJ because it does not cross the joint. However, it does play an assistive role in chewing by pressing the cheeks against the teeth. It forms the lateral

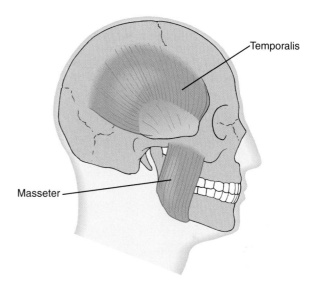

Figure 14-22. The temporalis and masseter muscles

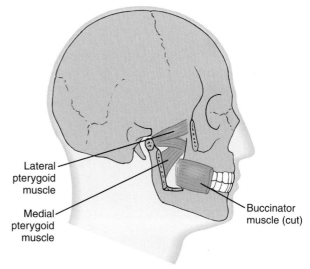

Figure 14-23. The pterygoid and buccinator muscles.

wall of the mouth and is better known as the "whistling" muscle, because it compresses the cheeks. The buccinator basically runs from the lips posteriorly to just below and above the molars on the mandible and maxilla, respectively (see Fig. 14-23).

There are two groups of assistive muscles: the suprahyoid and infrahyoid (see Fig. 14-20). These are deep muscles that work as a team to assist in mandibular depression. The infrahyoid group stabilizes the hyoid muscle. With the suprahyoid group's distal attachment stabilized, they can assist in mandibular depression.

Summary of Muscle Action

Table 14-1 summarizes the actions of the prime movers of the temporomandibular joint.

Summary of Muscle Innervation

Innervation of the TMJ muscles comes from cranial nerve V, the trigeminal nerve. If the assisting muscles of the suprahyoid and infrahyoid group are included, innervation additionally comes from cranial nerves VII and XII (the facial and hypoglossal nerves, respectively). The hypoglossal nerve communicates with the first three cervical nerves as well. Table 14-2 summarizes the innervation of all TMJ muscles.

Points to Remember
- The trigeminal nerve is the fifth cranial nerve, which has both sensory and motor components.
- The sensory component of the trigeminal nerves involves the facial area, while the motor component involves the chewing muscles.
- The facial nerve is the seventh cranial nerve, which also has sensory and motor components.
- The sensory component of the facial nerve involves the tongue area, whereas the motor component involves the muscles of the face.

Table 14-1 Prime Movers of the TMJ Joint

Mandibular Action	Muscle
Elevation	Temporalis, masseter, medial pterygoid
Depression	Lateral pterygoid
Protrusion	Lateral pterygoid, medial pterygoid
Retrusion	Temporalis (posterior)
Ipsilateral lateral deviation	Temporalis, masseter
Contralateral lateral deviation	Medial pterygoid, lateral pterygoid

Table 14-2 Innervation of TMJ Muscles

Muscle	Nerve	Cranial Nerve Number
Temporalis	Trigeminal	CN 5
Masseter	Trigeminal	CN 5
Lateral pterygoid	Trigeminal	CN 5
Medial pterygoid	Trigeminal	CN 5
Suprahyoid group		
Mylohyoid	Trigeminal	CN 5
Geniohyoid	C1, hypoglossal	CN 12
Stylohyoid	Facial	CN 7
Digastric	Trigeminal, facial	CN 5, 7
Infrahyoid group		
Sternohyoid	C1 to C3, hypoglossal	CN 12
Sternothyroid	C1 to C3, hypoglossal	CN 12
Thyrohyoid	C1, hypoglossal	CN 12
Omohyoid	C1 to C3, hypoglossal	CN 12

Review Questions

General Anatomy Questions

1. The zygomatic arch is made up of which two bones?

2. What are synonymous terms for the following TMJ motions?
   a. Opening the jaw
   b. Closing the jaw
   c. Moving the jaw posteriorly
   d. Moving the jaw anteriorly
   e. Moving the jaw toward the side

3. What two bones make up the temporomandibular joint?

4. What muscle can be palpated superior and anterior to the ear?

5. What muscle makes up the fullness of the posterior portion of the cheek?

6. What muscles work like a pulley?

7. If the fifth and seventh cranial nerves were damaged, which would impair function of the TMJ more?

8. Two motions occur during mandibular depression: (1) the disk and condyle glide forward and inferiorly, and (2) the mandible rotates anteriorly on the disk. Which occurs first?

9. Lateral deviation of the mandible to the left involves both spinning and gliding motions. Describe how that happens.

10. What is another term for "Adam's apple"?

Functional Activity Questions

1. Forming the letter *O* with your lips requires what motion of the TMJ?

2. Biting off a tough piece of bread is usually done by placing it in one side of the mouth.
   a. The biting action requires what motion of the TMJ?
   b. Which side of the jaw experiences some distraction?
   c. Which side of the jaw experiences some compression?

3. Grinding your teeth could involve motions in the sagittal plane and frontal plane. What are these motions?

4. Clenching your teeth requires what TMJ motion and involves what muscles?

Clinical Exercise Questions

1. Sit in a good posture position with your hands on each side of your jaw. Move your jaw from side to side against slight resistance.
   a. What is the joint motion?
   b. What type of contraction (isometric, concentric, or eccentric) is occurring?
   c. Name the muscles responsible for moving the jaw to the right.

2. Sit in a good posture position with your index and middle fingers on the anterior surface of your lower jaw in the midline. Without allowing your fingers to move, push against them with your lower jaw.
   a. What is the joint motion?
   b. What type of muscle contraction (isometric, concentric, or eccentric) is occurring?
   c. Name the muscles responsible for moving the jaw to the right.

3. Sit in a good posture position with your thumb beneath your chin. Open your mouth against slight pressure (Fig. 14-24).
   a. What is the joint motion?
   b. What type of muscle contraction (isometric, concentric, or eccentric) is occurring?
   c. Name the muscle responsible for moving the mouth.

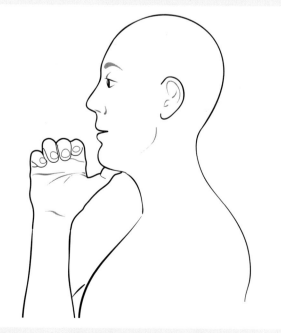

Figure 14-24.   Opening mouth against slight pressure.

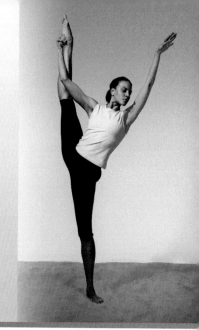

CHAPTER 15
Neck and Trunk

Vertebral Curves

Clarification of Terms

Joint Motions

Bones and Landmarks

Joints and Ligaments

Muscles of the Neck and Trunk

Muscles of the Cervical Spine

Muscles of the Trunk

Anatomical Relationships

Summary of Muscle Actions

Summary of Muscle Innervation

Common Vertebral Column Pathologies

Points to Remember

Review Questions

General Anatomy Questions

Functional Activity Questions

Clinical Exercise Questions

The vertebral column establishes and maintains the longitudinal axis of the body. Because it is a multijointed rod, the motions of the column occur due to the combined motions of individual vertebrae.

The spinal column provides a pivot point for motion and support of the head at the cervical region. The weight of the head, shoulder girdle, upper extremities, and trunk are transmitted through the vertebral column. The vertebral column encases the spinal cord and is therefore able to protect it. Not only does this multijointed rod provide movement, but also the arrangement of these segments provides effective shock absorption and transmission.

The skull sits atop the vertebral column. Divided into the bones of the cranium, the skull is the bony structure of the head, containing and protecting the brain and the facial bones. Because the sensory organs for sight, hearing, taste, and vestibular responses are located within the cranium and head, it is important that the head be able to move freely. This occurs through movements at various levels of the cervical spine.

Vertebral Curves

The vertebrae are arranged in a manner that forms anterior-posterior (concave-convex) curves in the vertebral column, which can be seen from the side (Fig. 15-1). These curves provide the vertebral column with much more strength and resilience, approximately 10 times more than if it were a straight rod. Table 15-1 summarizes the curves of the vertebral column.

Clarification of Terms

The term *spine* can be used in more than one way. The spinal cord, sometimes called the *spine*, is made of nervous tissue. The *spine, spinal column,* and *vertebral column* are synonymous terms referring to the bony components

211

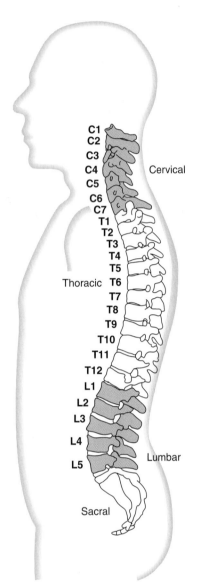

Figure 15-1. The anterior-posterior curves of the vertebral column (lateral view).

housing the spinal cord. This chapter discusses the spine as a bony structure.

Another term that needs clarification is *facet*. A **facet** is a small, smooth, flat surface on a bone. Facets, as will be discussed, are found on thoracic vertebrae at the

point of contact with a rib (see Fig. 15-9). A **facet joint** is the articulation between the superior articular process of the vertebra below with the inferior articular process of the vertebra above (see Fig. 15-5).

Joint Motions

The vertebral column as a whole is considered to be triaxial. Therefore, it has movement in all three planes (Fig. 15-2). **Flexion, extension,** and **hyperextension** occur in the sagittal plane around a frontal axis. **Lateral bending,** also called *side bending* or *lateral flexion,* occurs in the frontal plane around a sagittal axis. It always occurs toward the same side. **Rotation** occurs in the transverse plane around a vertical axis, except between the skull and the atlas (C1). No rotation occurs at this joint. Alignment of the facet joints will greatly determine the amount of rotation and other motions possible.

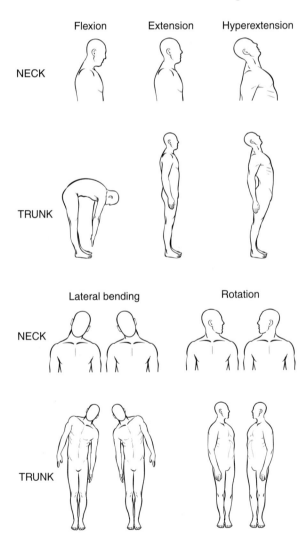

Figure 15-2. Motions of the neck and trunk.

Table 15-1	Vertebral Segments	
Segment	**Number**	**Anterior Curve**
Cervical	7	Convex
Thoracic	12	Concave
Lumbar	5	Convex
Sacral	5 (fused)	Concave

The cervical spine allows movement and positioning of the head, and it requires additional explanation. The articulation between the head and C1 (atlas) is often called the **atlanto-occipital joint.** The main motion here is **flexion** and **extension,** as when nodding your head in agreement. There is some lateral bending that also occurs between C1 and C2 (the atlantoaxial joint). Most **rotation** of the head on the neck, as in shaking your head in disagreement, occurs at the **atlantoaxial joint.** The muscles having the most control over moving the head on the neck are the prevertebral muscles anteriorly and the suboccipital muscles posteriorly. Obviously, to have the ability to move the head on the neck, a muscle must have an attachment on the head and on the cervical region. Tucking your chin in involves the head flexing on C1, as well as the neck (C2–C7) extending. This combined motion is sometimes referred to as **axial extension,** or *cervical retraction.* Conversely, extending the head on C1 and flexing the neck (C2–C7) is *cervical protraction.* A relaxed forward head posture or looking at a computer screen through bifocals tends to accentuate cervical protraction. "Standing up straight" emphasizes axial extension.

Bones and Landmarks

The skull is made up of 21 separate bones and is considered to be the skeleton of the head (Fig. 15-3A and B). We will discuss only those bones directly connected with the vertebral column:

Occipital Bone
Also called the occiput, it forms the posterior inferior part of the cranium.

Occipital Protuberance
The small prominence in the center of the occiput.

Nuchal Line
The ridge running horizontally along the back of the head from the occipital protuberance toward the mastoid processes.

Basilar Area
Refers to the base, or inferior, portion of the occiput.

Foramen Magnum
Opening in the occipital bone through which the spinal cord enters the cranium.

Occipital Condyles
Located lateral to the foramen magnum on the occiput; provides articulation with the atlas (C1).

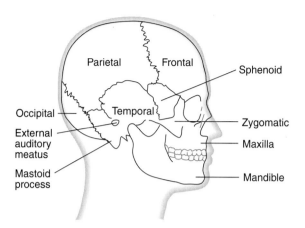

A

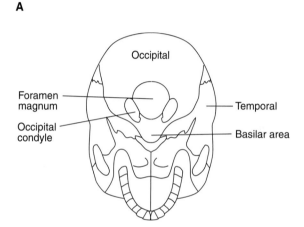

B

Figure 15-3.   The bones of the skull as viewed from **(A)** the lateral view and **(B)** below the base of the skull.

Temporal Bone
Forms part of the base and lateral inferior sides of the cranium.

Mastoid Process
Bony prominence behind the ear to which the sternocleidomastoid muscle attaches.

Vertebrae (plural of *vertebra*) differ in size and shape but generally have the same layout (Fig. 15-4). The typical parts of a vertebra are as follows:

Body
Being primarily a cylindrical mass of cancellous bone, it is the anterior portion of the vertebra and the major weight-bearing structure. It is not present in the atlas (C1) (see Fig. 15-7). Between C3 and S1, bodies become progressively larger, bearing progressively more weight (see Fig. 15-10).

Neural Arch
Also called the *vertebral arch,* it is the posterior portion of the vertebra with many different parts.

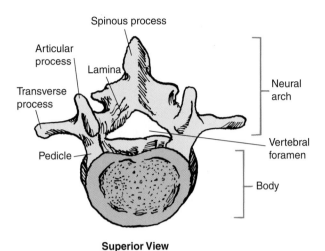

Superior View

Figure 15-4.   The body landmarks of the anterior and posterior portions of a typical vertebra.

Vertebral Foramen
Opening formed by the joining of the body and neural arch through which the spinal cord passes.

Pedicle
Portion of the neural arch just posterior to the body and anterior to the lamina.

Lamina
Posterior portion of the neural arch that unites from each side in the midline.

Transverse Process
Formed at the union of the lamina and pedicle, the lateral projections of the arch to which muscles and ligaments attach.

Vertebral Notches
Depressions located on the superior and inferior surfaces of the pedicle, and are so named (see Fig. 15-10).

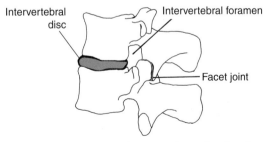

Figure 15-5.   Lateral view of two vertebrae showing the intervertebral foramen and the facet joint. Both are formed by parts from each vertebra. The vertebrae are separated anteriorly by the intervertebral disk.

Intervertebral Foramen (Fig. 15-5)
Opening formed by the superior vertebral notch of the vertebra below and the inferior vertebral notch of the vertebra above.

Articular Process
Projecting superiorly and inferiorly off the posterior surface of each lamina, and so named. Superior articular processes face posteriorly or medially, whereas inferior processes face anteriorly or laterally (see Fig. 15-10).

Spinous Process
The most posterior projection on the neural arch; located at the junction of the two laminae. It serves as a point of attachment for many muscles and ligaments and can be palpated throughout the length of the vertebral column.

Between vertebrae is an **intervertebral disk** that articulates with adjacent bodies (see Figs. 15-5 and 15-6). There are 23 disks beginning between C2 and C3. Their

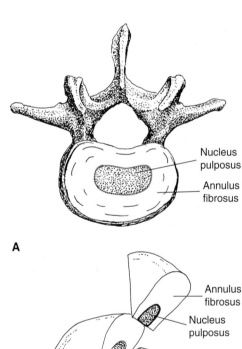

Figure 15-6.   The two parts of the intervertebral disk. **(A)** Viewed from above, the nucleus pulposus cannot be seen, as it is surrounded by the annulus fibrosus. Its approximate location is shown within the red line. **(B)** The longitudinal section view shows the relationship between the annulus fibrosus and the nucleus pulposus.

main function is to absorb and transmit shock and maintain flexibility of the vertebral column. The disks make up approximately 25% of the total length of the vertebral column.

Annulus Fibrosus
The outer portion of the disk consisting of several concentrically arranged fibrocartilaginous rings that serve to contain the nucleus pulposus (see Fig. 15-6).

Nucleus Pulposus
Pulpy, gelatinous substance with a high water content in the center of the disk (see Fig. 15-6). At birth, it is approximately 80% water, decreasing to less than 70% at 60 years of age. This is partially why an individual loses height with advanced age.

There are a few vertebrae with distinguishing characteristics that must be identified. They are as follows:

Atlas (C1)
The first cervical vertebra upon which the cranium rests (Fig. 15-7). Because it supports the globe of the head, it is named after the Titan in Greek mythology who held up the earth. The atlas is ring-shaped and has no body or spinous process.

Anterior Arch
The anterior portion of C1.

Axis (C2)
The second cervical vertebra (Fig. 15-8) is so named because it forms the pivot that allows rotation of the atlas (C1), which supports the head.

Dens
Also called the *odontoid process;* large vertical projection located anteriorly on the axis. Cervical rotation occurs through its articulation with the atlas.

C7
Also known as *vertebra prominens* because of its long and prominent spinous process. It resembles a

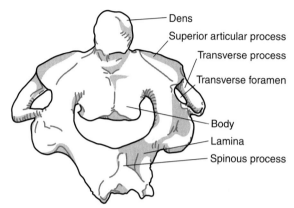

Figure 15-8.   The parts of the second cervical vertebra (C2), also called the *axis* (posterior view).

thoracic vertebra and can be easily palpated with the neck in flexion.

Transverse Foramen
Holes or openings in the transverse process of each of the cervical vertebra through which the vertebral artery passes (see Figs. 15-7 and 15-8)

Facet
Also called *costal facets,* they are located superiorly and inferiorly on the sides of the vertebral bodies and on the transverse processes of thoracic vertebrae (Fig. 15-9). It is here that the ribs articulate with the vertebrae.

Demifacet
In Latin, *demi* means "half," so a partial or half facet; located laterally on the superior and inferior edges of the vertebral body where ribs articulate with thoracic vertebrae. Depending on rib placement on the body, a facet or demifacet may be found on these edges.

Although the cervical, thoracic, and lumbar vertebrae have all the same parts, there are differences (Fig. 15-10; Table 15-2).

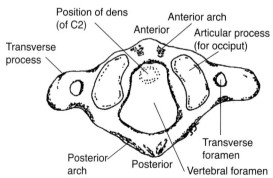

Figure 15-7.   The parts of the first cervical vertebra (C1), also called the *atlas* (superior view).

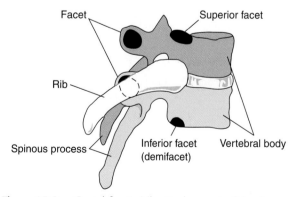

Figure 15-9.   Costal facets (rib attachments) of the thoracic vertebrae (lateral view).

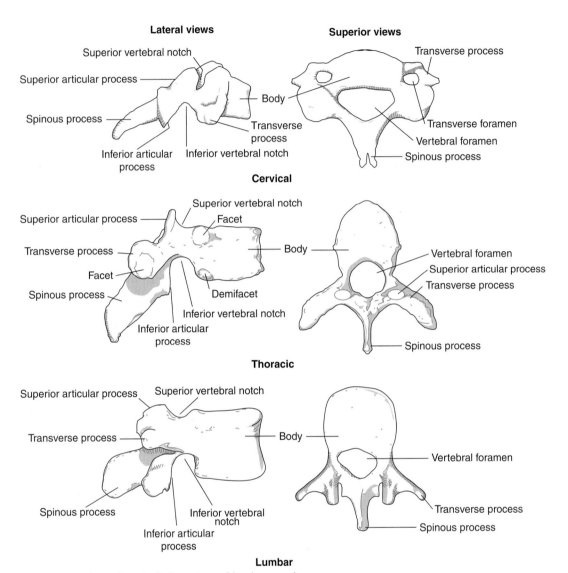

Figure 15-10. Comparison of cervical, thoracic, and lumbar vertebrae.

Table 15-2	Parts of the Vertebra		
	Cervical	Thoracic	Lumbar
Size	Smallest	Intermediate	Largest
Body shape	Small oval	Heart-shaped, with facets that connect with ribs	Large oval
Vertebral foramen	Large, triangular	Smallest	Intermediate
Transverse process	Foramen for vertebral artery; laterally	Facets that connect with ribs; long, thick, point posteriorly and laterally	No foramen or articulation
Spinous process	Short, stout, bifid	Long, slender, point inferiorly	Thick, point posteriorly
Superior articular process	Face upward, medially, and posteriorly	Face posteriorly and laterally	Face posteriorly
Inferior articular process	Face laterally	Face anteriorly and medially	Face anteriorly
Vertebral notches	Equal depth	Deeper inferior notches	Deeper inferior notches

Joints and Ligaments

The cervical spine begins with two very different articulations. The **atlanto-occipital joint** is formed by the condyles of the occiput that articulate with the superior articular processes of the atlas. This union is strong and supports the weight of the head. The anterior atlanto-occipital membrane is an extension of the anterior longitudinal ligament (see Fig. 15-14A and B), which is somewhat thin superiorly. The tectorial membrane is a continuation of the posterior longitudinal ligament. It serves as a sling to support the spinal cord as it enters the vertebral column. The posterior atlantoaxial ligament serves to secure the weight of the head on the neck. Each of the condyloid joints formed at the union of the occipital condyles and the superior articular processes of the atlas are synovial joints, with a synovial membrane enclosed in a joint capsule.

The articulations between the atlas and the axis are known as the **atlantoaxial joints,** of which there are three. The **median atlantoaxial joint** (Fig. 15-11) consists of a synovial articulation between the odontoid process (dens) of the axis and the anterior arch of the atlas anteriorly and the transverse ligament posteriorly. There are two synovial cavities present, one on each side of the dens. Each is enclosed in a joint capsule. The anterior atlantoaxial ligament and the posterior atlantoaxial ligament are continuations of the anterior and posterior longitudinal ligaments, which traverse the length of the vertebral column. The two **lateral atlantoaxial joints** are between the articular processes of the two vertebrae (see Fig. 15-11).

The articulations between C2 through S1 are all basically the same. The strong, weight-bearing articulations occur anteriorly on the vertebra between vertebral bodies. The posterior portion of the vertebrae has two articulations (one on each side), called **facet joints** (also known as *apophyseal* or *zygapophyseal joints*; see Fig. 15-5).

The facet joints are formed by the articulation between the superior articular processes of the vertebra below and the inferior articular processes of the vertebra above. Each facet joint is a synovial joint housing a synovial membrane and is enclosed in a joint capsular ligament. Each vertebra has two superior articular processes and two inferior articular processes. Therefore, each vertebra is involved with two facet joints. By the direction they face, these facet joints largely determine the type and amount of motion possible (Fig. 15-12) at that part of the vertebral column.

While processes in the lumbar area are located in the sagittal plane, processes in the thoracic area are in the frontal plane. Therefore, most flexion and extension of the vertebral column occurs in the lumbar spine, and most rotation and lateral bending occurs in the thoracic spine (Fig. 15-13). The attachment of ribs to the vertebra also

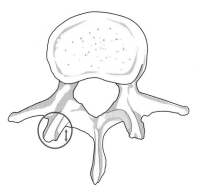
Lumbar orientation is in the sagittal plane

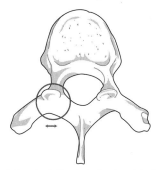
Thoracic orientation is in the frontal plane

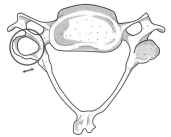
Cervical orientation is triplanar

Figure 15-12. A comparison of the orientation of the superior articular process (in circles) on the cervical, thoracic, and lumbar vertebrae (superior view).

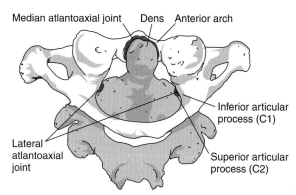

Figure 15-11. The relationship of C1 sitting on top of C2, showing the three atlantoaxial joints (posterior view).

contributes to the lack of flexion and extension in the thoracic spine. Because the processes are located diagonally between the sagittal and frontal planes, the cervical spine has a great deal of all three types of motion.

Many ligaments hold these vertebrae together (Fig. 15-14). The **anterior longitudinal ligament** runs down the vertebral column on the anterior surface of the bodies and tends to prevent excessive hyperextension. It is thin superiorly and thick inferiorly, where it fuses to the sacrum. It is found in the thoracic and lumbar regions just deep to the aorta. The **posterior longitudinal ligament** runs along the vertebral bodies posteriorly, inside the vertebral foramen. Its purpose is to prevent excessive flexion. It is thick superiorly, where it helps support the skull. It is thin inferiorly, which contributes to instability and increased disk injury in the lumbar region. The **supraspinal ligament** extends from the seventh cervical vertebra distally to the sacrum posteriorly along the tips of the spinous processes. The **interspinal ligament** runs between successive spinous processes. The very thick ligamentum nuchae (nuchal ligament) takes the place of the supraspinal and interspinal ligaments in the cervical region (Fig. 15-15). The **ligamentum flavum** connects adjacent laminae anteriorly.

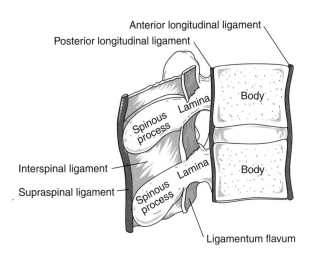

Sagittal Section View

A

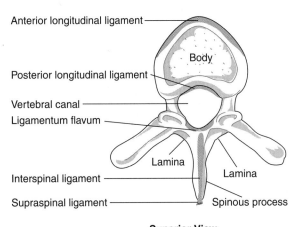

Superior View

B

Figure 15-14.   The vertebral ligaments. **(A)** Sagittal section view showing the ligaments inside and outside the vertebral canal. **(B)** Superior view showing the attachments of the ligaments on the vertebra.

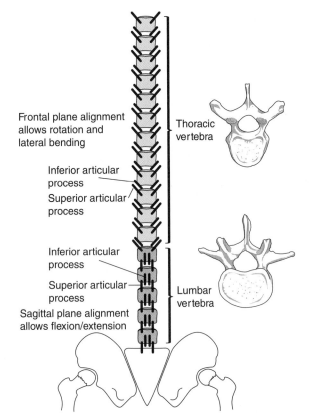

Figure 15-13.   The direction in which facet joints are aligned will determine the type of motions allowed (posterior view).

The lumbar spine is the most injured region of the human body. It absorbs the majority of our body weight plus any weight we carry. The center of gravity is located anterior to the second sacral vertebra. Most movement of the lumbar spine occurs between L4 and L5 and between L5 and S1; most disk herniations occur at these two levels.

The thoracic spine has much less motion than the cervical and lumbar regions due to its attachments to the rib cage. The shape of the vertebral bodies and the length of the spinous processes also limit thoracic motion.

The cervical spine moves freely. Unlike the lumbar spine, weight distribution is not its job. The cervical region supports the head and allows freedom of motion of the head on the neck, allows for the nervous tissue to

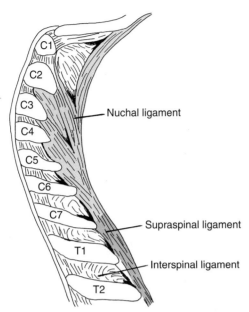

Figure 15-15. The nuchal ligament (ligamentum nuchae) becomes the supraspinal ligament in the cervical region (lateral view).

enter the vertebral canal, and allows for entrance and exit of the major blood vessels in the skull.

Muscles of the Neck and Trunk

Muscles of the neck and trunk are numerous and can be divided generally into anterior and posterior muscles (Table 15-3). (The quadratus lumborum muscle is the one exception; it is located in the midline of the frontal plane and is neither an anterior nor a posterior muscle.) The clinical significance of the anterior or posterior location is function. As with most other joints, anterior muscles flex and posterior muscles extend. Only those muscles that are clinically important from an exercise standpoint will be discussed here. Other muscles will be summarized in charts and illustrations.

Muscles of the Cervical Spine

Generally speaking, muscles located anterior to the cervical vertebral column are neck flexors. The largest flexor, the **sternocleidomastoid muscle,** is a long, superficial, straplike muscle that originates as two heads from the medial aspect of the clavicle and the superior end of the sternum (Fig. 15-16). It runs superiorly and posteriorly to insert on the mastoid process of the temporal bone. When it contracts bilaterally, it flexes the neck; when it contracts unilaterally, it laterally bends and rotates the face to the opposite side. For example, when the right sternocleidomastoid muscle contracts, your neck rotates so that you are looking over your left shoulder. Hence, it rotates to the opposite side. Because it attaches on the head, it can affect head motion. Looking at the muscle's line of pull from the side (posterior to the joint axis), you can see that in addition to flexing the neck, the sternocleidomastoid can also hyperextend the head. This accentuates the "forward

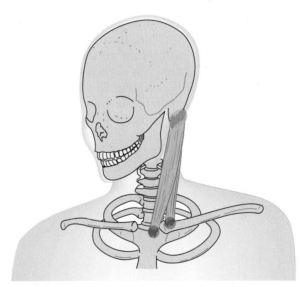

Figure 15-16. The sternocleidomastoid muscle (anterior view).

Table 15-3	Vertebral Muscles	
	Neck	**Trunk**
Anterior	Sternocleidomastoid	Rectus abdominis
	Scalenes (3)	External oblique
	Prevertebral group (4)	Internal oblique
		Transverse abdominis
Posterior	Erector spinae group (3)	Erector spinae group (3)
	Splenius capitis	Transversospinalis group (3)
	Splenius cervicis	Interspinales
	Suboccipital group (4)	Intertransversarii
Lateral		Quadratus lumborum

head" position common in faulty posture. To neutralize this action, one should always "tuck the chin" before doing such activities as sit-ups.

Sternocleidomastoid Muscle

O	Sternum and clavicle
I	Mastoid process
A	Bilaterally: flexes neck, hyperextends head Unilaterally: laterally bends the neck; rotates face to the opposite side
N	Accessory nerve (cranial nerve XI); second and third cervical nerves

Deep to the sternocleidomastoid muscle lie the three **scalene muscles** (Fig. 15-17). The **anterior scalene muscle** originates on the transverse processes of C3 through C6 and inserts into the superior surface of the first rib. The **middle scalene muscle** originates on the transverse processes of C2 through C7; it, too, inserts into the superior surface of the first rib. The **posterior scalene muscle,** the smallest and deepest muscle, originates from C5 through C7 and inserts into the second rib. Because they all perform the same action and are located close to each other, it is not necessary to differentiate between them. Located laterally at the neck, they are very effective in laterally bending the cervical spine. Because they are close to the axis, they are only assistive in flexion.

Scalene Muscles

O	Transverse processes of the cervical vertebrae
I	First and second ribs
A	Bilaterally: assists in neck flexion Unilaterally: neck lateral bending
N	Lower cervical nerves

There is an anterior group of muscles often referred to as the **prevertebral muscles.** They are located deep and run along the anterior portion of the cervical vertebrae (Fig. 15-18). These muscles have a role in flexing either the neck or the head. Because of their small size in relation to other neck flexors, perhaps their greatest role is maintaining postural control and "tucking" the chin. Table 15-4 summarizes their locations and actions.

Several small muscles in the neck serve as anchors for the hyoid bone and the tongue. Except for the platysma, these muscles are illustrated in Figures 15-19 through 15-21. The hyoid bone is unique in that it has no bony articulation. It functions as a primary support for the tongue and its numerous muscles. The influence of these muscles on motions of the cervical spine is assistive at best. These muscles approach the base of the skull

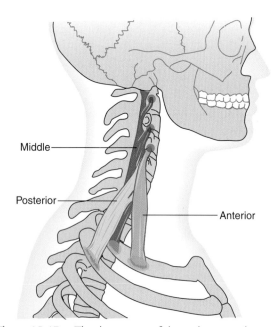

Figure 15-17. The three parts of the scalene muscles (lateral view).

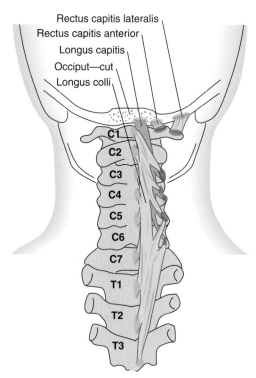

Figure 15-18. The prevertebral muscles (anterior view). Note that the anterior skull has been cut away to view the attachments on the occiput.

| Table 15-4 | Prevertebral Muscles (Anterior) | | |
Muscle	Origin	Insertion	Action
Longus colli	Bodies and transverse processes of C3–T2	Transverse processes and bodies of C1–C6	Flex neck
Longus capitis	Transverse processes of C3–C6	Occipital bone	Flex head
Rectus capitis anterior	Atlas (C2)	Occipital bone	Flex head
Rectus capitis lateralis	Transverse process of atlas	Occipital bone	Laterally bend head

from all directions. Table 15-5 summarizes the actions of these muscles.

The **suboccipital muscles** are clustered together below the base of the skull posteriorly and move only the head (see Fig. 15-19). The muscles work together to extend the head, with a rocking motion of the occipital condyles on the atlas, or to rotate it by pivoting the skull and atlas around the odontoid process of the axis. Table 15-6 summarizes these muscles.

The muscles located superficially along the posterior vertebral column are known as the **erector spinae group,** which will be discussed later in more detail with the trunk muscles. These muscles provide postural control over the gravitational pull of the head into flexion; they act as extensors to bring the head back from the flexed position. The deepest back muscles (transversospinalis, interspinales, and intertransversarii) will also be described in

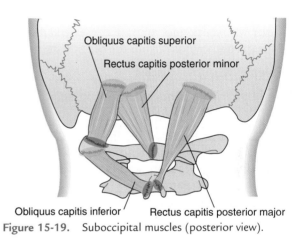

Figure 15-19.   Suboccipital muscles (posterior view).

| Table 15-5 | Muscles of the Mouth and Hyoid Bone | |
Group	Muscle	Action
Superficial cervical	Platysma	Draws lower lip down and out, tensing skin over neck
Suprahyoid	Digastric	Raises hyoid bone and/or tongue
	Stylohyoid	
	Mylohyoid	
	Geniohyoid	
Infrahyoid	Sternohyoid	Lowers hyoid bone
	Sternothyroid	
	Thyrohyoid	
	Omohyoid	

| Table 15-6 | Suboccipital Muscles (Posterior) | |
Muscle	Location	Head Motion
Obliquus capitis superior	Posterior	Extension
Obliquus capitis inferior	Posterior	Extension, lateral bending, rotation to the same side
Rectus capitis posterior minor	Posterior	Extension
Rectus capitis posterior major	Posterior	Extension, lateral bending, rotation to the same side

the trunk section, as that is where the majority of these muscles are located.

Deep to the erector spinae are the **splenius capitis** and **splenius cervicis muscles.** As their names imply, they attach to the head and to the cervical spine. The splenius capitis muscle is the more superficial of the two. They both attach from the spinous processes of the lower cervical and upper thoracic vertebrae, and they run superiorly and laterally to the lateral occiput (capitis) and transverse processes of the upper cervical vertebrae (cervicis), respectively (see Fig. 15-20). When the muscles on only one side contract, they rotate and laterally bend the face and neck to the same side. However, when both sides contract, they extend the neck and the splenius capitis extends the head on the neck.

Splenius Capitis Muscles

O	Lower half of nuchal ligament; spinous processes of C7 through T3
I	Lateral occipital bone; mastoid process
A	Bilaterally: extend head and neck Unilaterally: rotate and laterally bend the face to same side
N	Middle and lower cervical nerves

Splenius Cervicis Muscles

O	Spinous processes of T3 through T6
I	Transverse processes of C1 through C3
A	Bilaterally: extend neck Unilaterally: rotate and laterally bend the neck to same side
N	Middle and lower cervical nerves

It should be noted that the upper trapezius and levator scapula can assist the splenius capitis and cervicis under certain conditions. If the scapula is fixed, they can function in a reversal of muscle action. Instead of moving the scapula on the head and neck, the head and neck move on the scapula.

Muscles of the Trunk

Spanning the anterior trunk in the midline is the **rectus abdominis** muscle. The two sides are separated from each other by the linea alba. The rectus abdominis muscle arises from the crest of the pubis and inserts into the costal cartilages of the fifth, sixth, and seventh ribs. Three tendinous intersections divide the muscle horizontally into smaller units (see Figs. 15-21 and 15-22). Located in the anterior midline, the rectus abdominis muscle is a strong trunk flexor that, along with the other anterior trunk muscles, compresses the abdominal contents.

When doing a sit-up, note that the trunk moves on the hips. The hip flexor muscles, in a reversal of muscle action, are also involved in performing a sit-up if the ankles or legs are held down. Therefore, if the objective

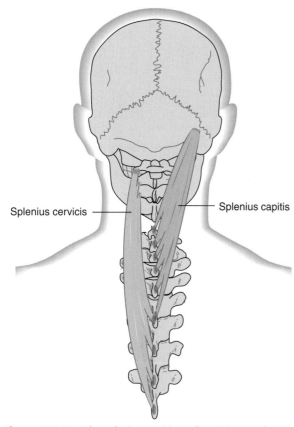

Figure 15-20.   The splenius capitis and cervicis muscles (posterior view).

Splenius cervicis — Splenius capitis

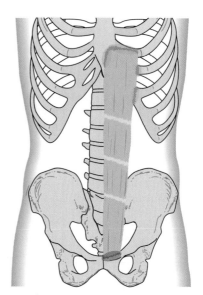

Figure 15-21.   The rectus abdominis muscle (anterior view). Note that the muscle is shown only on the left side.

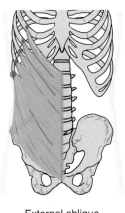
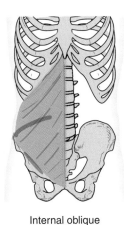

External oblique   Internal oblique

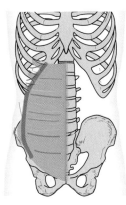

Transverse abdominis

Figure 15-22.   The three layers of abdominal muscles (anterior view). The external oblique is superficial, the internal oblique lies underneath it, and the transverse abdominis is the deepest layer.

is to strengthen the abdominals (not the hip flexors), the hips and knees should be flexed and the ankles should not be held down. Flexing the hips and knees will shorten the hip flexors, making them less efficient. The hip flexors cannot work in a reversal-of-muscle-action role when the distal segment (feet or legs) is not stabilized (held down).

Rectus Abdominis Muscles

O	Pubis
I	Xiphoid process and costal cartilages of fifth, sixth, and seventh ribs
A	Trunk flexion; compression of abdomen
N	Seventh through 12th intercostal nerves

The **external oblique muscle** is a large, broad, flat muscle (see Fig. 15-22) that lies superficially on the anterolateral abdomen. It originates laterally on the lower eight ribs, and it runs inferiorly and medially to

insert into the iliac crest and, via the abdominal aponeurosis, into the linea alba at the midline. Taken together, the fibers of the left and right external oblique muscles form the shape of a *V.* When both sides contract, they flex the trunk and compress the abdominal contents. When one side contracts, that external oblique bends laterally to the same side and rotates the trunk to the opposite side. This means that the right external oblique muscle rotates the right side of the trunk toward the midline. Visualize the right shoulder moving forward and toward the left.

Located deep to and running at right angles to the external oblique muscle is the **internal oblique muscle.** It originates from the inguinal ligament, iliac crest, and thoracolumbar fascia. It then runs superiorly and medially to insert into the last three ribs and, via the abdominal aponeurosis, into the linea alba (see Fig. 15-22). Taken together, the fibers of the left and right internal oblique muscles form the shape of an inverted *V.* Like the external oblique muscle, when both sides contract, they flex and compress the abdominal contents. When one side contracts, that internal oblique laterally bends the trunk to that side. However, the internal oblique muscle has the opposite action in rotation by rotating the trunk to the same side. This means that the right internal oblique muscle rotates the right side of the trunk away from the midline. Visualize the right shoulder moving back and toward the right. Therefore, the right external oblique and left internal oblique are agonists in rotating the trunk to the left. During the same action, the left external and right internal obliques are antagonists.

External Oblique Muscle

O	Lower eight ribs laterally
I	Iliac crest and linea alba
A	Bilaterally: trunk flexion; compression of abdomen Unilaterally: lateral bending; rotation to opposite side
N	Eighth through 12th intercostal, iliohypogastric, and ilioinguinal nerves

Internal Oblique Muscle

O	Inguinal ligament, iliac crest, thoracolumbar fascia
I	Tenth, eleventh, and twelfth ribs; abdominal aponeurosis
A	Bilaterally: trunk flexion; compression of abdomen Unilaterally: lateral bending; rotation to same side
N	Eighth through 12th intercostal, iliohypogastric, and ilioinguinal nerves

The deepest of the abdominal muscles is the **transverse abdominis** muscle, which lies deep to the internal oblique muscle. It is named for the transverse, or horizontal, direction of its fibers. It originates from the lateral portion of the inguinal ligament, the iliac crest, the thoracolumbar fascia, and the last six ribs. It spans the abdomen horizontally to insert into the abdominal aponeurosis and linea alba (see Fig. 15-22). Because of its horizontal line of pull, it plays no effective part in moving the trunk. However, it does work with the other abdominal muscles to compress and support the abdominal contents. This is important in activities such as coughing, sneezing, laughing, forced expiration, and "bearing down" during childbirth or while having a bowel movement.

Transverse Abdominis Muscle

O	Inguinal ligament, iliac crest, thoracolumbar fascia, and last six ribs
I	Abdominal aponeurosis and linea alba
A	Compression of abdomen
N	Seventh through 12th intercostal, iliohypogastric, and ilioinguinal nerves

There are many groups of posterior muscles, which are summarized in Table 15-7. Some general statements can be made regarding their attachments and actions (Fig. 15-23). Generally speaking, muscles attaching from spinous process to spinous process have a vertical line of pull; thus, they extend. Because they are located in the midline, there is only one set of them. Muscles that run from transverse process to transverse process have a vertical line of pull lateral to the midline. When acting unilaterally, they laterally bend; when acting bilaterally, they extend. Muscles attaching from rib to rib have the same line of pull as those attaching between transverse processes. Being more lateral, muscles attaching to ribs are even more effective at lateral bending. Muscles attaching

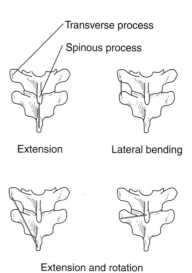

Figure 15-23.   The line of pull determines muscle action as summarized for posterior trunk muscles.

from spinous process to transverse process or from transverse process to spinous process have an oblique line and therefore extend bilaterally and rotate unilaterally. Of these, shorter muscles are more effective at rotation, and longer muscles are more effective at extension.

The intermediate layer of back extensors is a group of muscles called the **erector spinae muscles,** sometimes called the *sacrospinalis muscle group.* This muscle group can be subdivided into three groups that tend to run parallel to the vertebral column and that connect spinous processes, transverse processes, and ribs (Fig. 15-24). The most medial group is the **spinalis muscle group,** which primarily attaches to the nuchal ligament and spinous processes of the cervical and thoracic vertebrae. The portion of this group that attaches to the occiput also attaches to the transverse processes of the cervical vertebrae. Located in the midline, these muscles are prime movers in trunk extension.

Table 15-7	Posterior Trunk Muscles	
Attachments	**Action**	**Muscles**
Spinous process to spinous process	Extension	Spinalis (ES)
		Interspinales
Transverse process to transverse process	Extension, lateral bending	Longissimus (ES)
		Intertransversarii
Spinous to transverse process	Extension, rotation	Splenius cervicis
Transverse to spinous process	Extension, rotation	Semispinalis (T)
		Multifidus (T)
		Rotatores (T)
Transverse process to rib, or rib to rib	Extension, lateral bending	Iliocostalis (ES)

ES, erector spinae; T, transversospinalis.

Erector Spinae Muscles

O	Spinous processes, transverse processes, and posterior ribs from the occiput to the sacrum and ilium
I	Spinous processes, transverse processes, and posterior ribs from the occiput to the sacrum and ilium
A	Bilaterally: extend neck and trunk Unilaterally: laterally bend neck and trunk
N	Spinal nerves

The deepest of the back extensor muscles is a group of three muscles called the **transversospinalis (transverse spinal) muscle group** (Fig. 15-25). They get their name from their attachments. They have an oblique line of pull, essentially attaching

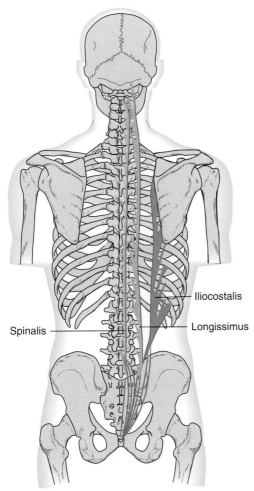

Figure 15-24. The three parts of the erector spinae muscle group (posterior view).

Spinalis — Iliocostalis — Longissimus

The intermediate muscles, the **longissimus muscle group,** are located lateral to the spinalis muscle group, attaching to the transverse processes from the occiput to the sacrum. Because these muscles are lateral to the midline and have a vertical line of pull, they produce lateral bending when contracting unilaterally and produce extension when contracting bilaterally. The **iliocostalis muscles** are the most lateral group, attaching primarily to the ribs posteriorly. Superiorly, they attach to transverse processes, and inferiorly they attach to the sacrum and ilium. Because of their lateral position, these muscles are excellent at lateral bending. Acting bilaterally, they are effective extensors. These three groups of muscles generally are referred to as the *erector spinae muscle group*; and, therefore, will be summarized as a group. However, it should be noted that the upper fibers of the spinalis and longissimus groups attach to the occiput and therefore can extend the head on the neck.

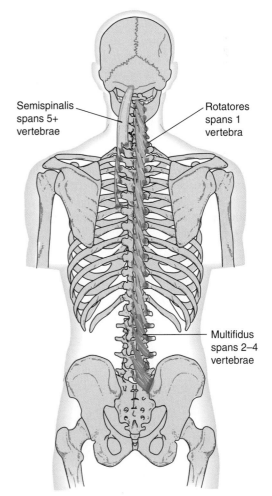

Semispinalis spans 5+ vertebrae

Rotatores spans 1 vertebra

Multifidus spans 2–4 vertebrae

Figure 15-25. The transversospinalis muscle group (posterior view). For illustration purposes, muscles are shown in different parts of the vertebral column. In fact, all run the entire vertebral column in layers.

from a transverse process to the spinous process of a vertebra above; therefore, they are very effective at rotation. The *semispinalis muscles* tend to span five or more vertebrae; the *multifidus* muscles tend to span two to four vertebrae; and the *rotatores* muscles, the shortest and deepest of this group, span only one vertebra. These muscles rotate to the opposite side and extend the spine. The semispinalis is the most superficial muscle of this group. The multifidus lies underneath it, and the rotators are the deepest of these muscles.

Transversospinalis Muscles

O	Transverse processes
I	Spinous processes of vertebra above
A	Bilaterally: extend neck and trunk Unilaterally: rotate neck and trunk to opposite side
N	Spinal nerves

Like the transversospinalis muscle group, these next two muscles are located deep, but they have a vertical, not oblique, line of pull. Therefore, they must be considered separately. The names of the interspinales and intertransversarii muscles indicate where they attach. The **interspinales muscles** attach from the spinous process below to the spinous process above throughout most of the vertebral column (Fig. 15-26). With this vertical line of pull in the midline, they are effective extensors. The **intertransversarii muscles** attach from the transverse process below to the transverse process above, and they appear throughout most of the vertebral column (Fig. 15-27). They are effective at lateral bending.

Interspinales Muscles

O	Spinous process below
I	Spinous process above
A	Neck and trunk extension
N	Spinal nerves

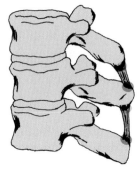

Figure 15-26.   The interspinales muscles (lateral view).

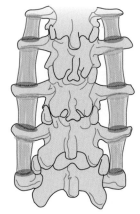

Figure 15-27.   Intertransversarii muscles (posterior view).

Intertransversarii Muscles

O	Transverse process below
I	Transverse process above
A	Neck and trunk lateral bending
N	Spinal nerves

The **quadratus lumborum muscle** is a deep muscle that originates from the iliac crest. It runs superiorly to insert into the last rib and transverse processes of all lumbar vertebrae (Fig. 15-28). Because it is located in the anterior-posterior midline, it does not have a function of flexion or extension; being vertical, it has no role in rotation. However, being lateral to the midline makes it effective at lateral bending. It has another function that occurs when its origin is pulled toward its insertion (reversal of muscle action). The action is

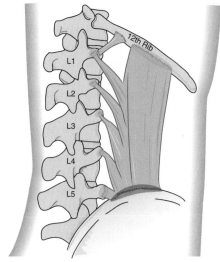

Figure 15-28.   The quadratus lumborum muscle (lateral view).

called *hip hiking,* or *elevation,* of one side of the pelvis. This is an important function to anyone with a long leg cast or fused knee, because it allows the foot to clear the floor without bending the knee.

Quadratus Lumborum Muscle

O	Iliac crest
I	Twelfth rib, transverse processes of all five lumbar vertebrae
A	Trunk lateral bending
N	12th thoracic and first lumbar nerves

Anatomical Relationships

Looking at the anterior neck, the most superficial muscle is the very broad, thin platysma muscle (Fig. 15-29). This muscle covers a large portion of the anterior and lateral neck. It participates in facial expression and has no function at the neck. Beneath the platysma and running diagonally from the medial clavicle out and up to the mastoid process behind the ear is the sternocleidomastoid muscle (Fig. 15-30). Deep to the sternocleidomastoid are the infrahyoid muscles, which align more vertically in the anterior neck region. Looking under the chin, you would see the suprahyoid muscles. The prevertebral muscles are the deepest muscle group, lying next to the vertebral column (not visible).

From a lateral view, the platysma covers all but the upper half of the sternocleidomastoid (see Fig. 15-29). Because the sternocleidomastoid runs diagonally from posterior-superior to anterior-inferior, it covers portions of the infrahyoid muscles anteriorly and the three

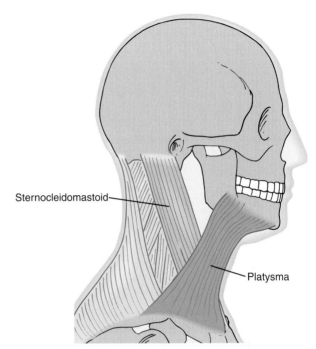

Figure 15-29. Platysma muscle (side view).

scalene muscles near the midline laterally (Fig. 15-31). The posterior scalene is not visible. Posteriorly, the sternocleidomastoid covers portions of the levator scapula and splenius capitus near their superior attachments. The upper trapezius is the most superficial muscle posteriorly.

There are several layers of muscles in the posterior neck (Fig. 15-32). As mentioned earlier, the most

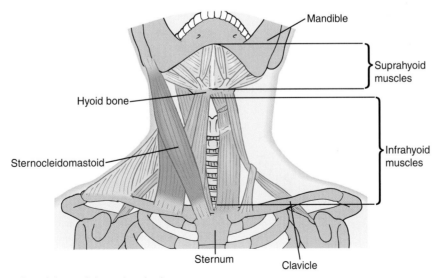

Figure 15-30.   Muscles of the neck (anterior view).

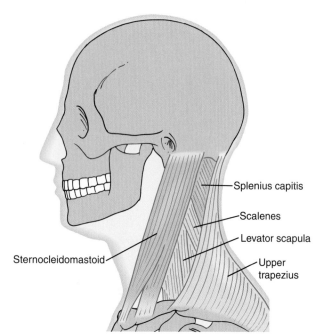

Figure 15-31.   Muscles of the neck (lateral view).

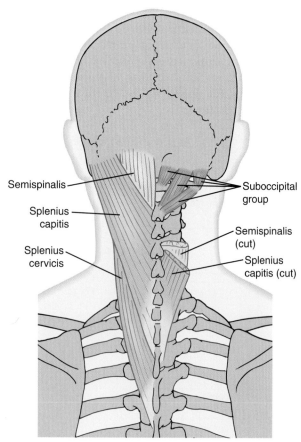

Figure 15-32.   Muscles of the neck (posterior view).

superficial muscle is the upper trapezius (see Fig. 9-12). This muscle has been removed in Figure 15-32 to show the splenius capitis partially covering the splenius cervicus. Beneath these muscles is the semispinalis portion of the transversospinalis group. This group covers the erector spinae (not visible). The deepest layer in the neck includes the shortest muscles: the suboccipital (near the head) and the interspinales and intertransversarii muscles. These last two muscles are not visible.

The trunk muscles are divided into anterior and posterior muscles. There are four layers of muscles on the abdominal, or anterior, trunk wall (Fig. 15-33). Rectus femoris lies the most superficial and is in the midline. The external oblique muscle is superficial on the sides of the abdominal wall and is just underneath the rectus femoris anteriorly. Directly under the external oblique muscle lies the internal oblique. The transverse abdominis is the deepest of the abdominal muscles; its fibers run in a horizontal direction.

The posterior trunk muscles are located deep to the shoulder girdle and shoulder joint muscles (see Fig. 9-21). As shown in Figure 15-34, the most superficial layer of back muscles are the erector spinae muscles: iliocostalis (lateral column), longissimus

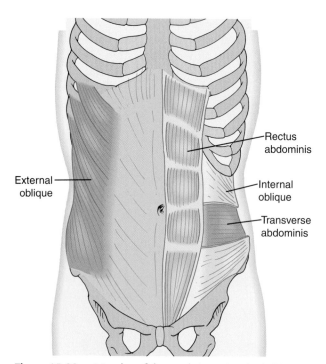

Figure 15-33.   Muscles of the trunk (anterior view). Note that the external oblique is shown only on one side, and that a portion of the internal oblique has been cut away to show the transverse abdominis deep to it.

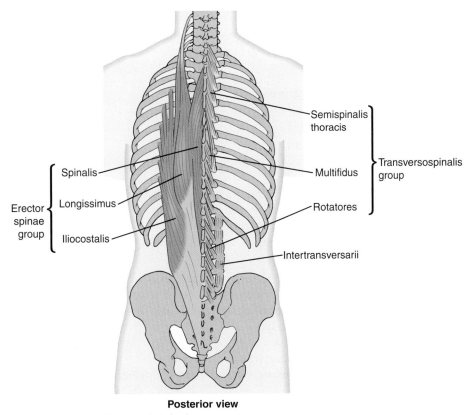

Posterior view

Figure 15-34.   Muscles of the trunk (posterior view).

(middle column), and spinalis (medial column). Deep to the erector spinae muscles are the intrinsic back muscles that belong to the transversospinalis group (semispinalis, multifidus, and rotators). These muscles lie vertically in the groove between the transverse and spinous processes. The deepest muscles of the trunk are the one-joint interspinal and intertransversarii muscles. The interspinal muscles are not visible in Figure 15-34.

Summary of Muscle Actions

Table 15-8 summarizes the muscle action of the prime movers of the neck and trunk.

Summary of Muscle Innervation

Most muscles of the neck and trunk do not receive innervation from branches or terminal nerves of a plexus. Because they tend to be groups that span several vertebral levels, their innervation typically reflects that. Generally speaking, they receive innervation from spinal nerves at various levels. For example, a spinal

cord injury at T12 will not cause paralysis of all erector spinae muscles but will cause paralysis of those located below that level.

Common Vertebral Column Pathologies

Thoracic outlet syndrome is a general term referring to compression of the neurovascular structures (brachial plexus and subclavian artery and vein) that run from the neck to the axilla. The thoracic outlet is located between the first rib, the clavicle, and the scalene muscles. The brachial plexus and subclavian artery pass between the anterior and middle scalene muscles, the first rib, and the clavicle. A variety of signs and symptoms can occur, depending on the structures involved. **Torticollis** (from the Latin *tortus*, meaning "twisted," and *collum*, meaning "neck") is a deformity of the neck in which the person's head is laterally bent to one side and rotated toward the other side. It is also known as *wry (twisted) neck*. **Cervical sprains** occur when the head suddenly and violently

Table 15-8	Prime Movers of the Neck and Trunk
Action	**Muscle**
Head (Occiput on C1)	
Flexion	Prevertebral group
Extension	Suboccipital group
Neck	
Flexion	Sternocleidomastoid
Extension	Splenius capitis, splenius cervicis, erector spinae, transversospinalis, interspinales
Lateral bending	Sternocleidomastoid, splenius capitis, splenius cervicis, scalenes, erector spinae, intertransversarii
Rotation (same side)	Splenius capitis, splenius cervicis
Rotation (opposite side)	Sternocleidomastoid, transversospinalis
Trunk	
Flexion	Rectus abdominis, external oblique, internal oblique
Extension	Erector spinae, transversospinalis, interspinales
Lateral bending	Quadratus lumborum, erector spinae, internal oblique, external oblique, intertransversarii
Rotation same side	Internal oblique
Rotation opposite side	External oblique, transversospinalis
Compression of abdomen	Rectus abdominis, external oblique, internal oblique, transverse abdominis

hyperextends and then flexes. *Whiplash* is the layman's term for this condition. **Sciatica** is pain that tends to run down the posterior thigh and leg. It is caused by pressure on the sciatic nerve roots and usually is symptomatic of an underlying pathology such as a herniated lumbar disc.

The vertebral column has a normal anterior-posterior curvature. In the cervical and lumbar regions, the curves are concave posteriorly; in the thoracic and sacral regions, they are convex posteriorly (see Fig. 15-1). **Lordosis** is an abnormally increased curve of the lumbar spine. The layman's term is *swayback*. **Flat back** is an abnormally decreased lumbar curve. **Kyphosis** is an abnormally increased thoracic curve. Any amount of lateral curve is a pathological condition known as **scoliosis.**

Spondylosis (spinal osteoarthritis) is a degenerative disorder of vertebral structure and function. It may result from bony spurs, thickening of ligaments, and decreased disk height that results from reduced water content of the nucleus pulposus, a normal part of the aging process. All of these problems may lead to nerve root and spinal cord compression. **Spinal stenosis** is a narrowing of the vertebral

canal that houses the spinal cord. It is also possible to have stenosis of the intervertebral foramen through which the nerve roots pass. **Herniated disks** occur when there is a weakness or degeneration of the annulus fibrosus (outer layer). This allows a portion of the nucleus pulposus to bulge, or herniate, through the annulus. It becomes symptomatic when the herniation puts pressure on the spinal cord or, more commonly, on the nerve root. L4 and L5 are the most common sites for disk lesions, and the fourth and fifth lumbar nerve roots are the most commonly affected. **Ankylosing spondylitis,** a chronic inflammation of the vertebral column and sacroiliac joints, leads to fusion. It is a progressive rheumatic disease; over time, it can lead to a total loss of spinal mobility.

Spondylolysis is a vertebral defect in the pars interarticularis (the part of the lamina between the superior and inferior articular processes). This defect is most commonly seen in L5 and less commonly in L4. **Spondylolisthesis** usually results from a fracture, or giving way, of a defective pars interarticularis. One vertebra slips forward in relation to an adjacent vertebra, usually L5 slipping anterior on S1.

Osteoporosis, meaning "porous bone," is a disease in which bone is removed faster than it can be laid down. This results in decreased bone mass and density, making the bone more prone to fracture. Common sites for fracture are the hip, the thoracic vertebral column, and the wrist.

Compression fractures typically result in the collapse of the anterior (body) portion of the vertebrae. They are usually caused by trauma in the lumbar region or by osteoporosis in the thoracic region. This type of fracture does not commonly cause spinal cord damage and paralysis, because the fracture is usually stable. A stable fracture does not have progressive displacement or dislocation. Unstable fractures, or **fractures with dislocation,** usually result in spinal cord injury and paralysis. A fracture involving C2, commonly called a **hangman's fracture,** typically occurs when there is a forceful, sudden hyperextension of the head. Striking the head against the windshield in a motor vehicle accident is often the cause. This is usually a stable fracture, but without proper care and handling, it could become unstable. Spinal cord paralysis at this level usually results in death because respiration stops.

> ## Points to Remember
> - When a muscle contracts, it knows no direction; it simply shortens.
> - When a muscle contracts, it usually moves its insertion (more movable end) toward its origin (more stable end).
> - A muscle insertion is usually the distal end and the more movable end.
> - A muscle origin is usually the proximal end and the more stable end.
> - Reversal of muscle action occurs when the origin becomes more movable and moves toward the insertion, which has become more stable.
> - Concentric contractions occur when the body part is moving against gravity.
> - Eccentric contractions occur when the body part is moving in the same direction as the pull of gravity.
> - Isometric contractions occur when a muscle contracts but no significant joint motion occurs.
> - The muscle group contracting isometrically is the same group as if the joint were contracting concentrically.

Review Questions

General Anatomy Questions

1. Describe neck and trunk motions in
   a. the frontal plane around the sagittal axis.
   b. the transverse plane around the vertical axis.
   c. the sagittal plane around the frontal axis.

2. You are handed a cervical, thoracic, and lumbar vertebra. What identifying features help you distinguish among them?

3. What structural features allow the thoracic vertebrae to rotate but not flex?

4. What structural features allow the lumbar vertebrae to flex but not rotate?

5. Name the ligament that extends over the spinous processes from the occiput to C7 and from C7 to the sacrum.

6. What is the name of the series of ligaments that connect the lamina above to the lamina below along the length of the vertebral column?

7. Name the ligaments that attach to the bodies of the vertebrae and run the length of the vertebral column.

8. Why doesn't the quadratus lumborum muscle play a role in trunk flexion, extension, or rotation?

9. Which posterior muscle groups are the most superficial?

10. You ask your patient, who is lying supine, to bring her left shoulder toward her right knee. What joint motion(s) and prime movers are involved?

Functional Activity Questions

Identify the main **cervical** positions in the following activities:

1. Sleeping on your stomach

2. Cradling the telephone between your ear and shoulder

(continued on next page)

Review Questions—cont'd

3. Looking at the top of a tall building from the street below

4. Lying supine on a sofa with your head propped up on a pillow or the sofa's arm

5. Painting the ceiling

Identify the main **trunk** action in the following activities:

6. Preparing to hit a tennis ball with a backhand swing with the racket in your right hand (Fig. 15-35)

7. Hitting the tennis ball with the backhand swing (Fig. 15-36)

8. Reaching down to pick up a suitcase beside you (Fig. 15-37)

9. The follow-through of punting a football

10. Doing a backward handstand

Clinical Exercise Questions

Head and Neck

1. Lie prone with your head and shoulders over the edge of the table and head down. Tuck

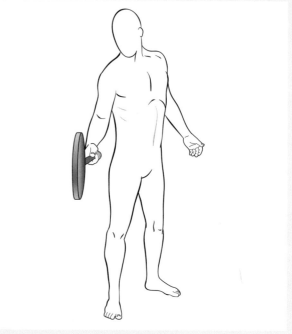

Figure 15-36.   Hitting with backswing.

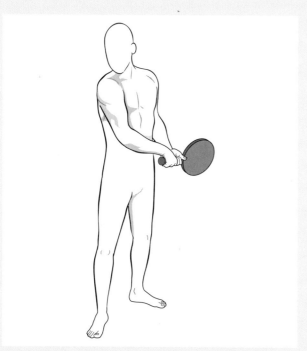

Figure 15-35.   Preparing to hit with tennis backswing.

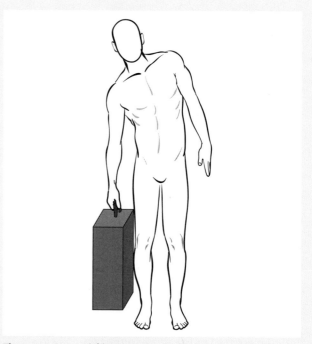

Figure 15-37.   Picking up suitcase.

Review Questions—cont'd

your chin in and raise your head to anatomical position.

  a. What joint motion is occurring in the neck as you tuck in your chin?

  b. What joint motion is occurring in the neck as you raise your head?

  c. What type of contraction (isometric, concentric, eccentric) occurs as you raise your head?

  d. What type of contraction (isometric, concentric, eccentric) occurs as you hold your head in anatomical position while in this prone position?

  e. What are the prime movers that are working to raise your head?

2. Sitting or standing with your head and neck in anatomical position, press your right hand against the right side of your head. Try to move your head but resist any motion with your hand.

  a. What joint motion is occurring (or attempting to occur)?

  b. What type of contraction (isometric, concentric, or eccentric) is occurring?

  c. What are the prime movers of this joint motion?

3. While lying supine, lean your head toward your right shoulder. Do not raise your right shoulder. Both stretching and strengthening are occurring here. In answering the questions below, be sure to indicate whether you are referring to the right or left side.

  a. What joint motion is occurring (or attempting to occur)?

  b. What muscle group is being stretched?

  c. What are the prime movers of this joint motion?

  d. What muscle group is being strengthened?

  e. What are the prime movers of this joint motion?

4. Which muscle would be stretched if you leaned your head toward the right shoulder and rotated your head to the left?

5. From a supine position, tuck your chin and raise your head off the mat, hold for the count of 5, then return to the starting position.

  a. Is the head flexing or extending on C1 as you tuck in your chin?

  b. What type of contraction (isometric, concentric, or eccentric) is occurring?

  c. What is the muscle group involved in tucking your chin?

  d. Is your neck flexing or extending as you raise your head?

  e. What type of contraction is occurring as you raise your head?

  f. What muscles are prime movers in this joint motion?

  g. What type of contraction is occurring as you hold your head for the count?

  h. What muscles are prime movers in this action?

  i. Is neck flexion or extension occurring in the neck as you return to the starting position?

  j. What type of contraction is occurring with this motion?

  k. What muscles are involved with this action?

Trunk

1. Sit in a chair with your legs abducted. Drop your head and shoulders forward, bending at hips and trunk until your shoulders are between your knees.

  a. Is trunk flexion or extension occurring in this activity?

  b. Are the trunk flexors or extensors being stretched?

  c. What muscles are being stretched?

2. Lie supine with your knees extended and your arms at your sides. First, press your lower back to the mat, and then curl your trunk. Lift your head and shoulders up (keeping your chin down) until your scapulae leave the floor.

  a. Is trunk flexion or extension occurring in this activity?

  b. What type of contraction (isometric, concentric, or eccentric) is occurring?

  c. What muscles are prime movers in this trunk motion?

3. Repeat the action of the exercise in question 2, except this time have someone hold down your feet. In this exercise, the hip flexors are contracting.

  a. Is the trunk motion still the same as in question 1?

  b. Are the hips flexing or extending?

  c. Is the hip muscle moving its origin toward its insertion or its insertion toward its origin?

  d. What is the kinesiology term for a muscle that contracts in this direction?

(continued on next page)

Review Questions—cont'd

e. What is the main one-joint hip muscle that is contracting in this motion?

f. Describe how holding the feet down allows certain hip muscles to contract.

4. Lie supine with your knees bent and feet flat. Put your right hand behind your head. Lift your right shoulder and scapula off the mat toward your left knee.

a. What two trunk motions are occurring (flexion, extension, right rotation, left rotation, right lateral bending, or left lateral bending)?

b. What type of contraction (isometric, concentric, or eccentric) is occurring?

c. What muscles are causing these trunk motions? Be sure to indicate which side the muscle is on that is contracting.

5. Lie prone with your face in the mat and your arms at your side. Tuck your chin in and raise your head and shoulders up off the mat. Be sure to keep your chin tucked and eyes looking down at the mat.

a. Is the head flexing or extending on C1 as you tuck in your chin?

b. What type of contraction (isometric, concentric, or eccentric) is occurring as you tuck in your chin?

c. What type of contraction is occurring as you hold your chin tucked in?

d. What is the muscle group involved in tucking your chin?

e. Is your neck in flexion or extension as you raise your head and shoulders from the mat?

f. What type of contraction is occurring at the neck as you raise your shoulders from the mat?

g. What are the prime movers at the neck as you raise your shoulders from the mat?

h. Is your trunk flexing, extending, or hyperextending as you raise your shoulders from the mat?

i. What type of trunk muscle contraction is occurring as you raise your shoulders?

j. What muscles are causing the trunk motion that raises your shoulders?

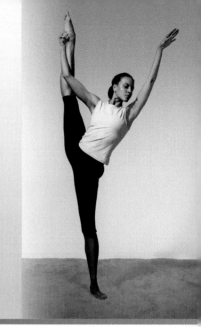

CHAPTER 16
Respiratory System

The Thoracic Cage

    Joints and Articulations

    Movements of the Thorax

Structures of Respiration

    Mechanics of Respiration

Phases of Respiration

Muscles of Respiration

    Diaphragm Muscle

    Intercostal Muscles

    Accessory Inspiratory Muscles

    Accessory Expiratory Muscles

    Anatomical Relationships

    Diaphragmatic Versus Chest Breathing

    Summary of Innervation of the Muscles of Respiration

    Valsalva's Maneuver

    Common Respiratory Conditions or Pathologies

Review Questions

    General Anatomy Questions

    Functional Activity Questions

    Clinical Exercise Questions

Simply stated, the main function of the respiratory system is to supply oxygen to and eliminate carbon dioxide from the lungs. The respiratory organs are the conduits through which air enters and exits the lungs. The thorax provides bony protection to the lungs and assists in the air exchange. Although a brief description of the passage of air through the respiratory organs will be given, the main focus of this chapter will be the bony and muscular mechanisms that make air exchange possible.

The Thoracic Cage

The thorax consists of the sternum, the ribs and costal cartilages, and the thoracic vertebrae (Fig. 16-1). It is bounded anteriorly by the sternum, posteriorly by the bodies of the 12 thoracic vertebrae, superiorly by the clavicle, and inferiorly by the diaphragm. The thorax is wider from side to side than it is from front to back. The thoracic, or chest, cavity lies inside the thorax. It is within this cavity that the lungs, heart, and other vital structures are located.

The **rib cage** serves to attach the vertebral column posteriorly to the sternum anteriorly. Due to these attachments, movement within the thoracic spine is very limited. The chest organs (heart, lungs, aorta, thymus gland, portion of trachea, esophagus, lymph nodes, and important nerves) are housed within and protected by the rib cage. Each side has 12 ribs, for a total of 24. The upper 7 ribs (also called **true ribs**) attach directly to the sternum anteriorly. Ribs 8 through 10 are called **false ribs,** because they attach indirectly to the sternum via the costal cartilage of the 7th rib. The 11th and 12th ribs are called **floating ribs,** because they have no anterior attachment.

The **sternum** is the long, flat bone in the midline of the anterior chest wall. Its shape resembles a dagger, and it consists of three parts: manubrium, body, and xiphoid process (see Fig. 16-1).

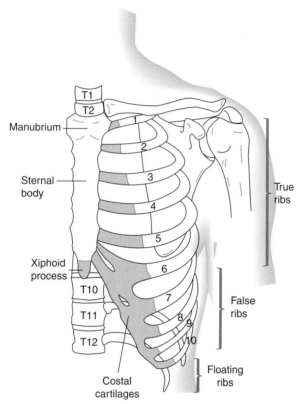

Figure 16-1.   The thoracic cage (anterior view).

The *manubrium* (Latin for "handle") is the superior part, the *body* is the middle and longest part, and the *xiphoid process* (Greek for "sword") is the inferior tip portion. The ribs, sternum, and vertebral bodies form the thorax.

Joints and Articulations

The ribs mainly articulate with the vertebrae in two areas: (1) the bodies of the vertebrae and (2) the transverse processes. These joints are called **costovertebral joints** (Fig. 16-2). The articulating surface on the vertebral body, the **facet,** is located laterally and posteriorly on the body near the beginning of the neural arch. Some ribs articulate partially with two adjacent bodies. These articulations are with the superior part of the vertebral body below and the inferior part of the vertebral body above. These facets are often called **demifacets,** because they articulate with only about half of the rib. In other words, the rib articulates with a demifacet on the vertebra above plus a demifacet on the vertebra below. A facet that articulates with the tubercle and neck of the rib is located on the anterior tip of the transverse process of the vertebra. Figure 16-3 shows the facets and demifacets.

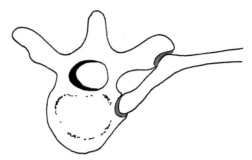

Figure 16-2.   Costovertebral joints (superior view).

Movements of the Thorax

Like the costovertebral articulations, the articulations of the ribs and the sternum, with the costal cartilage in between, are nonaxial, diarthrodial, gliding joints. Because most of the ribs attach anteriorly and posteriorly, there is little movement, but **elevation** and **depression** of the rib cage do occur. These movements are associated with inspiration and expiration, respectively.

As you inhale, the rib cage moves up and out, increasing the medial-lateral diameter of the chest. Accordingly, as you exhale, the rib cage returns to its starting position by moving down and in, decreasing the medial-lateral chest diameter. This type of movement has been compared with the up and down movement of a bucket handle (Fig. 16-4A). When the handle is resting against the side of the bucket, it is comparable to the lowered position of the rib cage during expiration. As the handle (the lateral aspect of the ribs) moves up and away from the bucket (the vertebral column and sternum), it is comparable to the increased mediolateral diameter of the rib cage during inspiration.

In addition to a change in medial-lateral diameter, there is a change in the anterior-posterior diameter of the chest. This is called the *pump-handle effect* (Fig. 16-4B). As

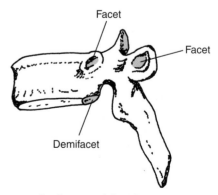

Figure 16-3.   The facets and demifacets on the thoracic vertebra (lateral view).

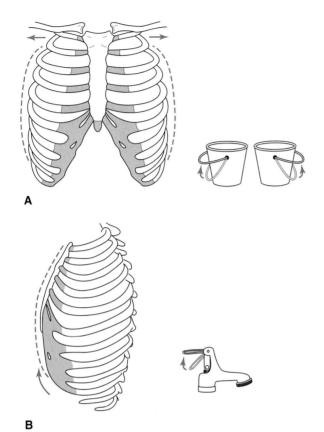

A

B

Figure 16-4.   Comparison of thorax movements during breathing with movements of bucket and pump handles. **(A)** Medial-lateral chest diameter and **(B)** anterior-posterior chest diameter.

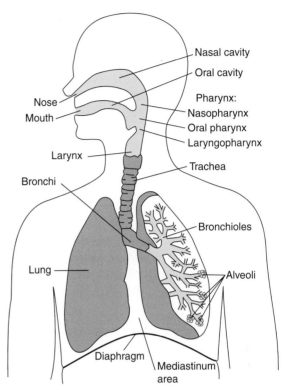

Figure 16-5.   The respiratory structures are divided into the upper and lower airway tracts (anterior view). Note that the left lung is cut in cross section to show terminal structures.

Structures of Respiration

you inhale, the sternum and ribs move upward and outward (forward), increasing the anterior-posterior diameter of the chest. This is comparable to the pump handle moving up. Conversely, as the ribs and sternum are lowered, the diameter of the anterior-posterior thorax decreases, resulting in expiration. This movement is comparable to the pump handle moving back down.

Respiratory structures can be divided into upper and lower airway tracts (Fig. 16-5). The **upper respiratory tract** consists of the nasal cavity, oral cavity, pharynx, and larynx. The **lower respiratory tract** is made up of the trachea and bronchial tree. To allow the airways to remain open, all structures, down to the smallest bronchi, are made up of cartilaginous material. The **nose** is mostly made up of relatively soft cartilage and consists of the two nostrils, also called *nasal nares.* Only the upper part, or bridge, is bony. The two nostrils lead

into the **nasal cavity.** The nasal septum, formed by the vomer and part of the ethmoid bones, separates the nasal cavity into two fairly equal chambers. The ethmoid, sphenoid, and a small part of the frontal bone form the roof of the nasal cavity, whereas the palatine and part of the maxillae bones form the floor. These bones also make up the hard palate of the mouth. The functions of the nasal cavity are to warm, filter, and moisten the air you breathe in.

If you breathe through your mouth, air enters the **oral cavity,** moving over the lips and tongue and into the pharynx. The roof of the mouth consists of the bony hard palate and the fibrous soft palate. The uvula is the soft tissue structure that hangs down in the middle at the back of the mouth; it is part of the soft palate. The function of the soft palate is to close off the opening between the nasal and oral pharynx during such activities as swallowing, blowing, and certain speech sounds. This forces food and liquids down into the throat during swallowing and forces air out through the mouth when blowing and speaking.

Once air passes through the nasal cavity, it enters the pharynx through the nasopharynx. The **pharynx,** or throat, has three parts: the nasal pharynx, which has primarily a respiratory function; the oral pharynx, which receives food from the mouth; and the laryngopharynx. This last part is located between the base of the tongue and the entrance to the esophagus. Next, air passes into the **larynx,** or voice box. The larynx is located between the pharynx and the trachea, anterior to vertebrae C4 through C6. Anteriorly, it is fairly easy to locate by the laryngeal prominence, or *Adam's apple,* which tends to be more prominent in men than in women. The larynx consists of cartilage, ligaments, muscles, and the vocal cords. Its function is to (1) act as a passageway for air between the pharynx and trachea, (2) prevent food or liquid from passing into the trachea, and (3) generate speech sounds. When you swallow, the epiglottis, which is one of the cartilaginous structures of the larynx, closes over the vocal cords, allowing food or liquids to pass into the esophagus but not into the trachea, thus preventing aspiration of food or drink into the lungs. The glottis is the opening between the vocal cords and the area where sound is produced. It is also an important part of the cough mechanism, which is important for keeping the airways clear.

Passing out of the larynx, air then enters the **trachea,** commonly called the *windpipe.* It is located anterior to the esophagus and vertebrae C6 through T4. To keep the airway open, the trachea is made up of C-shaped cartilage on all sides, except posteriorly. It divides into right and left **main stem bronchi.** The right bronchus is shorter and wider and subdivides into three **lobar bronchi** (upper, middle, and lower), with one going to each lobe of the lung. The longer, narrower left bronchus subdivides into two lobar bronchi (upper and lower). As the bronchi continue to divide, they become progressively smaller, narrower, and more numerous. The trachea, bronchi, and their subdivisions are sometimes referred to as the *bronchial tree.* The smallest bronchi, which are less than 1 mm in diameter, are called **bronchioles.** It is at this point that the airway becomes noncartilaginous. The **alveolus** (plural, *alveoli*) is at the very end of the bronchial tree subdivision. These saclike alveoli cluster around the terminal bronchioles much like grapes on their stem. The alveoli exchange oxygen for carbon dioxide and vice versa.

When the trachea divides into the right and left bronchi, they each enter a lung. The **lungs** are somewhat triangular, being wider and concave at the bottom. This concave shape fits with the convex dome shape of the diaphragm located below. The right lung has an upper, middle, and lower lobe, whereas the left lung has an upper and lower lobe. A double-walled sac, called the **pleura,** encases each lung. The outer wall of the pleura lines the chest wall and covers the diaphragm, and the inner wall adheres to the lung. The pleural cavity lies between the two walls, and the **mediastinum** lies between the lungs. The mediastinum contains several structures, including the heart, esophagus, and several vital blood vessels and nerves.

Mechanics of Respiration

The lungs are passive during the process of breathing. Although the pleural cavities around the lungs are closed, the inside of the lungs are in communication with the outside atmosphere and are subject to its pressure. It is important to remember that air flows from higher pressure to lower pressure until pressure is equalized. During inspiration, the thoracic cavity increases, causing the pressure within the thorax to decrease and forcing air into the lungs. You can simulate this inspiration action by pulling apart the handles of a bellows (Fig. 16-6A). When the handles are pulled apart, the bellows become larger as air rushes into them. The reverse happens during expiration. Similarly, the thoracic cavity returns to its smaller size, pressure in the thorax increases, and air is forced out of the lungs. You can simulate expiration by pushing the handles of the bellows together, making them smaller and forcing air out of them (Fig. 16-6B).

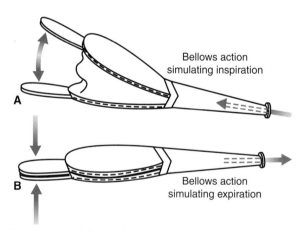

Bellows action simulating inspiration

Bellows action simulating expiration

Figure 16-6.   **(A)** Simulation of inspiration. As the handles of the bellows are pulled apart, air is brought into the bellows. As the ribs elevate and the diaphragm moves down, the thoracic cavity gets larger and air is pulled into the lungs. **(B)** Simulation of expiration. As the handles of the bellows are pushed together, air is pushed out of the bellows. Similarly, as the ribs move downward and the diaphragm moves upward, the thoracic cavity gets smaller and air is pushed out of the lungs.

Using the Heimlich maneuver to dislodge a foreign object from the pharynx or larynx of someone who is choking demonstrates the mechanics of expiration. To perform the Heimlich, stand behind the choking victim and put both arms around the victim's waist. With one hand curled into a fist, place it between the umbilicus and the rib cage. Cover your fist with the other hand, and perform a quick, forceful, upward thrust (Fig. 16-7). This forces the diaphragm upward and compresses the lungs, forcing air and the foreign object out of the victim's trachea. This action can be compared to a forceful artificial cough.

Phases of Respiration

Inspiration is commonly divided into three phases of increasing effort: quiet, deep, and forced. **Quiet inspiration** occurs when an individual is resting or sitting quietly. The diaphragm and external intercostal muscles are the prime movers. The actions of quiet inspiration increase during **deep inspiration.** A person needs more oxygen and therefore breathes harder. Muscles that can pull the ribs up are being called into action. **Forced inspiration** occurs when an individual is working very hard, needs a great deal of oxygen, and is in a state of "air hunger." The muscles of quiet and deep

inspiration are working, as are muscles that stabilize or elevate the shoulder girdle; this directly, or indirectly, elevates the ribs.

Expiration is divided into two phases: quiet and forced. **Quiet expiration** is mostly a passive action. It occurs through relaxation of the diaphragm and the external intercostal muscles, the elastic recoil of the thoracic wall and tissue of the lungs and bronchi, and gravity pulling the rib cage down from its elevated position. Essentially, no muscle action occurs. **Forced expiration** uses muscles that can pull down on the rib as well as muscles that can compress the abdomen, forcing the diaphragm upward.

Muscles of Respiration

Respiration is the result of changes in thoracic volume, hence thoracic pressure. There are two ways of changing thoracic volume: (1) moving the ribs and (2) lowering the diaphragm. Either action requires muscles. The primary muscles during respiration are the diaphragm and the intercostal muscles. The role of accessory muscles, which come into play during forced respiration, can be determined by noting whether a muscle's action pulls the ribs up (inspiration) or pulls them down (expiration). There has been a great deal of controversy over which muscles are active during which phases of respiration. In recent years, more refined electromyographic (EMG) instruments and techniques may have helped to clarify the roles of various muscles. Because there have been numerous studies conducted, many of which disagree, the waters are still cloudy.

Diaphragm Muscle

The thoracic cavity is separated from the abdominal cavity by the diaphragm muscle, a large, sheetlike, dome-shaped muscle (Fig. 16-8). It has a somewhat circular origin on the xiphoid process anteriorly, on the lower six ribs laterally, and on the upper lumbar vertebra posteriorly. Its insertion is rather unique. Because the muscle is somewhat circular, it inserts into itself at the broad central tendon. Three openings in the diaphragm muscle allow passage of the esophagus, the aorta, and the inferior vena cava. Because the insertion (central tendon) is higher than the origin, the diaphragm muscle descends when it contracts (Fig. 16-9). This makes the thoracic cavity larger and the abdominal cavity smaller, causing inspiration. Very forced inspiration may lower the dome as much as 4 inches.

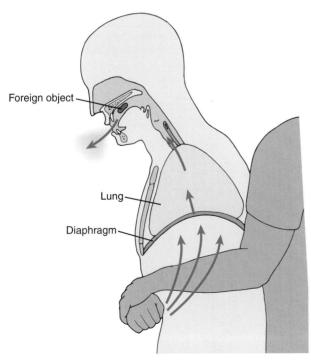

Foreign object

Lung

Diaphragm

Figure 16-7.　Heimlich maneuver.

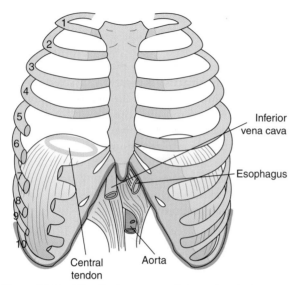

Figure 16-8.   The diaphragm muscle (anterior view).

Intercostal Muscles

The intercostal muscles are located between the ribs and run at right angles to each other (Fig. 16-10). The most superficial muscles are the **external intercostal muscles,** which run inferiorly and medially from the rib above to the rib below (Fig. 16-11). They elevate the ribs below by pulling up on them from their attachment on the rib above. The fibers of the **internal intercostal muscles,** which lie deep and at a 90-degree angle to the external intercostal muscles, perform the opposite action. They run superiorly and medially from the rib below to the rib above (Fig. 16-12). They depress the ribs by pulling down on the rib above.

Anteriorly, the external intercostal muscles run in the same direction as the external oblique muscles of the abdomen. The fibers of the left and right external intercostals form a *V*. Similarly, the internal intercostal muscles, which run in the opposite direction, form the shape of an inverted *V*.

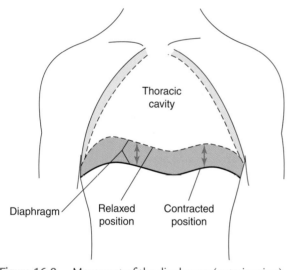

Figure 16-9.   Movement of the diaphragm (anterior view). When the diaphragm contracts, it descends, making the thoracic cavity larger. As in the bellows example, this allows air to be pulled into the lungs. When it relaxes, it moves upward, decreasing the size of the thoracic cavity and forcing air out of the lungs.

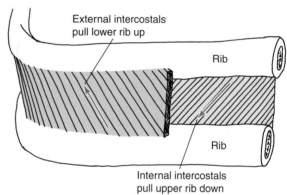

Figure 16-10.   The direction of the fibers of the external and internal intercostal muscles (anterior view).

Diaphragm Muscle

O	Xiphoid process, ribs, lumbar vertebrae
I	Central tendon
A	Inspiration
N	Phrenic nerve (C3, C4, C5)

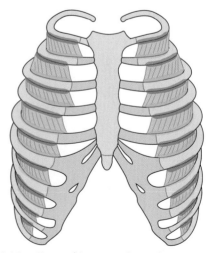

Figure 16-11.   External intercostal muscles (anterior view).

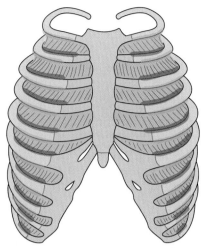

Figure 16-12. Internal intercostal muscles (anterior view).

If you view these two sets of muscles posteriorly, the direction of their fibers is just the opposite from their direction anteriorly. Posteriorly, the external intercostals on the right and left sides are in the shape of an inverted *V*, while the internal intercostals on both sides are now in the shape of a *V*. To clearly understand how this change occurs, take a pencil and place it diagonally next to the sternum of a skeleton (or your partner). Next, move the pencil around the rib cage posteriorly toward the vertebral column without changing the *direction* of the pencil. Notice that the pencil (muscle fibers) direction posteriorly is opposite to what it was in front. Although the fibers have not changed direction, the ribs have curved 180 degrees, causing this apparent change in direction.

External Intercostal Muscles

O	Rib above
I	Rib below
A	Elevate ribs
N	Intercostal nerve (T2 through T6)

Internal Intercostal Muscles

O	Rib below
I	Rib above
A	Depress ribs
N	Intercostal nerve (T2 through T6)

Accessory Inspiratory Muscles

Accessory muscles of inspiration assist the diaphragm and external intercostals in pulling up on the rib cage. These muscles demonstrate reversal of muscle action by pulling from origin toward insertion, not from insertion toward origin. For example, the sternocleidomastoid usually pulls from its insertion on the skull toward the sternum, causing the head to move. During inspiration, other muscles stabilize the head and neck, and the sternocleidomastoid now pulls from the origin on the sternum toward insertion on the head (Fig. 16-13). Pulling in this direction will elevate the rib cage.

Athletes who have just completed a sprint commonly put their hands on their hips while trying to "catch their breath." This posture makes breathing a closed-chain activity. With the arms braced, the pectoralis major can now pull the sternum toward the humerus, thus increasing the diameter of the rib cage. Individuals with chronic obstructive pulmonary disease commonly brace their arms against the arms of a chair to accomplish the same thing (Fig. 16-14).

The scalenes usually move the head and neck. However, when they act as accessory breathing muscles, they elevate the first and second ribs, assisting in inspiration.

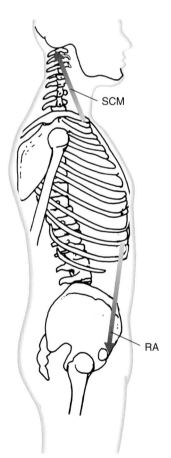

Figure 16-13. Sternocleidomastoid (SCM) muscle pulling up and rectus abdominis (RA) pulling down (lateral view).

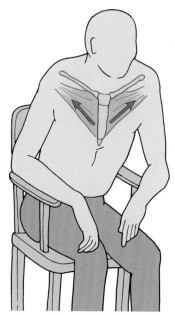

Figure 16-14.   The pectoralis major muscle assisting with inspiration in a reversal of muscle action by pulling the sternum toward the humerus, which is stabilized by resting the forearms on the arms of the chair (closed-chain action).

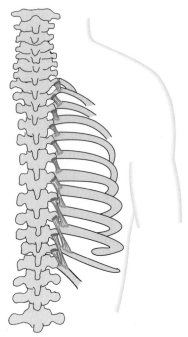

Figure 16-15.   The levator costarum muscles (posterior view).

Accessory Expiratory Muscles

Accessory expiratory muscles operate in much the same fashion, except that they pull down on the rib cage. For example, the rectus abdominis, which usually flexes the trunk, now pulls the sternum toward the pubis in a reversal of muscle action, assisting expiration (see Fig. 16-13). The quadratus lumborum pulls the lower ribs toward the iliac crest in the same fashion.

Many of the accessory breathing muscles have already been discussed with the vertebral column (see Chapter 15) or the shoulder girdle (see Chapter 9). Those that have not been discussed here or in previous chapters are illustrated in Figures 16-15 and 16-16 and listed in Table 16-1.

Table 16-2 summarizes the phases of respiration.

Anatomical Relationships

Many muscles attach to the rib cage, including those of the neck and trunk, the shoulder girdle, the shoulder, and the respiratory muscles. The main respiratory muscles are the deepest, while the accessory muscles lie more superficial. As described earlier, any muscle that attaches to the rib cage, even indirectly (as is the case with the levator scapula), and exerts an upward pull can perform as an accessory inspiratory muscle. Figure 16-17 shows

most of the muscles listed in Table 16-2. Posteriorly, the shoulder girdle muscles that attach on the vertebral column and the scapula, such as the levator scapula, upper trapezius, and rhomboids, can exert an upward pull on the rib cage in a reversal of muscle action via the scapula's and clavicle's connection.

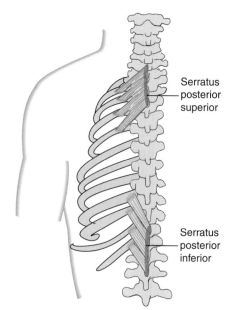

Serratus posterior superior

Serratus posterior inferior

Figure 16-16.   The serratus posterior superior and inferior muscles (posterior view).

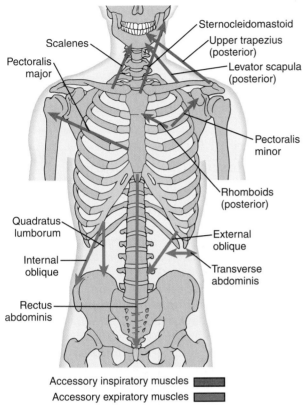

Figure 16-17. Muscles of respiration (anterior view).

Accessory inspiratory muscles
Accessory expiratory muscles

Table 16-1	Accessory Muscles of Respiration
Accessory Inspiratory Muscles	**Accessory Expiratory Muscles**
Deep Inspiration Muscles	**Forced Expiration Muscles**
Sternocleidomastoid	Rectus abdominis
Pectoralis major	External oblique
Scalenes	Internal oblique
Levator costarum (see Fig. 16-15)	Transverse abdominis superior
Serratus posterior superior (see Fig. 16-16)	Quadratus lumborum
	Serratus posterior inferior (see Fig. 16-15)
Forced Inspiration Muscles	
Levator scapula	
Upper trapezius	
Rhomboids	
Pectoralis minor	

Table 16-2	Phases of Respiration

Inspiration

Elevation (raising) of ribs and increase in size of thoracic cavity via descent of the diaphragm muscle and expansion of the thoracic cavity.

Phase	Muscles
Quiet inspiration	Diaphragm
	External intercostals
Deep inspiration	Muscles of quiet inspiration *plus:*
	Sternocleidomastoid
	Scalenes
	Pectoralis major
	Levator costarum
	Serratus posterior superior
Forced inspiration	Muscles of quiet and deep inspiration *plus:*
	Levator scapula
	Upper trapezius
	Rhomboids
	Pectoralis minor

Expiration

Depression (lowering) of ribs and decrease in size of the thoracic cavity

Phase	Muscles
Quiet expiration	Relaxation of diaphragm and external intercostals
	Elastic recoil of thoracic wall, lungs, and bronchi
	Gravity
	(Internal intercostals)
Forced expiration	Internal intercostals *plus:*
	Rectus abdominis
	External oblique
	Internal oblique
	Quadratus lumborum
	Transverse abdominis
	Serratus posterior inferior

Anteriorly, the pectoralis minor, rectus abdominus, external and internal obliques, and quadratus lumborum have attachments on the ribs and can pull down in a similar reversal of muscle action. The transverse abdominis does not exert a pull on the ribs as much as it compresses the abdominal cavity, forcing air out of the lungs. The serratus posterior superior and inferior muscles assist in pulling the ribs up and down, respectively. They are the intermediate muscle layer in the back between the more superficial shoulder girdle muscles and the deeper trunk muscles (see Fig. 16-16).

Diaphragmatic Versus Chest Breathing

Diaphragmatic breathing is the most efficient method of breathing and requires the least amount of energy. Normally, the diaphragm lowers when it contracts, causing the abdomen to move out, the lungs to expand, and air to flow into the lungs. When the diaphragm relaxes, it raises, the abdomen moves in, the lungs recoil, and air flows out of the lungs. When sitting or standing, the gravitational pull on the abdominal viscera also tends to lower the diaphragm. However, when lying down, gravity's effect on the abdominal viscera tends to push the diaphragm up into the thoracic cavity, making the diaphragm work harder. This gravitational effect provides the rationale for elevating the head of the bed of an individual with respiratory difficulty. The elevated position allows easier breathing.

Certain habits, conditions, or pathologies will not allow the diaphragm to work effectively. In those cases, the upper chest and rib cage must play a major role. **Chest breathing** requires greater effort and is much less efficient than diaphragmatic breathing. As described earlier, during inspiration, the rib cage moves up and out (both in a medial-lateral direction and in an anterior-posterior direction), the lungs expand, and air flows into the lungs. During expiration, the rib cage relaxes, the lungs recoil, and air flows out of the lungs. Chest breathing draws a much smaller volume of air into the lungs. With shorter breaths, the individual must breathe more rapidly. A person who chest breathes is more prone to hyperventilate and faint.

To increase your awareness of the two methods of breathing, lie supine in a comfortable position with pillows under your knees and head. Place one hand on your upper chest and the other hand on your stomach just below your ribs. Breathe in slowly through your nose with your mouth closed. With diaphragmatic breathing, you will notice that the hand on your stomach moves up and down as you breathe in and out. There should be little or no movement of the hand on your chest. With chest breathing, the opposite occurs. You will notice movement of the hand on your chest instead of the one on your stomach.

A century ago, it was considered fashionable for women to wear dresses with tightly laced corsets. Aesthetically, this made for a small waist, but functionally it forced the internal organs up against the diaphragm, greatly restricting its effectiveness and forcing women to become chest breathers. No wonder the literature is full of accounts of women "swooning" or fainting. Today, we have the "designer jeans syndrome." Tight-fitting clothing, belts, and waistbands restrict diaphragmatic breathing and force a person to chest breathe. Extremely obese people and women in the later stages of pregnancy cannot effectively contract the diaphragm; therefore, they also tend to chest breathe.

Summary of Innervation of the Muscles of Respiration

Muscles of respiration, like other trunk muscles, receive innervation from spinal nerves at various levels, primarily in the thoracic region. The notable exception is the diaphragm muscle, which is innervated by the phrenic nerve. The phrenic nerve arises from the third, fourth, and fifth cervical nerves. This is functionally significant because an individual with a spinal cord injury at C3 or above cannot breathe unassisted. They will be dependent on a respirator. Inspiration in individuals with a cervical spinal cord injury below C3 will have impaired respiration, but they can breathe unassisted, although activities such as coughing, yelling, or taking deep breaths will be limited. Not only are the intercostal muscles involved, but other accessory breathing muscles are necessary as well. Activities requiring forced inspiration or expiration are affected to the degree that the accessory breathing muscles are involved.

Valsalva's Maneuver

Valsalva's maneuver occurs when people hold their breath and attempt to exhale. Several things can happen. Forcibly exhaling while keeping the mouth closed and nose pinched shut forces air into the eustachian tubes and increases pressure inside the eardrum. This is sometimes helpful in "clearing your ears," which may have become blocked from diving or quickly descending from a high elevation.

Prolonged breath-holding and straining forces exhalation against the closed glottis. This increases intrathoracic pressure, which traps blood in veins and prevents it from entering the heart. When the breath is released, intrathoracic pressure drops and the trapped blood is quickly propelled through the heart, increasing the heart rate (tachycardia) and blood pressure. Immediately, a reflex bradycardia (slowed heart rate) follows. This event can have no consequences, or it can lead to cardiac arrest.

Young children having a temper tantrum sometimes take several deep, fast breaths, then stick their thumb in their mouth and blow hard without releasing any air. This can cause them to get dizzy and pass out. During exertion, adults may take a deep breath and blow hard or "bear down" without exhaling. Because this maneuver helps to create intraabdominal pressure and strong contraction of the abdominal muscles that help to stabilize the spine and keep the trunk tight during a heavy lift, it may be done purposefully during exercise. It is also commonly done during birth delivery, moving up in bed, straining when urinating, defecating, vomiting, coughing, or sneezing.

A healthy heart can usually withstand these sudden and changing demands. However, in a weakened heart, it can lead to cardiac arrest. Therefore, when exercising, it is a good general rule to breathe out slowly and avoid holding your breath.

Common Respiratory Conditions or Pathologies

An **upper respiratory infection (URI)** is any infection confined to the nose, throat, and larynx. The larynx marks the transition between the upper and lower airways. The common cold is perhaps the most frequent URI. Other URIs include influenza (flu), laryngitis, rhinitis (inflammation of the nasal mucosa), and hay fever.

Lower respiratory infections (LRIs) involve structures from the trachea to the alveoli. **Pneumonia** is perhaps the most common LRI. It is an inflammation of the alveoli caused by a bacterial or viral infection. Pneumonia can affect an entire lobe (lobar pneumonia) or can be scattered throughout the entire lung (bronchopneumonia). Bronchopneumonia is more common in the very young and very old. "Walking pneumonia" is

so named because, in most cases, the disease is not severe enough to confine the individual to bed or to be hospitalized. Bronchitis, emphysema, and asthma are other common LRIs. **Bronchitis** involves the bronchi and their many subdivisions. In **emphysema,** the walls of the alveoli become distended and lose their elasticity due to chronic bronchial obstruction. **Asthma** symptoms are usually due to a spasm of the bronchial walls, which makes exhalation very difficult.

Hyperventilation occurs commonly during rapid breathing when more carbon dioxide is removed from the system than is being produced metabolically. A common treatment for hyperventilation involves breathing into a paper bag to "rebreathe" carbon dioxide. A **stitch** is a temporary condition common in runners. It is a localized, sharp pain, usually felt just below the rib cage and commonly caused by a cramp in the diaphragm. **Hiccups** are involuntary spasms of the diaphragm accompanied by rapid closure of the glottis, producing short, sharp, inspiratory sounds.

Pleurisy is a quiet, painful condition caused by an inflammation of the pleura. A **pneumothorax,** or *collapsed lung,* occurs by introducing air into or otherwise destroying the vacuum of the pleural cavity, thereby reducing ventilation capacity.

Rib separation refers to a dislocation between the rib and its costal cartilage. A **rib dislocation** is the displacement of the costal cartilage from the sternum. A **flail chest** occurs when four or more ribs are fractured in two places (comminuted). This causes that part of the chest wall to collapse rather than expand during inspiration. Conversely, the chest wall will also expand during expiration.

Review Questions

General Anatomy Questions

1. What bony structures make up the thorax?
2. Costovertebral articulations involve what bony structures?
3. What type of movement is allowed at the costovertebral articulations?
4. How do (a) movements of the thorax, and (b) movements of the diaphragm affect inspiration and expiration?
5. What is the muscle origin of all accessory inspiratory muscles in relation to the rib cage?
6. The line of pull of the right and left external intercostal muscles forms a V shape in front similar to the right and left external obliques. However, in the back, they have the opposite line of pull. Why?
7. The diaphragm has only one bony attachment. How is the other end attached? How does the muscle work?
8. When you talk, are you doing so during inspiration, expiration, or both?
9. How do the accessory muscles assist with breathing?

(continued on next page)

Review Questions—cont'd

10. Movement of the rib cage is often compared mechanically to what? Movement of the thoracic cavity (lung expansion/deflation) is often compared to what?

11. What is the functional significance with regard to respiration between a person with a C3 spinal cord injury and a person with an injury at C5?

Functional Activity Questions

Identify the phase(s) of respiration occurring during the following activities:

1. Blowing up a balloon
2. Holding your breath for the count of 15
3. Sneezing
4. Whistling a tune
5. Sitting quietly

Clinical Exercise Questions

1. Lie supine in a comfortable position with a pillow under your knees and head. Place your right hand on your upper chest and your left hand on your stomach just below your ribs. Breathe in slowly through your nose with your mouth closed.
   a. What type of breathing is occurring if your *right* hand is moving up and down?
   b. What type of breathing is occurring if your *left* hand is moving?

2. Lying in the same position, place one hand on your stomach and the other hand over your mouth. Cough. What muscles do you feel contract?

3. Place one hand on your chest and the other on the anterior lateral side of your neck. Sniff strongly (as if you had a runny nose).
   a. What movement occurs at your chest?
   b. Did you feel any muscle contraction at your neck?
   c. What phase of respiration occurs when sniffing, and what neck muscles in a reversal of muscle action produced the sniffing?

4. Sit in a chair with your elbows supported on the armrests. Place your right hand on the left side of your chest with your fingers pointing up toward the left shoulder. Take a deep breath.
   a. What rib movement occurred, and in what phase of respiration did it occur?
   b. What accessory breathing muscle is working?
   c. What type of chain activity is occurring?

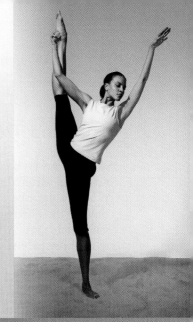

CHAPTER 17
Pelvic Girdle

Structure and Function

False and True Pelvis

Sacroiliac Joint

Pubic Symphysis

Lumbosacral Joint

Pelvic Girdle Motions

Muscle Control

Review Questions

General Anatomy Questions

Functional Activity Questions

Clinical Exercise Questions

Structure and Function

Four bones make up the **pelvic girdle:** the sacrum; the coccyx; and the two hip bones, which are comprised of the ilium, the ischium, and the pubis. The joints or articulations in the pelvic girdle include the right and left **sacroiliac joints** posterolaterally, the **symphysis pubis** anteriorly, and the **lumbosacral joint** superiorly (Fig. 17-1).

The pelvic girdle, also referred to as the **pelvis,** performs several functions. Perhaps most important to movement and posture is that it supports the weight of the body through the vertebral column and passes that force on to the hip bones. Conversely, it receives the ground forces generated when the foot contacts the ground and transmits them upward toward the vertebral column. During walking, the pelvic girdle moves as a unit in all three planes, allowing relatively smooth motion. In addition, the pelvic girdle supports and protects the pelvic viscera, provides attachment for muscles, and makes up the bony portion of the birth canal in females.

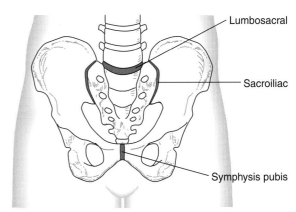

Figure 17-1. Joints of the pelvic girdle (anterior view).

False and True Pelvis

Several terms are commonly used when referring to the birth canal within the pelvis. Therefore, it is appropriate to briefly describe a few of these terms and identify some of the differences between the male and female bony pelvis.

The **false pelvis,** also called the *greater* or *major pelvis,* is the bony area between the iliac crests and is superior to the pelvic inlet. The **pelvic inlet** can be seen by drawing a line between the sacral promontory posteriorly and the superior border of the symphysis pubis anteriorly (Fig. 17-2). There are no pelvic organs within the false pelvis.

The **true pelvis,** also called the *lesser* or *minor pelvis,* lies between the pelvic inlet and the pelvic outlet. The **pelvic outlet** can be seen by drawing a line from the tip of the coccyx to the inferior surface of the pubic symphysis (see Fig. 17-2). The true pelvis area makes up the **pelvic cavity.** It contains portions of the gastrointestinal (GI) tract, the urinary tract, and some reproductive organs. In females, it forms the *birth canal.*

There are several differences between the male and female pelvis (Fig. 17-3). The superior opening into the pelvic cavity is more oval in females and more heart-shaped in males. The pelvic cavity is also shorter and less funnel-shaped in females, and the sacrum is shorter and less curved. The walls are not as vertical, and the

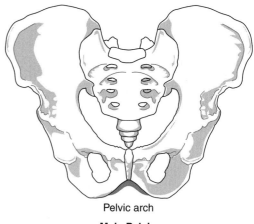

Pelvic arch

Male Pelvis

A

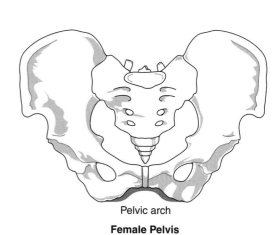

Pelvic arch

Female Pelvis

B

Figure 17-3. Comparison of the male and female pelvis (anterior view). **(A)** Male pelvis. **(B)** Female pelvis.

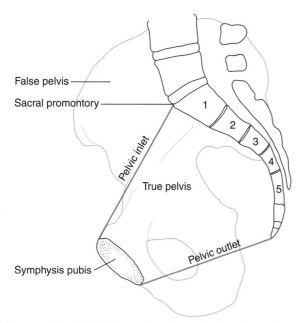

False pelvis

Sacral promontory

1

2

3

4

5

Pelvic inlet

True pelvis

Pelvic outlet

Symphysis pubis

Figure 17-2. Pelvic inlet and outlet, sagittal section. The bony area between them is called the *true pelvis,* which makes up the pelvic cavity. The bony area above the pelvic inlet is called the *false pelvis.*

acetabula (plural of acetabulum) and ischial tuberosities are farther apart. These features make the area within the female pelvic cavity greater than the longer, funnel-shaped cavity of the male pelvis. In addition, the pelvic arch is wider and more rounded in females. The differences in these arches can be represented visually with your hand: form an arch by extending the thumb and index finger on one hand (in females) or by extending the index and middle finger (in males).

Sacroiliac Joint

Joint Structure and Motions

The **sacroiliac joint,** commonly referred to as the **SI joint,** is a synovial, nonaxial joint between the sacrum and the ilium. It is described as a plane joint, but its articular surfaces are very irregular. It is this irregularity that helps to lock the two surfaces together.

The function of the sacroiliac joint is to transmit weight from the upper body through the vertebral column to the hip bones. It is designed for great stability and has very little mobility. Like other synovial joints, its articular surface is lined with hyaline cartilage. Synovial membrane lines the nonarticular portions of the joint. It has a fibrous capsule reinforced by ligaments.

SI Joint Motion

The actual type and amount of movement occurring at the SI joint is the subject of considerable controversy. However, it is generally accepted that the motions that do occur at the SI joint are nutation and counternutation (Fig. 17-4).

Nutation, sometimes referred to as *sacral flexion,* occurs when the base of the sacrum (on the superior end) moves anteriorly and inferiorly. This causes the inferior portion of the sacrum and the coccyx to move posteriorly. The pelvic outlet becomes larger and can be visualized by drawing a line from the tip of the coccyx to the bottom surface of the pubic symphysis.

Counternutation, sometimes called *sacral extension,* refers to the opposite motion. The base of the sacrum moves posteriorly and superiorly, causing the tip of the coccyx to move anteriorly. The pelvic inlet becomes larger. The pelvic inlet can be visualized by drawing a line from the base of the sacrum across to the top of the symphysis pubis.

The amount of motion that occurs in nutation and counternutation is minimal, and it can occur only in conjunction with other joint motions. Nutation occurs with trunk flexion or hip extension. Conversely, counternutation occurs with trunk extension or hip flexion. These motions are also important during childbirth. When the baby moves through the pelvic inlet during the early stages of labor, the anterior-posterior (A-P) diameter needs to be larger. Therefore, the SI joints are in counternutation. In the later stages of labor, when the baby passes through the pelvic outlet, it is important that this A-P diameter has increased. Putting the SI joints in nutation increases the A-P diameter.

Bones and Landmarks

The two bones of the SI joint are the sacrum and the ilium, the latter of which is the superior portion of the hip bone. The **sacrum** is wedge-shaped and consists of five fused sacral vertebrae. It is located between the two hip bones and makes up the posterior border of the bony pelvis. Its anterior surface, often called the *pelvic surface,* is concave (Fig. 17-5). Because it is tilted, the sacrum articulates with the fifth lumbar vertebra at an angle referred to as the *lumbosacral angle.* The significant landmarks are as follows (Figs. 17-5 and 17-6):

Base
Superior surface of S1.

Promontory
Ridge projecting along the anterior edge of the body of S1.

Superior Articular Process
Located posteriorly on the base, it articulates with the inferior articular process of L5.

Ala
Lateral flared wings that are actually fused transverse processes.

Foramina
Located on the anterior (pelvic) and dorsal surfaces are four pair of foramina. They serve as the exit for the anterior and posterior divisions of the sacral nerves. The anterior foramina are larger.

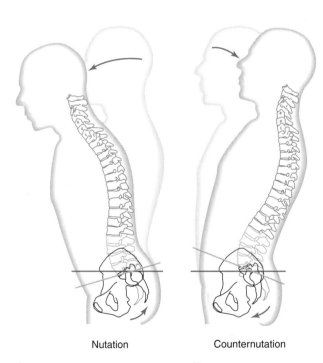

Nutation   Counternutation

A   **B**

Figure 17-4.   Sacroiliac joint motions. **(A)** Nutation occurs when the sacral promontory moves anteriorly and inferiorly while the tip of the coccyx moves in the opposite direction. **(B)** Counternutation occurs when the sacral promontory moves posteriorly and superiorly while the tip of the coccyx moves in the opposite direction.

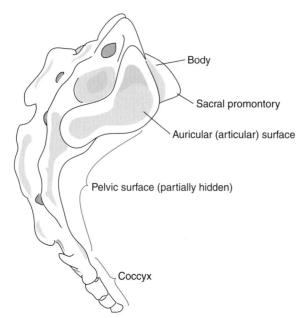

Figure 17-5.   Sacrum (lateral view).

Auricular Surface
Named because its shape is similar to the external ear (*auricular* is Latin for "earlike"). It is located on the lateral surface of the sacrum and articulates with the ilium. The irregular surface assists in locking the two surfaces together, providing greater stability.

Pelvic Surface
Concave axnterior surface.

The **ilium** will be described in more detail in Chapter 18. The ilium makes up the superior part of

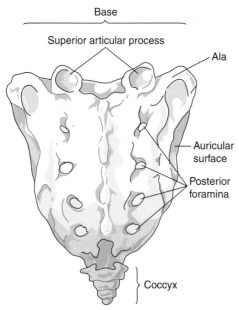

Figure 17-6.   Sacrum (posterior view).

the hip bone. Landmarks relevant to the sacroiliac joint are as follows (Fig. 17-7):

Tuberosity
Large, roughened area between the posterior portion of the iliac crest and the auricular surface. It serves as an attachment for the interosseous ligament.

Auricular Surface
Named for its earlike shape, it is the articular surface of the ilium with the sacrum. It is located inferior and anterior to the iliac tuberosity.

Iliac Crest
Superior ridge of the ilium, the bony area felt when you place your hands on your hips.

Posterior Superior Iliac Spine
Often abbreviated PSIS, it is the posterior projection of the iliac crest and serves as an attachment for the posterior sacroiliac ligaments.

Posterior Inferior Iliac Spine
Often abbreviated as PIIS, it lies inferior to the PSIS and serves as an attachment for the sacrotuberous ligament.

Greater Sciatic Notch
Formed by the ilium superiorly and the ilium and ischium inferiorly.

Greater Sciatic Foramen
Formed from the greater sciatic notch by ligamentous attachments. The sacrotuberous ligament forms the posterior medial border of the foramen, and the sacrospinous ligament forms the inferior border (Figs. 17-8 and 17-9). The sciatic nerve passes through this opening.

The **ischium** will also be described in more detail in Chapter 18. The portions of the ischium pertaining to the sacroiliac joint are as follows (see Fig. 17-7):

Body
Makes up all of the ischium superior to the tuberosity.

Lesser Sciatic Notch
Smaller concavity located on the posterior body between the greater sciatic notch and the ischial tuberosity.

Spine
Located on the posterior body and between the greater sciatic and lesser sciatic notches. It provides attachment for the sacrospinous ligament.

Tuberosity
The blunt, rough projection on the inferior part of the body. It is a weight-bearing surface when you are sitting.

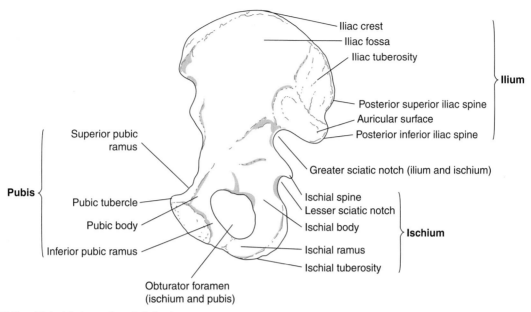

Figure 17-7. Right hip bone (medial view).

Ligaments

Because the sacroiliac joint is meant to absorb a great deal of stress while providing great stability, it is heavily endowed with ligaments. The **anterior sacroiliac ligament** is a broad, flat ligament on the anterior (pelvic) surface connecting the ala and pelvic surface of the sacrum to the auricular surface of the ilium (see Fig. 17-8). It holds together the anterior portion of the joint. The **interosseous sacroiliac ligament** is the deepest, shortest, and strongest of the sacroiliac ligaments (see Fig. 17-9). It fills the roughened area immediately above and behind the auricular surfaces and the anterior sacroiliac ligament. It also connects the tuberosities of the ilium to the sacrum.

The posterior sacroiliac ligament is comprised of two parts (Fig. 17-10). The **short posterior sacroiliac**

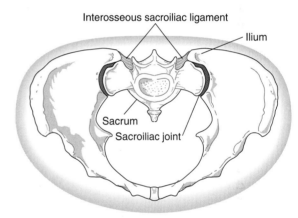

Figure 17-9. Cross section of the sacroiliac joints (superior view).

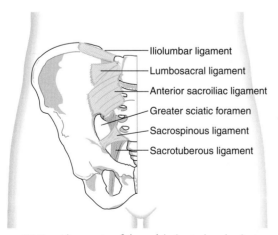

Figure 17-8. Ligaments of the pelvis (anterior view).

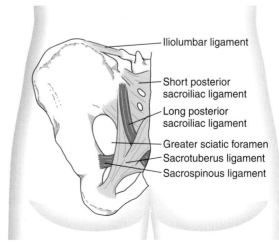

Figure 17-10. Ligaments of the pelvis (posterior view).

ligament runs more obliquely between the ilium and the upper portion of the sacrum on the dorsal surface. It prevents forward movement of the sacrum. The **long posterior sacroiliac ligament** runs more vertically between the posterior superior iliac spine and the lower portion of the sacrum. It prevents downward movement of the sacrum.

Three accessory ligaments further reinforce the sacroiliac joint and are seen in Figures 17-8 and 17-10. The **sacrotuberous ligament** is a very strong, triangular ligament running from between the PSIS and PIIS of the ilium, from the posterior and lateral side of the sacrum inferior to the auricular surface, and from the coccyx. These fibers come together to attach on the ischial tuberosity. It serves as an attachment for the gluteus maximus and prevents forward rotation of the sacrum. The **sacrospinous ligament** is also triangular and lies deep to the sacrotuberous ligament. It has a broad attachment from the lower lateral sacrum and coccyx on the posterior side. It then narrows to attach to the spine of the ischium. These two ligaments convert the greater sciatic notch into a foramen through which the sciatic nerve passes. The **iliolumbar ligament** connects the transverse process of L5 with the ala of the sacrum. It is described in more detail in the "Lumbosacral Joint" section.

Pubic Symphysis

The pubic symphysis joint is located in the midline of the body (Fig. 17-11). The right and left pubic bones are joined anteriorly and form the pubic symphysis. A fibrocartilage disk lies between the two bones. Because

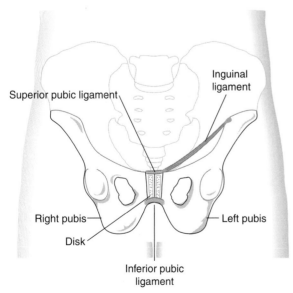

Figure 17-11.   Pubic symphysis, frontal view with pubic bone cut away.

it is an amphiarthrodial joint, there is little movement. However, it becomes much more moveable in women during childbirth.

The pubic symphysis is held together primarily by two ligaments (see Fig. 17-11). The **superior pubic ligament** attaches to the pubic tubercles on each side of the body and strengthens the superior and anterior portions of the joint. The **inferior pubic ligament** attaches between the two inferior pubic rami. It strengthens the inferior portion of the joint.

Landmarks

The **pubis** will be described in greater detail in Chapter 18. The landmarks relevant to the pubic symphysis are the following (see Fig. 17-7):

Body
Main portion of the pubic bone, between the two projections (rami)—superior and inferior.

Superior Ramus
Superior projection of the pubic body.

Inferior Ramus
Inferior projection of the pubic body that provides attachment for the inferior pubic ligament.

Tubercle
Projects anteriorly on the superior ramus near the midline and provides attachment for superior pubic ligament.

Lumbosacral Joint

Joint Structure and Ligaments

The lumbosacral joint is made up of the fifth lumbar vertebra and the first sacral vertebra. The articulation between these vertebrae is the same as that for all other vertebrae. The bodies of these two bones are separated by an intervertebral disk and are held together at the bodies by the anterior and posterior longitudinal ligaments. The vertebrae articulate at the articular processes (inferior articular process of L5 and superior articular process of S1). The ligaments holding together this portion of the joint are the supraspinal, interspinal, and ligamentum flava. All of these ligaments are described in Chapter 15.

Two additional ligaments specifically hold the lumbosacral joint together (see Fig. 17-8). The **iliolumbar ligament** attaches on the transverse process of L5 and runs laterally to the inner lip of the posterior portion of the iliac crest. This ligament limits the rotation of L5 on S1, and it assists the articular processes in preventing L5 from moving anteriorly on S1. The **lumbosacral ligament** also attaches on the transverse process of L5. It

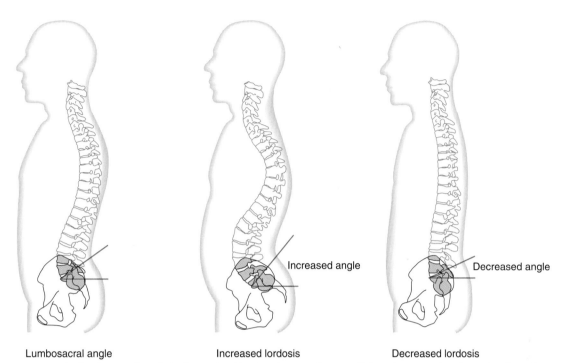

Lumbosacral angle   Increased lordosis   Decreased lordosis

Figure 17-12. The lumbosacral angle is determined by drawing one line parallel to the ground and another line along the base of the sacrum. The angle increases or decreases as lumbar lordosis increases or decreases, respectively.

runs inferiorly and laterally to attach on the ala of the sacrum, where its fibers intermingle with the fibers of the anterior sacroiliac ligament.

Lumbosacral Angle

The lumbosacral angle (Fig. 17-12) is determined by drawing one line parallel to the ground and another line along the base of the sacrum. This angle will increase as the pelvis tilts anteriorly and will decrease as the pelvis tilts posteriorly. The optimal lumbosacral angle is approximately 30 degrees. As the lumbar lordosis increases, the angle increases. This causes the shearing stresses of L5 on S1 to increase. Forward movement of L5 on S1 is prevented by ligamentous restraint, and the shape and fit of the inferior articular process of L5 is seated inside and behind the superior articular process of S1. Conversely, as the lumbar lordosis decreases, lumbosacral angle decreases.

Pelvic Girdle Motions

The joints directly involved in pelvic girdle movement include the two hip joints and the lumbar joints, particularly the lumbosacral articulation between L5 and S1. Pelvic motions occur in all three planes. When you stand in an upright position, the pelvis should be level; in the sagittal plane, the anterior superior iliac spine

(ASIS) and the pubic symphysis should be in the same vertical plane (Fig. 17-13). **Anterior tilt** occurs when the pelvis tilts forward, moving the ASIS anterior to the pubic symphysis. **Posterior tilt** occurs when the pelvis tilts backward, moving the ASIS posterior to the pubic symphysis. These motions are shown in Figure 17-13.

Keeping the body upright when the pelvis tilts forward requires the joints above and below the pelvis to move in the opposite direction. Therefore, when the pelvis tilts anteriorly, the lumbar portion of the vertebral column goes into hyperextension and the hip joints flex. Thus, when a person with a hip flexion contracture stands in the upright position, the pelvis tilts anteriorly and the lumbar region hyperextends. Conversely, a person with tight hamstrings may stand with the pelvis tilted posteriorly and the lumbar curve flattened.

In the frontal plane, the iliac crests should be level (Fig. 17-14). You can assess this by placing your thumbs on the ASISs and determining if your thumbs are at the same level. **Lateral tilt** occurs when the two iliac crests are not level. Because the pelvis moves as a unit, one side moves up as the other side moves down (Fig. 17-15). Therefore, a point of reference must be used. *The side that is unsupported will be the point of reference.* Another way of identifying the reference point is to identify the *side of the pelvis farthest from the joint axis.* For example, in right unilateral stance, the joint axis is the right hip. The side of the pelvis farthest away is the left side. When you

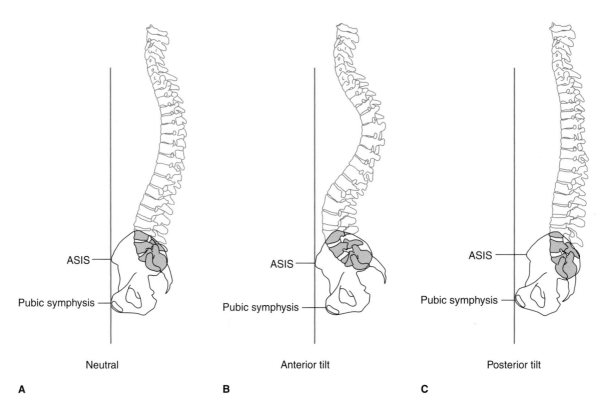

ASIS

Pubic symphysis

Neutral

ASIS

Pubic symphysis

Anterior tilt

ASIS

Pubic symphysis

Posterior tilt

A   B   C

Figure 17-13.   Pelvic movement in the sagittal plane. **(A)** The anterior superior iliac spine (ASIS) and the pubic symphysis should be in the same vertical plane. **(B)** Anterior tilt occurs when the pelvis tilts forward, moving the ASIS anterior to the pubic symphysis. **(C)** Posterior tilt occurs when the pelvis tilts backward, moving the ASIS posterior to the pubic symphysis.

walk, the pelvis is level when both legs are in contact with the ground. However, when one leg leaves the ground (swing phase), it becomes unsupported, and the pelvis on that side drops slightly. It is impossible to drop the pelvis on the weight-bearing side. Therefore, the point of reference for lateral tilt is the unsupported or less supported side, or the side farthest from the weight-bearing joint axis. Figure 17-16 illustrates a left lateral tilt. The person bears weight on the right leg while lifting the left leg from the ground. The left side of the pelvis becomes unsupported and drops, or laterally tilts to the left.

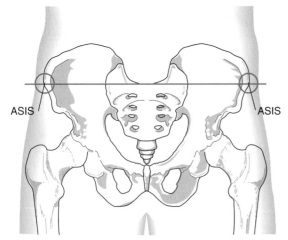

ASIS   ASIS

Figure 17-14.   Pelvic movement in the frontal plane. When standing upright on both feet, the iliac crests and the ASISs should be level.

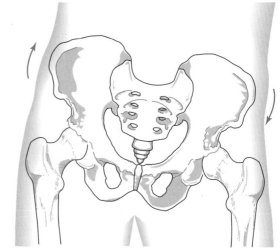

Figure 17-15.   Lateral tilt (anterior view). One side of the pelvis moves up while the other side moves down.

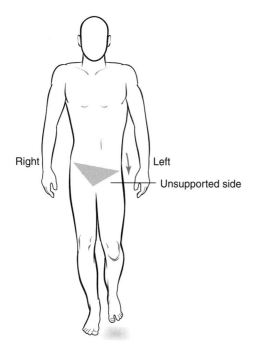

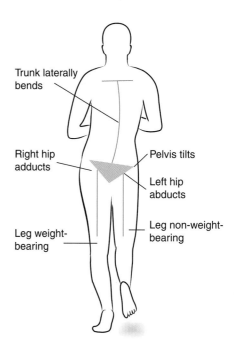

Figure 17-16. Left lateral tilt (anterior view). When one leg leaves the ground, the pelvis on that side becomes unsupported. This causes the pelvis on that side to drop slightly. Therefore, lateral tilt is named by the unsupported side.

Posterior View

Figure 17-17. Other joint motions affected by pelvic tilting. As the pelvis tilts to the right, the vertebral column laterally bends to the left. The left hip (the weight-bearing side) adducts and the right hip (the non-weight-bearing side) abducts.

To keep the body balanced, joints directly above and below will shift in the opposite direction. Notice in Figure 17-17 that as the pelvis tilts (drops) to the right, the vertebral column laterally bends to the left. While the weight-bearing hip joint (left) adducts, the unsupported hip (right) becomes more abducted.

Although this discussion has centered on one side of the pelvis dropping below the level of the other side, it is possible to raise the pelvis on the unsupported side. This is commonly called *hip hiking*. When a person walks with a long leg cast or a brace, hip hiking helps

the foot clear the floor during the swing phase. Shifting from one ischial tuberosity to the other also involves raising the pelvis on one side. This motion is useful in allowing some pressure relief while sitting.

Pelvic rotation occurs in the transverse plane around a vertical axis when one side of the pelvis moves forward or backward in relation to the other side. Looking down on the pelvis, the significant landmarks again are the ASISs. In the anatomical (neutral) position (Fig. 17-18A), both ASISs should be in the same plane. With forward rotation of the pelvis (Fig. 17-18B),

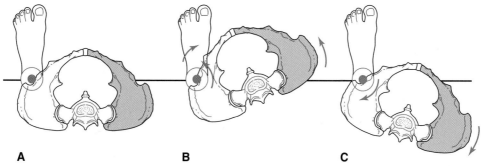

A **B** **C**

Figure 17-18. Pelvic rotation in the transverse plane (superior view). **(A)** In the anatomical (neutral) position, both ASISs are in the same plane. **(B)** With forward rotation, the pelvis on the right moves forward. This causes the left pelvis to rotate around the femoral head, resulting in hip medial rotation. **(C)** With backward rotation, the pelvis on the right moves backward. This causes the left pelvis to rotate on the femoral head, resulting in hip lateral rotation.

the left leg is weight-bearing and the right leg is swinging forward. Once again, *the unsupported side is the point of reference.* This action causes the right side of the pelvis to rotate forward, moving the right ASIS in front of the left ASIS. If the right leg swung backward (Fig. 17-18C), the pelvis would rotate backward. Stated another way, if you bear weight on your left leg and swing your right leg backward, the right side of your pelvis rotates backward.

This pelvic rotation occurs because the pelvis moves on the weight-bearing hip joint. If there is right forward rotation of the pelvis, there is left hip medial rotation (see Fig. 17-18B). Remember that hip medial rotation occurs because the pelvis moves on the femoral head rather than, more commonly, the other way around. With right backward rotation of the pelvis, there is left hip lateral rotation (see Fig. 17-18C). The combinations of joint motions that occur during walking are described in greater detail in Chapter 22. However, a summary of some of the associated joint motions are listed in Table 17-1.

Muscle Control

The pelvis is moved and controlled by groups of muscles acting as force couples. As the pelvis tilts in the anterior/posterior direction, the opposing muscle groups provide movement and control (Fig. 17-19). To tilt the pelvis anteriorly, the lumbar trunk extensors, primarily the erector spinae, pull up posteriorly while the hip flexors pull down anteriorly. Conversely, to tilt the pelvis posteriorly, the abdominals pull up anteriorly while the gluteus maximus and hamstrings pull down posteriorly (Fig. 17-20). In both cases, these muscle groups are acting as a force couple by pulling in opposite directions and causing the pelvis to tilt.

Without any muscle action, the force of gravity can tilt the pelvis laterally when that leg becomes unsupported. However, to control or limit the amount of lateral tilting, muscle groups on opposite sides of the body also work as a force couple. Using the example shown in Figure 17-21, in a reversal of muscle action, the left trunk lateral benders (primarily the erector spinae and quadratus lumborum) pull up on the left side of the

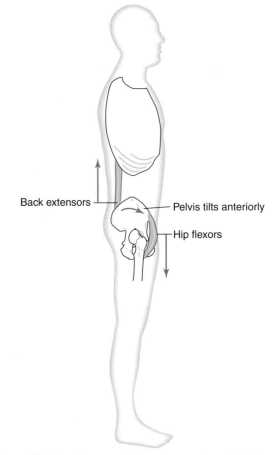

Back extensors — Pelvis tilts anteriorly — Hip flexors

Figure 17-19. Force couple causing anterior pelvic tilt (lateral view). The trunk extensors pulling up (posteriorly) and the hip flexors anterior pulling down (anteriorly) cause the pelvis to tilt anteriorly.

pelvis, while the right hip abductors (gluteus medius and minimus) pull down on the right side to keep the pelvis fairly level.

By preventing pelvic motion, all of these same muscle groups can work together to provide stability. Pelvic and trunk control are necessary to provide the stable foundation upon which the head and extremities can move.

Table 17-1	Associated Motions of the Pelvic Girdle, Vertebral Column, and Hip Joints	
Pelvic Girdle	**Vertebral Column**	**Hip**
Anterior tilt	Hyperextension	Flexion
Posterior tilt	Flexion	Extension
Lateral tilt (unsupported side)	Lateral bending (to supported side)	Adduction: weight-bearing side
		Abduction: non-weight-bearing side
Rotation (forward)	Rotation: to opposite side	Medial rotation: weight-bearing side
Rotation (backward)	Rotation: to opposite side	Lateral rotation: weight-bearing side

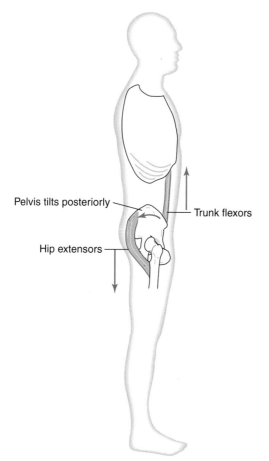

Pelvis tilts posteriorly

Trunk flexors

Hip extensors

Figure 17-20.   Force couple causing posterior pelvic tilt (lateral view). The trunk flexors pulling up (anteriorly) and the hip extensors pulling down (posteriorly) cause the pelvis to tilt posteriorly.

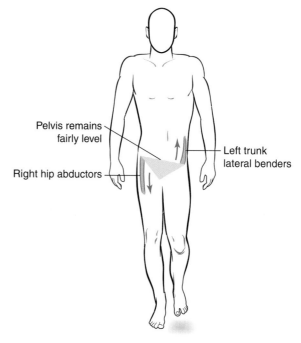

Pelvis remains fairly level

Left trunk lateral benders

Right hip abductors

Anterior View

Figure 17-21.   Force couple keeps the pelvis level in the frontal plane. In a reversal of muscle action, the left trunk lateral benders pull up while the right hip abductors pull down. This keeps the pelvis fairly level as opposed to letting the pelvis drop on the unsupported side.

Review Questions

General Anatomy Questions

1. What pelvic girdle motions occur in the following?
   a. The sagittal plane around the frontal axis
   b. The frontal plane around the sagittal axis
   c. The transverse plane around the vertical axis

2. Concentric contraction of the right quadratus lumborum would cause the pelvis to laterally tilt to which side?

3. Motion occurs at the lumbosacral joint when the pelvis tilts anteriorly and posteriorly and at what other distal joint?

4. What associated hip motion occurs when the pelvis tilts
   a. anteriorly?
   b. posteriorly?
   c. laterally?

5. What associated hip motions occur when the left side of the pelvis rotates
   a. forward?
   b. backward?

(continued on next page)

Review Questions—cont'd

6. What associated lumbar motion occurs when the pelvis tilts
   a. anteriorly?
   b. posteriorly?
   c. laterally?

7. If a person maintained a posture in which the pelvis were tilted excessively in an anterior position, what muscle groups would tend to be tight?

Functional Activity Questions

Identify the position of the pelvis in the following activities:

1. Lying supine, bring your right leg up to your chest.

2. Kneeling on your hands and knees, let your trunk sag downward.

3. Kneeling on your hands and knees, arch your back.

4. Stand with your left foot on a telephone book and your right foot on the floor with weight on both feet. Identify the position of right and left hips in terms of abducted or adducted positions (Fig. 17-22).

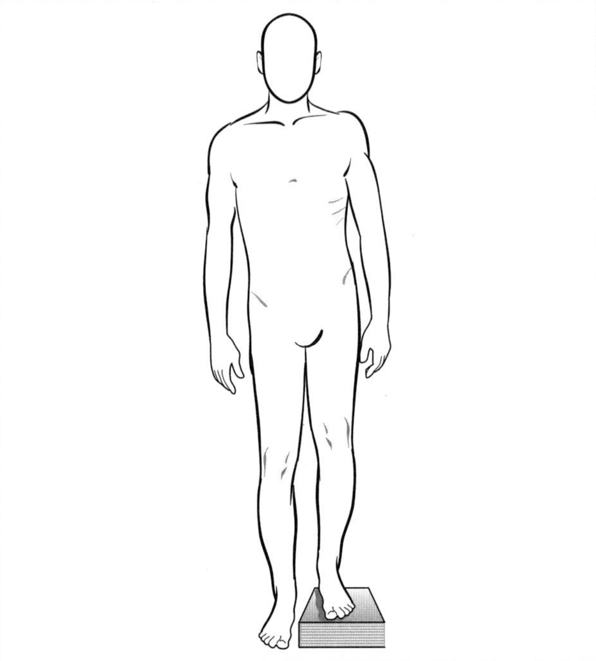

Clinical Exercise Questions

1. Lie supine with your knees flexed and the soles of your feet flat on the mat. Place your hand in the small of your back (lumbar curve). Push your back against your hand. Identify the main trunk, pelvic, and hip motions. Which muscles contribute to this force couple action?
   Motions:
   Muscles:

2. Standing in anatomical position, lift your left foot off the ground while keeping your hip and knee extended. Identify the main pelvic and hip motions. Which muscles contribute to this force couple action?
   Motions:
   Muscles:

Figure 17-22. Standing with one foot on a telephone book and the other foot on the floor.

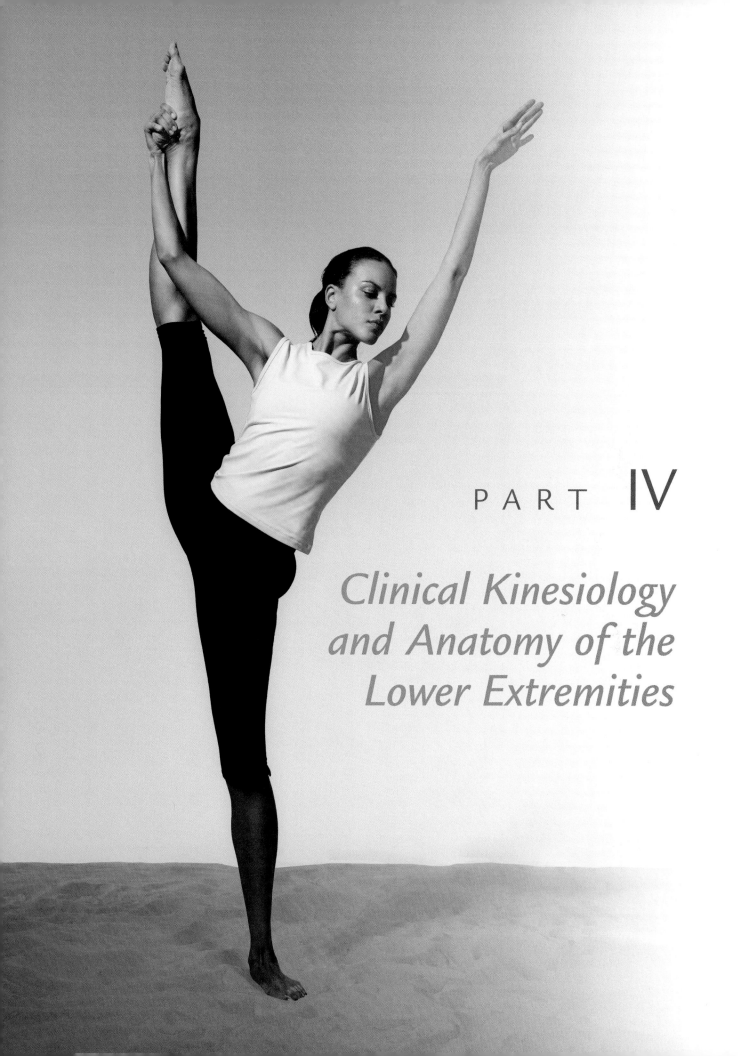

PART IV

Clinical Kinesiology and Anatomy of the Lower Extremities

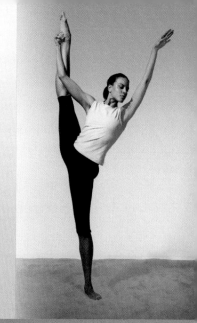

CHAPTER 18
Hip Joint

Joint Structure and Motions

Bones and Landmarks

Ligaments and Other Structures

Muscles of the Hip

    Anatomical Relationships

    Common Hip Pathologies

    Summary of Muscle Action

    Summary of Muscle Innervation

Points to Remember

Review Questions

    General Anatomy Questions

    Functional Activity Questions

    Clinical Exercise Questions

The lower extremity includes the pelvis, thigh, leg, and foot (Fig. 18-1). Bones of the pelvis are the two hip bones (os coxae bones), the sacrum, and the coccyx. The hip bone consists of three bones (ilium, ischium, and pubis) fused together. The thigh contains the femur and the patella. The leg includes the tibia and fibula, and

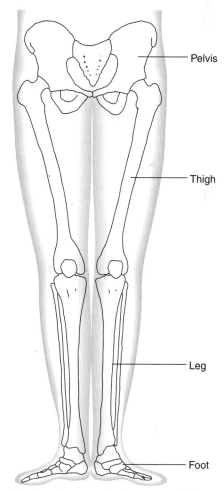

Figure 18-1. The bones of the lower extremities (anterior view).

the foot includes seven tarsal bones, 5 metatarsals, and 14 phalanges. Table 18-1 summarizes the bones of the lower extremity.

Joint Structure and Motions

The **hip** is the most proximal of the lower extremity joints. It is very important in weight-bearing and walking activities. Like the shoulder, it is a ball-and-socket joint. The rounded or convex-shaped femoral head fits into and articulates with the concave-shaped acetabulum (Fig. 18-2). The convex femoral head slides in the direction opposite the movement of the thigh. Unlike the shoulder, the hip is a very stable joint and therefore sacrifices some range of motion. Conversely, the shoulder, which allows a great deal of motion, is not as stable.

Being a triaxial joint, the hip has motion in all three planes (Fig. 18-3). Flexion, extension, and hyperextension occur in the sagittal plane, with approximately 120 degrees of flexion and 15 degrees of hyperextension. Extension is the return from flexion. Abduction and adduction occur in the frontal plane, with about 45 degrees of abduction. Adduction is usually thought of as the return to anatomical position, although there is approximately an additional 25 degrees of motion possible beyond the anatomical position. In the transverse plane, medial and lateral rotations are sometimes referred to as *internal* and *external rotation,* respectively. There are approximately 45 degrees of rotation possible in each direction from the anatomical position.

The two hip bones are connected to each other anteriorly and to the sacrum posteriorly. The sacrum is also

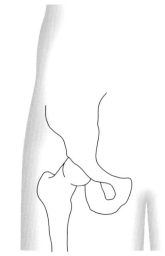

Figure 18-2.   The hip joint (anterior view).

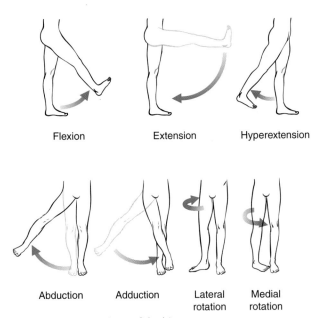

Flexion   Extension   Hyperextension

Abduction   Adduction   Lateral rotation   Medial rotation

Figure 18-3.   Motions of the hip.

connected distally to the coccyx. These four bones (the two hip bones, the sacrum, and the coccyx) are collectively known as the **pelvis,** or **pelvic girdle** (Fig. 18-4). Note that the pelvis does not include the femur.

Bones and Landmarks

As mentioned earlier, the hip joint is made up of the hip bone and the femur. The hip bone, also known as the *os coxae,* is irregularly shaped and actually consists of three bones—the ilium, the ischium, and the pubis (Fig. 18-5). By adulthood, these bones fuse together.

Table 18-1	Bones of the Lower Extremity	
Region	**Bones**	**Individual Bones**
Pelvis	Os coxae	Ilium, ischium, pubis
	Sacrum	
	Coccyx	
Thigh	Femur	
	Patella	
Leg	Tibia	
	Fibula	
Foot	Tarsals (7)	Calcaneus, talus, cuboid, navicular, cuneiform (3)
	Metatarsals (5)	First through fifth
	Phalanges (14)	Proximal (5), middle (4), distal (5)

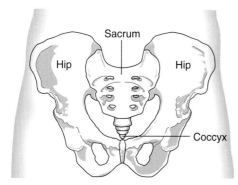

Figure 18-4.   The bones of the pelvis (anterior view).

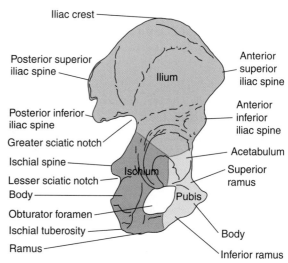

Figure 18-6.   Right hip bone (lateral view).

The fan-shaped **ilium** makes up the superior portion of the hip bone. Its significant landmarks are as follows (Figs. 18-5 and 18-6):

Iliac Fossa
Large, smooth, concave area on the internal surface to which the iliac portion of the iliopsoas muscle attaches

Iliac Crest
Bony part that your hands rest on when you put your hands on your hips. Its borders are the anterior superior iliac spine (ASIS) and the posterior superior iliac spine (PSIS).

Anterior Superior Iliac Spine
Abbreviated as ASIS. The projection on the anterior end of the iliac crest. The tensor

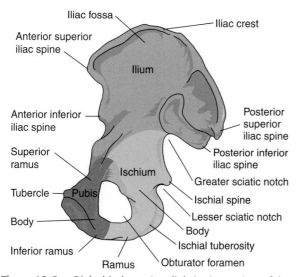

Figure 18-5.   Right hip bone (medial view), consists of the ilium, ischium, and pubis. The greater sciatic notch, acetabulum, and obturator foramen are formed by different combinations of these bones.

fascia latae, sartorius, and inguinal ligament attach here.

Anterior Inferior Iliac Spine
Abbreviated as AIIS. The projection is just inferior to the ASIS, to which the rectus femoris muscle attaches.

Posterior Superior Iliac Spine
Abbreviated as PSIS. It is the posterior projection on the iliac crest.

Posterior Inferior Iliac Spine
Abbreviated as PIIS; located just below the PSIS.

The **ischium** is the posterior inferior portion of the hip bone. Its significant landmarks are as follows (see Fig. 18-6):

Body
Makes up about two-fifths of the acetabulum.

Ramus
Extends medially from the body to connect with the inferior ramus of the pubis. The adductor magnus, obturator externus, and obturator internus muscles attach here.

Ischial Tuberosity
Rough, blunt projection of the inferior part of the body, which is weight-bearing when you are sitting. It provides attachment for the hamstring and adductor magnus muscles.

Spine
Located on the posterior portion of the body between the greater and lesser sciatic notches. It provides attachment for the sacrospinous ligament.

The **pubis** forms the anterior inferior portion of the hip. It can be divided into three parts—the body and its two rami (see Figs. 18-5 and 18-6):

Body
Externally forms about one-fifth of the acetabulum and internally provides attachment for the obturator internus muscle.

Superior Ramus
Lies superior between the acetabulum and the body and provides attachment for the pectineus muscle.

Inferior Ramus
Lies posterior, inferior, and lateral to the body. Provides attachment for the adductor magnus and brevis and gracilis muscles.

Symphysis Pubis
A cartilaginous joint connecting the bodies of the two pubic bones at the anterior midline

Pubic Tubercle
Projects anteriorly on the superior ramus near the symphysis pubis and provides attachment for the inguinal ligament

The following are made up of combinations of the hip bones (see Fig. 18-5):

Acetabulum
A deep, cup-shaped cavity that articulates with the femur. It is made up of nearly equal portions of the ilium, ischium, and pubis.

Obturator Foramen
A large opening surrounded by the bodies and rami of the ischium and pubis and through which pass blood vessels and nerves

Greater Sciatic Notch
Large notch just below the PIIS that is actually made into a foramen by the sacrospinous and sacrotuberous ligaments (see Fig. 17-8). The sciatic nerve, piriformis muscle, and other structures pass through this opening.

The **femur** is the longest, strongest, and heaviest bone in the body. A person's height can roughly be estimated to be four times the length of the femur (Moore, 1985). It articulates with the hip bones to form the hip joint and has the following significant landmarks (Fig. 18-7):

Head
The rounded portion covered with articular cartilage articulating with the acetabulum.

Neck
The narrower portion located between the head and the trochanters.

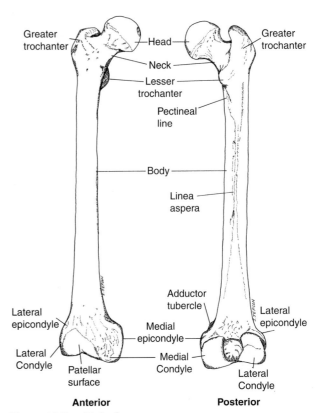

Figure 18-7.   Right femur.

Greater Trochanter
Large projection located laterally between the neck and the body of the femur, providing attachment for the gluteus medius and minimus and for most deep rotator muscles.

Lesser Trochanter
A smaller projection located medially and posteriorly just distal to the greater trochanter, providing attachment for the iliopsoas muscle.

Body
The long, cylindrical portion between the bone ends; also called the *shaft.* It is bowed slightly anteriorly.

Medial Condyle
Distal medial end.

Lateral Condyle
Distal lateral end.

Lateral Epicondyle
Projection proximal to the lateral condyle.

Medial Epicondyle
Projection proximal to the medial condyle.

Adductor Tubercle

Small projection proximal to the medial epicondyle to which a portion of the adductor magnus muscle attaches.

Linea Aspera

Prominent longitudinal ridge or crest running most of the posterior length.

Pectineal Line

Runs from below the lesser trochanter diagonally toward the linea aspera. It provides attachment for the adductor brevis.

Patellar Surface

Located between the medial and lateral condyle anteriorly. It articulates with the posterior surface of the patella.

The **tibia** will be discussed in more detail in Chapter 19, but it is important to identify one landmark now (Fig. 18-8):

Tibial Tuberosity

Large projection at the proximal end in the midline. It provides attachment for the patellar tendon.

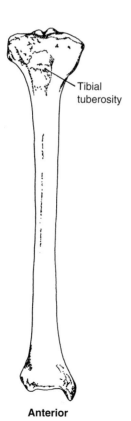

Tibial tuberosity

Anterior

Figure 18-8. Right tibia (anterior view).

Ligaments and Other Structures

Like all synovial joints, the hip has a fibrous **joint capsule.** It is strong and thick, and it covers the hip joint in a cylindrical fashion. It attaches proximally around the lip of the acetabulum and distally to the neck of the femur (Fig. 18-9). It forms a cylindrical sleeve that encloses the joint and most of the femoral neck.

Three ligaments reinforce the capsule: the iliofemoral, the pubofemoral, and the ischiofemoral ligaments (Fig. 18-10). The most important of these ligaments is the **iliofemoral ligament.** It reinforces the capsule anteriorly by attaching proximally to the anterior inferior iliac spine and crossing the joint anteriorly. It splits into two parts distally to attach to the intertrochanteric line of the femur. Because it resembles an inverted Y, it is often referred to as the *Y ligament.* It is also known as the *ligament of Bigelow.* Its main function is to limit hyperextension.

The **pubofemoral ligament** spans the hip joint medially and inferiorly. It attaches from the medial part of the acetabular rim and superior ramus of the pubis, and runs down and back to attach on the neck of the femur. Like the iliofemoral ligament, it limits hyperextension. In addition, it limits abduction.

The **ischiofemoral ligament** covers the capsule posteriorly. It attaches on the ischial portion of the acetabulum, crosses the joint in a lateral and superior direction, and attaches on the femoral neck. Its fibers limit hyperextension and medial rotation.

All three of these ligaments attach along the rim of the acetabulum and cross the hip joint in a spiral fashion to attach on the femoral neck. The combined effect of this spiral attachment is to limit motion in one direction (hyperextension) while allowing full motion (flexion) in the other direction. Therefore, these ligaments are slack in flexion and become taut as the hip moves into hyperextension. If you thrust your hips forward so

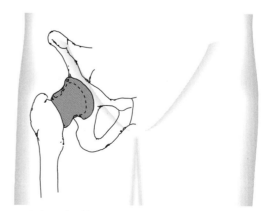

Figure 18-9.   The hip joint capsule (anterior view).

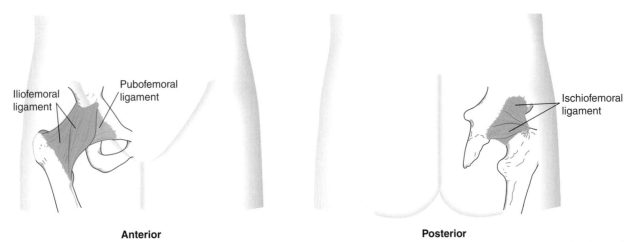

Anterior   **Posterior**

Figure 18-10.   The hip joint capsule is reinforced by three ligaments: the iliofemoral, the pubofemoral, and the ischiofemoral ligaments.

that they are in front of the shoulders and knees, you can stand in the upright position without using any muscles by essentially resting on the iliofemoral ligament. This is the basis for the standing posture of an individual with paralysis following spinal cord injury (Fig. 18-11).

The **ligamentum teres** is a small intracapsular ligament of debatable importance (Fig. 18-12). It attaches proximally in the acetabulum and distally in the fovea of the femoral head. Some sources indicate that it becomes taut during adduction or lateral rotation, when the hip is semiflexed. However, given its size, it is

doubtful that it adds significantly to the joint's strength. Its other feature is that it contains a blood vessel that supplies the head of the femur. However, this vessel alone cannot supply enough blood to the head to keep it viable.

The depth of the acetabulum is increased by the fibrocartilaginous **acetabular labrum,** which is located around the rim. The free end of the labrum surrounds the femoral head and helps to hold the head in the acetabulum.

Although the **inguinal ligament** has no function at the hip joint, it should be identified because of its presence. It runs from the anterior superior iliac spine to the pubic tubercle and is the landmark that separates the anterior abdominal wall from the thigh (Fig. 18-13). When the external iliac artery and vein pass under the inguinal ligament, their names change to the *femoral artery* and *vein.*

The **iliotibial band** or **tract** is the very long, tendinous portion of the tensor fascia latae muscle (see Fig. 18-26). It attaches to the anterior portion of the iliac crest and runs superficially down the lateral side of the thigh to attach to the tibia. Both the gluteus

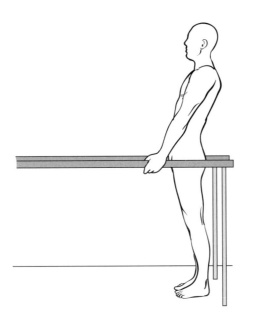

Figure 18-11.   The spiral attachment of the hip ligaments tends to limit hyperextension. Therefore, an individual who is paraplegic can stand in the upright position by thrusting the hips forward of the shoulders and knees.

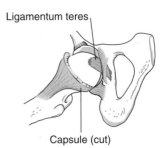

Figure 18-12.   The ligamentum teres. Oblique view with femur laterally rotated and capsule cut away.

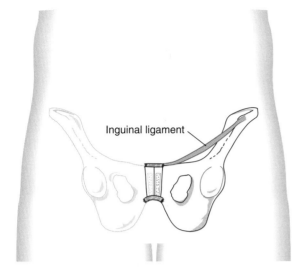

Figure 18-13. The inguinal ligament (anterior view).

Table 18-2	Muscles of the Hip	
Muscle Group	One-Joint Muscles	Two-Joint Muscles
Anterior	Iliopsoas	Rectus femoris Sartorius
Medial	Pectineus Adductor magnus Adductor longus Adductor brevis	Gracilis
Posterior	Gluteus maximus Deep rotators (6)	Semimembranosus Semitendinosus Biceps femoris (long head)
Lateral	Gluteus medius Gluteus minimus	Tensor fascia latae

maximus and tensor fascia latae muscles have fibers attaching to it.

The end feel of all hip joint motions except flexion is firm (soft tissue stretch) because of tension in the capsule, ligaments, and muscles. For hip flexion, the end feel is soft (soft tissue approximation) because of contact between the anterior thigh and the abdomen.

Iliopsoas Muscle

O	Iliac fossa, anterior and lateral surfaces of T12 through L5
I	Lesser trochanter
A	Hip flexion
N	Iliacus portion: femoral nerve (L2, L3) Psoas major portion: L2 and L3

Muscles of the Hip

There are many similarities between the shoulder and hip joints. Like the shoulder, the hip has a group of one-joint muscles that provide most of the control, and it has a group of longer, two-joint muscles that provide the range of motion. These muscles can also be grouped according to their location and somewhat by their function. For example, the anterior muscles tend to be flexors, lateral muscles tend to be abductors, posterior muscles tend to be extensors, and medial muscles tend to be adductors. Table 18-2 classifies the hip muscles by location and function.

The **iliopsoas muscle** is actually two muscles with separate proximal attachments and a common distal attachment (Fig. 18-14). The iliacus muscle portion arises from the iliac fossa, and the psoas major muscle portion comes from the transverse processes, bodies, and intervertebral disks of the T12 through L5 vertebrae. These muscles blend together to attach on the lesser trochanter of the femur. The iliopsoas muscle is a prime mover in hip flexion. Because of its attachment on the vertebrae, the psoas muscle portion contributes to trunk flexion when the femur is stabilized.

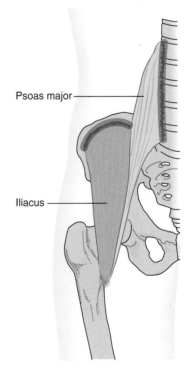

Figure 18-14. The iliopsoas muscle is made up of the psoas major and the iliacus (anterior view).

The **rectus femoris muscle** is part of the quadriceps muscle group and is the only one of that group to cross the hip (Fig. 18-15). Its proximal attachment is on the AIIS. It runs almost straight down the thigh, where it is joined by the three vasti muscles to blend into the quadriceps tendon (also called the *patellar tendon*). This tendon encases the patella, crosses the knee joint, and attaches to the tibial tuberosity. The rectus femoris muscle is a prime mover in hip flexion and knee extension.

Rectus Femoris Muscle

O	Anterior inferior iliac spine
I	Tibial tuberosity
A	Hip flexion, knee extension
N	Femoral nerve (L2, L3, L4)

The **sartorius muscle** is the longest muscle in the body (Fig. 18-16). This straplike muscle arises from the anterior superior iliac spine. It runs diagonally across the thigh from lateral to medial and proximal to distal to cross the medial knee joint posteriorly. Because of its line of pull, it is capable of flexing, abducting, and laterally rotating the hip and flexing the knee. However, it is not considered a prime mover in any one of these motions. It is most efficient when doing all four motions at the same time. An example of this motion is

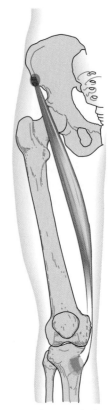

Figure 18-16.   The sartorius muscle (anterior view).

when you cross your legs by putting one foot on the opposite knee.

Sartorius Muscle

O	Anterior superior iliac spine
I	Proximal medial aspect of tibia
A	Combination of hip flexion, abduction, lateral rotation, and knee flexion
N	Femoral nerve (L2, L3)

Located medial to the iliopsoas muscle and lateral to the adductor longus muscle is the **pectineus muscle.** Its origin is on the superior ramus of the pubis, and its insertion is on the pectineal line of the femur (Fig. 18-17). Because it spans the hip anteriorly and medially, it provides hip flexion and adduction.

Pectineus Muscle

O	Superior ramus of pubis
I	Pectineal line of femur
A	Hip flexion and adduction
N	Femoral nerve (L2, L3, L4)

There are three other one-joint hip adductors, all with the same first name (Fig. 18-18). The **adductor**

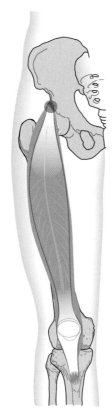

Figure 18-15.   The rectus femoris muscle (anterior view).

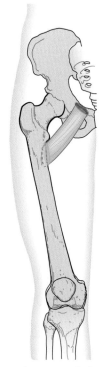

Figure 18-17. The pectineus muscle (anterior view). Note that the distal attachment is on the posterior femur.

longus muscle, the most superficial of the three, originates from the anterior surface of the pubis near the tubercle and inserts on the middle third of the linea aspera of the femur. Because it is superficial, its tendon can easily be felt in the anterior-medial groin. Being able to palpate this tendon is important when checking for correct fit of the quadrilateral socket of an above-knee prosthesis. It is a prime mover in hip adduction.

Adductor Longus Muscle

O	Pubis
I	Middle third of the linea aspera
A	Hip adduction
N	Obturator nerve (L3, L4)

The **adductor brevis muscle** implies by its name that it is shorter than the other adductor muscles. It lies deep to the adductor longus muscle but superficial to the adductor magnus muscle. It arises from the inferior ramus of the pubis and inserts on the pectineal line and proximal linea aspera above the adductor longus muscle. It is a prime mover in hip adduction.

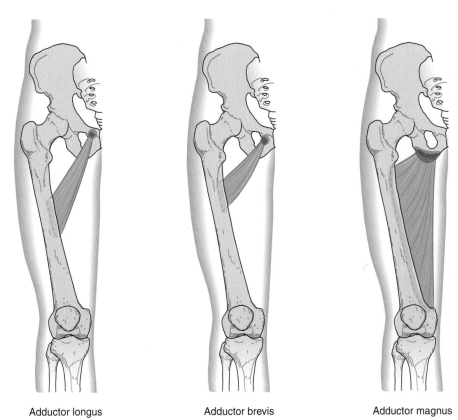

Adductor longus   Adductor brevis   Adductor magnus

Figure 18-18. The three adductor muscles (anterior view). Note that the distal attachments are on the posterior femur.

Adductor Brevis Muscle

O	Pubis
I	Pectineal line and proximal linea aspera
A	Hip adduction
N	Obturator nerve (L3, L4)

The largest and deepest of the adductors is the **adductor magnus muscle.** It arises from the ischial tuberosity and ramus of the ischium and inferior ramus of the pubis. It makes up most of the bulk on the medial thigh. It inserts along the entire linea aspera and adductor tubercle. There is an interruption, or hiatus, in the distal attachment between the linea aspera and adductor tubercle. The femoral artery and vein pass through this opening. After these structures have passed through to the posterior surface, their names become the *popliteal artery* and *vein,* respectively. Because of its size, the adductor magnus muscle is a very strong hip adductor.

Adductor Magnus Muscle

O	Ischium and pubis
I	Entire linea aspera and adductor tubercle
A	Hip adduction
N	Obturator and sciatic nerve (L3, L4)

The only hip adductor that is a two-joint muscle is the **gracilis muscle** (Fig. 18-19). It arises from the symphysis and inferior ramus of the pubis and descends the thigh medially and superficially. It crosses the knee joint posteriorly and curves around the medial condyle to attach distally on the anteromedial surface of the proximal tibia. It assists with knee flexion.

Gracilis Muscle

O	Pubis
I	Anterior medial surface of proximal end of tibia
A	Hip adduction
N	Obturator nerve (L2, L3)

The **gluteus maximus muscle** can be described as a large, thick, one-joint, quadrilateral muscle located superficially on the posterior buttock (Fig. 18-20). It arises from the general area of the posterior sacrum, coccyx, and ilium, and it runs in a diagonal direction distally and laterally to the posterior femur, inferior to the greater trochanter. Some fibers also attach to the iliotibial band. Because it spans the hip posteriorly in this diagonal direction, it is very strong in hip extension, hyperextension, and lateral rotation.

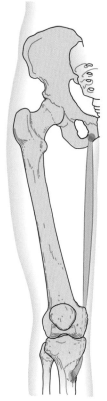

Figure 18-19. The gracilis muscle (anterior view). Note that it passes behind the knee but attaches anteriorly.

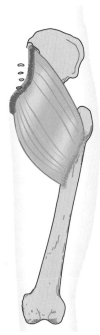

Figure 18-20. The gluteus maximus muscle (posterior view).

Gluteus Maximus Muscle

O	Posterior sacrum and ilium
I	Posterior femur distal to greater trochanter and to iliotibial band
A	Hip extension, hyperextension, lateral rotation
N	Inferior gluteal nerve (L5, S1, S2)

There are six small, deep, mostly posterior muscles that span the hip joint in a horizontal direction, and they all laterally rotate the hip. Because they all work together to produce the same motion, their individual attachments are not functionally important; therefore, they can be grouped together as the **deep rotator muscles** (Fig. 18-21). However, the piriformis is the best known of this group, perhaps because of its close relationship to the sciatic nerve. Table 18-3 summarizes their attachments and innervation.

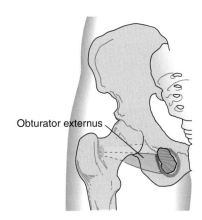

Obturator externus

Anterior

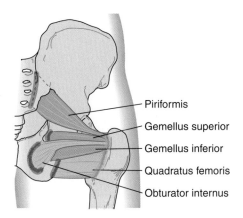

— Piriformis

— Gemellus superior

— Gemellus inferior

— Quadratus femoris

— Obturator internus

Posterior

Figure 18-21. The deep rotator muscles.

Deep Rotator Muscles

O	Posterior sacrum, ischium, pubis
I	Greater trochanter area
A	Hip lateral rotation
N	Numerous (see Table 18-3)

Three muscles that are known collectively as the **hamstring muscles** cover the posterior thigh. They consist of the semimembranosus, the semitendinosus, and the biceps femoris muscles (Fig. 18-22). They have a common site of origin on the ischial tuberosity.

The **semimembranosus muscle** runs down the medial side of the thigh, deep to the semitendinosus muscle, and inserts on the posterior surface of the medial condyle of the tibia. The **semitendinosus muscle** has a much longer and narrower distal tendon that spans the knee joint posteriorly and then moves anteriorly to attach to the anteromedial surface of the tibia with the gracilis and sartorius muscles. The **biceps femoris muscle** has two heads and runs down the thigh laterally on the posterior side. The long head arises with the other two muscles on the ischial tuberosity, but the short head arises from the lateral lip of the linea aspera. Both heads join together, spanning the knee posteriorly to attach laterally on the head of the fibula and, by a small slip, to the lateral condyle of the tibia. Because they span the knee posteriorly, they flex the knee. The long head, because it spans the hip posteriorly, extends the hip.

Semimembranosus Muscle

O	Ischial tuberosity
I	Posterior surface of medial condyle of tibia
A	Extend hip and flex knee
N	Sciatic nerve (L5, S1, S2)

Semitendinosus Muscle

O	Ischial tuberosity
I	Anteromedial surface of proximal tibia
A	Extend hip and flex knee
N	Sciatic nerve (L5, S1, S2)

Biceps Femoris Muscle

O	Long head: ischial tuberosity Short head: lateral lip of linea aspera
I	Fibular head
A	Long head: extend hip and flex knee Short head: flex knee
N	Long head: sciatic nerve (S1, S2, S3) Short head: common peroneal nerve (L5, S1, S2)

Table 18-3	Deep Rotator Muscles		
Muscle	**Proximal Attachment**	**Distal Attachment**	**Innervation**
Obturator externus	Rami of pubis and ischium	Trochanteric fossa	Obturator nerve
Obturator internus	Rami of pubis and ischium	Greater trochanter	Nerve to obturator internus
Quadratus femoris	Ischial tuberosity	Intertrochanteric crest	Nerve to quadratus femoris
Piriformis	Sacrum	Greater trochanter	S1, S2 segments
Gemellus superior	Ischium	Greater trochanter	Nerve to obturator internus
Gemellus inferior	Ischial tuberosity	Greater trochanter	Nerve to quadratus femoris

The other two gluteal muscles are more laterally located. The **gluteus medius muscle** is triangular, much like the deltoid muscle of the shoulder (Fig. 18-23). It attaches proximally to the outer surface of the ilium and distally to the lateral surface of the greater trochanter. Because it spans the hip laterally, the gluteus medius muscle can abduct the hip. Its anterior fibers are able to assist the gluteus minimus muscle in medially rotating the hip.

Gluteus Medius Muscle

O	Outer surface of the ilium
I	Lateral surface of the greater trochanter
A	Hip abduction
N	Superior gluteal nerve (L4, L5, S1)

Proximally, the **gluteus minimus muscle** lies deep and inferior to the gluteus medius muscle on the lateral ilium (Fig. 18-24). The distal attachment is on the anterior aspect of the greater trochanter. This gives the gluteus minimus muscle a somewhat diagonal line of pull, making it able to medially rotate the hip. Because it spans the hip laterally, it also abducts the hip.

Gluteus Minimus Muscle

O	Lateral ilium
I	Anterior surface of the greater trochanter
A	Hip abduction, medial rotation
N	Superior gluteal nerve (L4, L5, S1)

Attaching to the ilium and the femur and spanning the hip laterally, these two gluteal muscles have another very important function. When you stand on one leg, the distal segment (femur) becomes more stable than the proximal segment (pelvis); therefore, the origin moves toward the insertion. Another term for this change is **reversal of muscle function.** If these

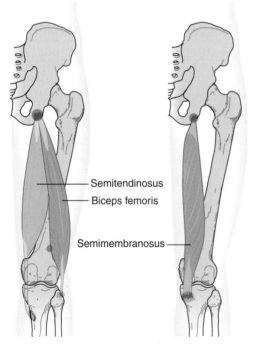

Figure 18-22.   The hamstring muscles (posterior view).

Semitendinosus
Biceps femoris
Semimembranosus

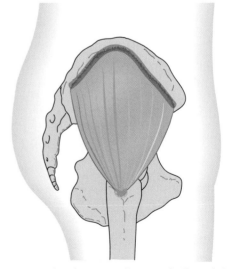

Figure 18-23.   The gluteus medius muscle (lateral view).

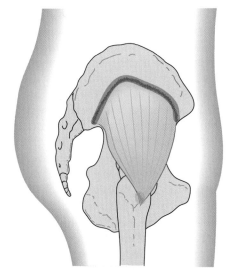

Figure 18-24. The gluteus minimus muscle (lateral view).

occurs every time you pick up one leg, as when walking. Weakness or loss of these muscles results in a "Trendelenburg gait." For example, if your right hip abductors are weak, the left side of your pelvis will drop significantly when you stand on your right leg and lift your left leg off the ground.

The **tensor fascia latae muscle** is a very short muscle with a very long tendinous attachment (Fig. 18-26). It arises from the ASIS, crosses the hip laterally and slightly anteriorly, and then attaches to the long fascial band called the *iliotibial band,* which proceeds down the lateral thigh and attaches to the lateral condyle of the tibia. It is a hip abductor, but due to its slight anterior position, it is perhaps strongest when performing a combination of flexion and abduction. Stated another way, it is most efficient when abducting in a slightly anterior direction.

muscles did not contract when you stood on one leg, the opposite side of your pelvis would drop (Fig. 18-25). Therefore, the gluteus medius and minimus muscles contract to keep the pelvis fairly level and to prevent the opposite side of the pelvis from dropping too much when you stand on one leg. This

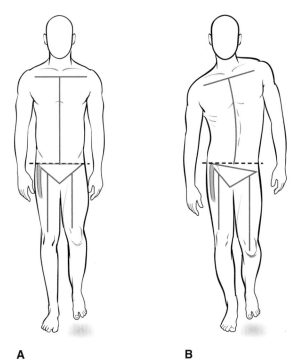

A   **B**

Figure 18-25. Anterior view. **(A)** In reversal of muscle function, the right hip abductors contract to keep the pelvis steady when the left leg is lifted. **(B)** When right hip abductors are weak, the left side of the pelvis drops.

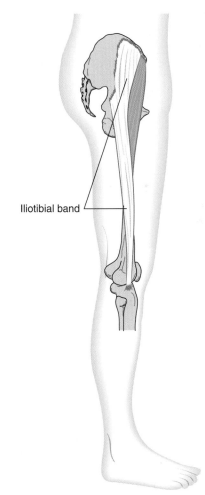

Iliotibial band

Figure 18-26. The tensor fascia latae muscle (lateral view). The very long, tendinous portion of this muscle is known as the *iliotibial band.*

Tensor Fascia Latae Muscle

O	Anterior superior iliac spine
I	Lateral condyle of tibia
A	Combined hip flexion and abduction
N	Superior gluteal nerve (L4, L5)

Anatomical Relationships

Table 18-2 organizes the hip muscles into four groups based on location. Using this grouping, the anatomical relationships of the hip muscles can be easily discussed by adding one other factor: superficial muscles versus deep muscles.

Starting anteriorly, there are two superficial muscles: the tensor fascia latae and the sartorius, which have their origin on the anterior superior iliac spine (Fig. 18-27). They make an inverted V from their common attachment. The tensor fascia latae runs down toward the knee and slightly lateral, while the sartorius runs down in a medial direction. Between these two muscles lies the rectus femoris, which runs straight down toward the knee. Moving medially from the sartorius are the iliopsoas, pectineus, adductor longus, and gracilis. Deep to the adductor longus near the hip is the adductor brevis, and deep to the adductor brevis is the large, wide adductor magnus. More distally on the thigh, the adductor magnus lies deep to the adductor longus (Fig. 18-28).

Viewing the hip region from the medial side superficially, the sartorius, the upper portion of the adductor longus, the gracilis, and the upper half of the adductor magnus can be seen from front to back, followed by the medial hamstrings (Fig. 18-29). From this medial view, you can see that most of the adductor longus and much of the adductor brevis and adductor magnus lie deep.

On the posterior side, the gluteus maximus covers the proximal posterior hip region (Fig. 18-30). Distal to the gluteus maximus, and taking up most of the posterior

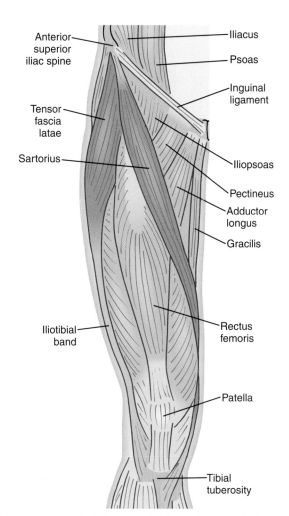

Figure 18-27.   Anterior superficial muscles (right leg).

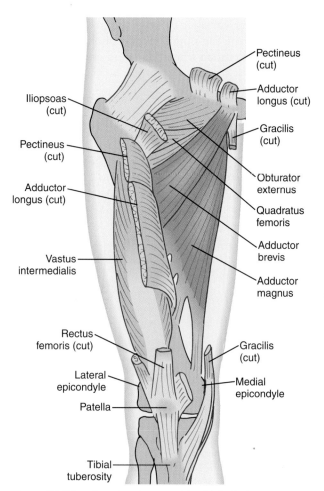

Figure 18-28.   Anterior deep muscles (right leg).

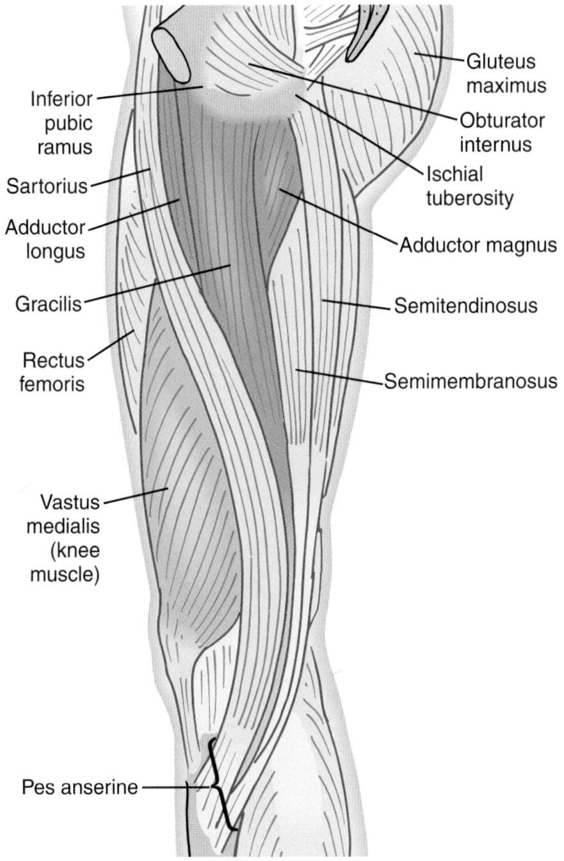

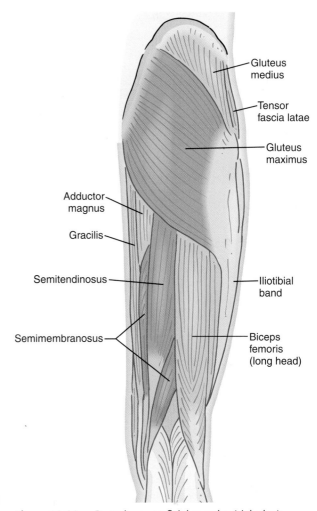

Figure 18-29.   Medial muscles (right leg).

Figure 18-30.   Posterior superficial muscles (right leg).

thigh, are the hamstring muscles. Deep to the gluteus maximus and slightly more lateral is the gluteus medius, and deeper still is the gluteus minimus (Fig. 18-31). The deep rotators are the deepest muscles; you can see five of the six deep rotators in the figure. The hamstring muscles are deep to the gluteus maximus at their proximal attachment on the ischial tuberosity.

Viewing the proximal hip from the lateral side in Figure 18-32, you can see the gluteus maximus posteriorly, the iliotibial band laterally, and the tensor fascia latae anteriorly. The gluteus medius lies deep to these structures, and the gluteus minimus lies deep to the gluteus medius.

Common Hip Pathologies

The hip joint is the site of many orthopedic conditions that occur throughout life and can affect lower extremity alignment. **Congenital hip dislocation,** or **dysplasia,** occurs when an unusually shallow acetabulum causes the femoral head to slide upward. The joint capsule remains intact, though stretched. **Legg-Calvé-Perthes disease,** or **coxa plana,** is a condition in which the

femoral head undergoes necrosis. It is usually seen in children between the ages of 5 and 10 years. During the course of the disease, it may take about 2 to 4 years for the head to die, revascularize, and then remodel. **Slipped capital femoral epiphysis** is seen in children during the growth-spurt years. The proximal epiphysis slips from its normal position on the femoral head.

The angle between the shaft and the neck of the femur in the *frontal plane* is referred to as the **angle of inclination,** which normally is 125 degrees. This angle varies from birth to adulthood. At birth, the angle may be as great as 170 degrees, but by adulthood the angle decreases significantly. However, factors such as congenital deformity, trauma, or disease may affect the angle. **Coxa valga** is characterized by a neck-shaft angle greater than 125 degrees (Fig. 18-33). Because this angle is "straighter," it tends to make the limb longer, thus placing the hip in an adducted position during weight-bearing. **Coxa vara** is a deformity in

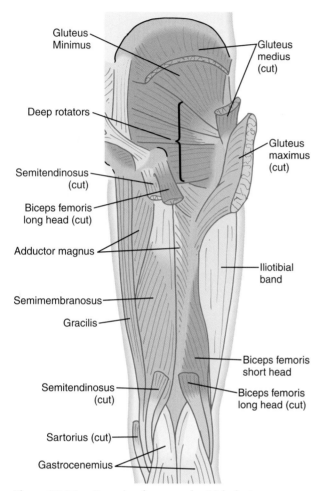

Figure 18-31. Posterior deep muscles (right leg).

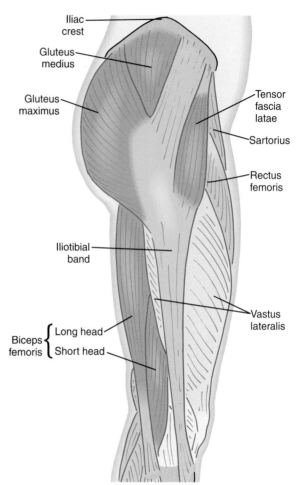

Figure 18-32. Lateral muscles (right leg).

which the neck-shaft angle is less than the normal 125 degrees. Because it is "more bent," it tends to make the involved limb shorter, dropping the pelvis on that side during weight-bearing.

The angle between the shaft and the neck of the femur in the *transverse plane* is called the **angle of torsion,** which normally has the head and neck rotated outward from the shaft approximately 15 to 25 degrees. Looking down on the femur (Fig. 18-34A), you can see the femoral head and neck superimposed on the shaft. The shaft is best shown here by a line through the femoral condyles, which attach to the shaft distally. As the shaft rotates, so do the condyles. An increase in this angle is called **anteversion,** which forces the hip joint into a more medially rotated position (Fig. 18-34B). This causes a person to walk more "toed in." A decrease in the angle of torsion is called **retroversion.** This forces the hip joint into a more laterally rotated position, causing the person to walk more "toed out" (Fig. 18-34C).

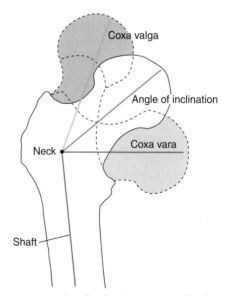

Figure 18-33. Angle of inclination is normally about 125 degrees. Coxa valga is an angle greater than 125 degrees, and coxa vara is an angle less than 125 degrees.

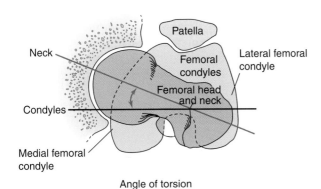

A

Angle of torsion

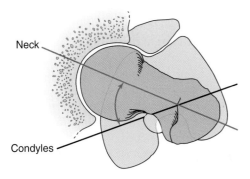

Anteversion is an increased angle and results in toed-in gait

B

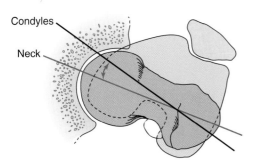

Retroversion is a decreased angle and results in toed-out gait

C

Figure 18-34. Superior view. **(A)** Angle of torsion normally has the head and neck rotated outward from the shaft approximately 15 to 25 degrees. An increase in this angle is called *anteversion* **(B)**, and a decrease in this angle is called *retroversion* **(C)**.

Osteoarthritis is a degeneration of the articular cartilage of the joint. It may result from trauma or wear and tear, and is typically seen later in life. It is commonly treated with a total joint replacement. **Hip fractures** tend to be of two types: intertrochanteric and femoral neck. These are very common among the elderly, usually resulting from falls. High-impact trauma such as motor vehicle accidents may cause hip fractures in younger individuals.

Iliotibial band syndrome is an overuse injury causing lateral knee pain. It is commonly seen in runners and bicyclists. This syndrome is believed to result from repeated friction of the band that slides over the lateral femoral epicondyle during knee motion. It is caused by such factors as muscle tightness, worn-down shoes, and running on uneven surfaces. Because many muscles insert at the greater trochanter, there are many bursae providing a friction-reducing cushion between the muscles and bone. **Trochanteric bursitis** is the result of either acute trauma or overuse. It can be seen in runners or bicyclists or in someone with a leg-length discrepancy, or it can be caused by other factors that put repeated stress on the greater trochanter. A **hamstring strain,** also called *"pulled hamstring,"* is probably the most common muscle problem in the body. Unfortunately, it is often recurrent. It may result from an overload of the muscle or trying to move the muscle too fast. Therefore, this is a common injury among sprinters and in sports that require bursts of speed or rapid acceleration, such as soccer, track and field, football, and rugby. Hamstring strains can occur at one of the attachment sites or at any point along the length of the muscle.

Hip pointer is a misnomer because it occurs at the pelvis, not the hip. It is a severe bruise caused by direct trauma to the iliac crest of the pelvis. It is most commonly associated with football but can be seen in almost any contact sport. Spearing the hip/pelvis with a helmet while tackling may be the most common cause.

Summary of Muscle Action

Table 18-4 summarizes the actions of the prime movers of the hip joint.

Summary of Muscle Innervation

Generally speaking, the femoral nerve innervates muscles on the anterior surface of the hip and thigh region (hip flexors). The obturator nerve innervates hip adductors on the medial side. The superior gluteal nerve supplies the hip abductors on the lateral side. The hamstring muscles, which are hip extensors and are located posteriorly, receive innervation from the sciatic nerve.

There are, of course, exceptions to all generalizations. The gluteus maximus, a posterior muscle, receives innervation from the inferior gluteal nerve. The deep rotators do not fit neatly into any sort of category; therefore, they are included individually in the summary of hip joint

Table 18-4	Action of Hip Prime Movers
Action	**Muscle**
Combination of flexion and abduction	Tensor fascia latae
Combination of flexion, abduction, and lateral rotation	Sartorius
Flexion	Rectus femoris, iliopsoas, pectineus
Extension	Gluteus maximus, semitendinosus, semimembranosus, biceps femoris (long head)
Hyperextension	Gluteus maximus
Abduction	Gluteus medius, gluteus minimus
Adduction	Pectineus, adductor longus, adductor brevis, adductor magnus, gracilis
Medial rotation	Gluteus minimus
Lateral rotation	Gluteus maximus, deep rotators

muscle innervation in Table 18-3 and 18-5 instead of as a group. Table 18-6 summarizes the segmental innervation. As has been stated in previous chapters, there is variation among sources regarding some segmental innervation. The deep rotators are included here as a group.

Points to Remember

- In determining the leverage, the muscle's point of attachment to the bone is used.
- With a second-class lever, resistance is between the axis and the force. With a third-class lever, force is in the middle.
- End feel is the quality of the feel when applying slight pressure at the end of the joint's passive range.
- A closed kinetic chain requires that the distal segment is fixed and the proximal segment(s) move.
- To stretch a one-joint muscle, it is necessary to put any two-joint muscles on a slack over the joint not crossed by the one-joint muscle.
- To contract a two-joint muscle most effectively, start with it being stretched over both joints.
- When determining whether a concentric or eccentric contraction is occurring, decide
  - if the activity is accelerating against gravity or slowing down gravity, or
  - if a weight greater than the pull of gravity is affecting the activity.

Table 18-5	Innervation of the Muscles of the Hip	
Muscle	**Nerve**	**Spinal Segment**
Iliopsoas		
Psoas part	Anterior rami	L2, L3
Iliacus part	Femoral	L2, L3
Rectus femoris	Femoral	L2, L3, L4
Sartorius	Femoral	L2, L3
Pectineus	Femoral	L2, L3, L4
Gracilis	Obturator	L2, L3
Adductor longus	Obturator	L3, L4
Adductor brevis	Obturator	L3, L4
Adductor magnus	Obturator	L3, L4
Gluteus maximus	Inferior gluteal	L5, S1, S2
Gluteus medius	Superior gluteal	L4, L5, S1
Gluteus minimus	Superior gluteal	L4, L5, S1
Tensor fascia latae	Superior gluteal	L4, L5
Semitendinosus	Sciatic	L5, S1, S2
Semimembranosus	Sciatic	L5, S1, S2

Table 18-5   Innervation of the Muscles of the Hip—cont'd

Muscle	Nerve	Spinal Segment
Biceps femoris (long head)	Sciatic	S1, S2, S3
Obturator externus	Obturator	L3, L4
Obturator internus	Nerve to the obturator internus	L5, S1
Gemellus superius	Nerve to the obturator internus	L5, S1
Quadratus femoris	Nerve to the quadratus femoris	L5, S1
Gemellus inferior	Nerve to the quadratus femoris	L5, S1
Piriformis	Anterior rami	S1, S2

Table 18-6   Segmental Innervation of Hip Muscles

Spinal Cord Level	L2	L3	L4	L5	S1	S2	S3
Iliopsoas	X	X					
Sartorius	X	X					
Gracilis	X	X					
Rectus femoris	X	X	X				
Pectineus	X	X	X				
Adductor longus		X	X				
Adductor brevis		X	X				
Adductor magnus		X	X				
Tensor fascia latae			X	X			
Gluteus medius			X	X	X		
Gluteus minimus			X	X	X		
Semitendinosus				X	X	X	
Semimembranosus				X	X	X	
Biceps femoris (long head)					X	X	X
Deep rotators		X	X	X	X	X	

Review Questions

General Anatomy Questions

1. List the bones that make up the
   a. pelvis.
   b. hip bone.
   c. hip joint.
   d. acetabulum.
   e. obturator foramen.
   f. greater sciatic notch.

2. If you were handed an unattached hip bone, what landmarks would you use to determine if it was a right or left hip bone?

3. How would you determine if an unattached femur is a right or left one?

4. Describe the hip joint:
   a. Number of axes:
   b. Shape of joint:
   c. Type of motion allowed:

5. What hip motions occur in
   a. the transverse plane around the vertical axis?
   b. the sagittal plane around the frontal axis?
   c. the frontal plane around the sagittal axis?

6. What is referred to as the *Y ligament*? Why?

7. Why is the hip joint not prone to dislocation?

8. What is the direction of the line of attachment of the hip ligaments—vertical, horizontal, or spiral? What does this line of attachment allow for?

(continued on next page)

Review Questions—cont'd

9. Which two-joint hip muscles attach below the knee?

10. Which hip joint muscles are not prime movers in any single action but are effective in a combination of movements? List the movements.

11. What muscle(s) keeps your pelvis from dropping on one side when you lift one foot off the floor? Describe what happens.

12. Does the femoral head surface glide in the same or opposite direction as the thigh during hip flexion/extension?

13. What is the end feel of hip flexion? Hip extension?

Functional Activity Questions

1. A right-handed tennis player strikes a ball with a forehand swing and follows through. The left hip is moving into what positions (Fig. 18-35)?

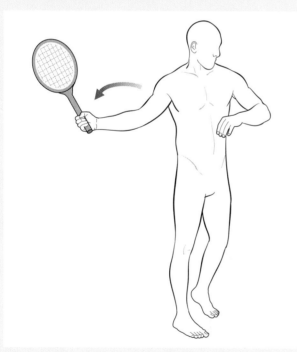

Figure 18-35.　Position of tennis player when hitting a forehand swing.

2. a. How is hip flexion affected by sitting on a low surface versus a higher one (e.g., a regular versus a raised toilet seat)?

   b. What accompanying hip motions or positions may occur if a person has her feet apart, knees together, and hands on her knees, and she pushes down to assist when standing (Fig. 18-36)?

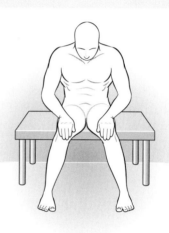

Figure 18-36.　Position of hips when beginning to stand.

3. Standing in anatomical position and keeping your pelvis fairly level, shift your weight to your right foot.
   a. What hip joint motion has occurred at your right hip?
   b. What muscle group initiates this action?
   c. Is this an open- or closed-chain activity?

4. While weight-bearing on the left leg, note the motions of your right hip as you swing your right leg in the following activities:
   a. Walking
   b. Stepping up onto a curb
   c. Getting into a car
   d. Getting on what is commonly called a boy's bicycle (bar between handlebars and seat)

5. Lie supine on a table with knees bent and your feet flat. Note the position of your pelvis and determine if you can put your hand on the small of your back.
   a. If you cannot, what is the position of your pelvis?
   b. If you can, what is the position of your pelvis and lumbar spine?

6. From the position described in question 5, slowly slide your feet down the table until your hips and knees are extended. Again, note the position of your pelvis and determine if you can put your hand

Review Questions—cont'd

on the small of your back. Repeat this again, keeping your right knee and hip flexed with your foot flat, while you move your left foot down until your left hip and knee are extended.

  a. What is accomplished at the pelvis by keeping your right hip and knee flexed?

  b. What can be said about left hip muscle length if you cannot rest your left thigh completely on the table? In other words, why wouldn't you be able to extend your left hip?

  c. What is the one-joint hip muscle attaching on the pelvis and lumbar spine that may be responsible for this limitation?

  d. What difference does the position of the pelvis have on anterior hip muscle length?

7. Pretend that you cannot completely extend your hip due to tight hip flexors. How might you compensate for this when standing?

8. You are seated at a table. Stand up while turning to the right. Stop halfway through this motion (before you move your feet).

  a. The right hip is in what positions? (1) flexed/extended, (2) abducted/adducted, or (3) medially rotated/laterally rotated

  b. The left hip is in what positions? (1) flexed/extended, (2) abducted/adducted, or (3) medially rotated/laterally rotated

9. When a tennis player hits the ball (see Fig. 18-35), what type of kinetic chain activity is occurring at the hip? At the shoulder?

Clinical Exercise Questions

1. While lying prone with your right knee flexed, raise your right leg straight up, keeping your pelvis flat on the table. Describe what has occurred in terms of

  a. hip joint motion.

  b. whether stretching or strengthening is occurring.

  c. muscle(s) involved.

2. In the position shown in Figure 18-37, move your right leg forward until your right knee is directly over your right ankle. Your left hip is hyperextended and your left knee is flexed and resting on the floor. Rock your weight forward onto the front (right) leg

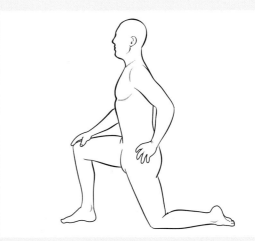

Figure 18-37.   Starting position.

without moving your right foot. Describe what has occurred at the left hip in terms of

  a. joint motion.

  b. whether stretching or strengthening is occurring.

  c. muscle(s) involved.

3. If the position in Figure 18-37 was changed by holding the left knee in more flexion (difficult to achieve comfortably, but pretend), do you think this a good position in which to stretch the rectus femoris? Why?

4. Lying on your right side with your left hip and knee in extension, raise your left leg toward the ceiling about 2 feet. Describe what has occurred in terms of

  a. joint motion.

  b. whether stretching or strengthening is occurring.

  c. muscle(s) involved.

5. Repeat the exercise in question 4 with your left hip in approximately 30 degrees of flexion. Describe what has occurred in terms of

  a. joint motion.

  b. whether stretching or strengthening is occurring.

  c. muscle(s) involved.

(continued on next page)

Review Questions—cont'd

6. Lie on your back with your hips and knees in extension. Raise your right leg toward the ceiling.
   a. Is a concentric or eccentric contraction occurring at the hip?
   b. The hip flexors are demonstrating what class of lever?

7. While lying prone with your left knee flexed, raise your left leg straight up, keeping your pelvis flat on the table.
   a. Are the hamstrings contracting at their strongest?
   b. Why?

8. Sitting on the floor with your legs far apart, lean forward from the hips while keeping your back straight. Describe what has occurred in terms of
   a. hip joint motion.
   b. whether stretching or strengthening is occurring.
   c. muscle(s) involved.

9. Figure 18-38 shows an individual doing hip flexion exercises two different ways. The starting position in both exercises is hip extension and knee extension. In exercise A, the person flexes the hips with the knees flexed. In exercise B, the person performs the same hip flexion motion but with the knees extended.
   a. Which exercise is more difficult?
   b. Why?

10. Starting in a supine position with the knees flexed, move into the position shown in Figure 18-39.
    a. What type of kinetic chain activity is this?
    b. What hip motion is occurring?
    c. What type of contraction is occurring?
    d. What hip muscle group is the agonist?
    e. If this motion could not be completed because a muscle was passively insufficient, what muscle would that be?

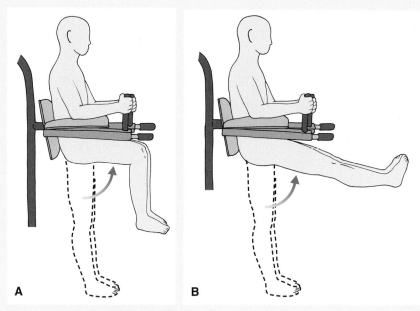

A   B

Figure 18-38.   Hip flexion exercise.

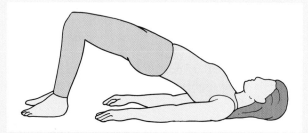

Figure 18-39.   Ending position.

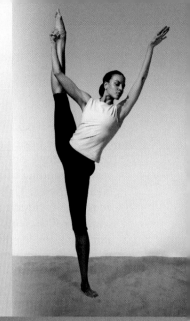

CHAPTER 19

Knee Joint

Joint Structure and Motions

Bones and Landmarks

Ligaments and Other Structures

Muscles of the Knee

Anterior Muscles

Posterior Muscles

Anatomical Relationships

Summary of Muscle Action

Summary of Muscle Innervation

Common Knee Pathologies

Points to Remember

Review Questions

General Anatomy Questions

Functional Activity Questions

Clinical Exercise Questions

Joint Structure and Motions

At first glance, the knee joint appears to be relatively simple. However, it is one of the more complex joints in the body. The knee is supported and maintained entirely by muscles and ligaments with no bony stability, and it frequently is exposed to severe stresses and strains. Therefore, it should be no surprise that it is one of the most frequently injured joints in the body.

The knee joint is the largest joint in the body, and it is classified as a synovial hinge joint (Fig. 19-1). The motions possible at the knee are flexion and extension (Fig. 19-2). From 0 degrees of extension, there are approximately 120 to 135 degrees of flexion. Due to some ligament laxity, the knee may have a few degrees of hyperextension beyond 0; beyond 5 degrees of hyperextension is considered genu recurvatum. Unlike the elbow, the knee joint is not a true hinge, because it has a rotational component. This rotation is not a free motion but rather an accessory motion that accompanies flexion and extension.

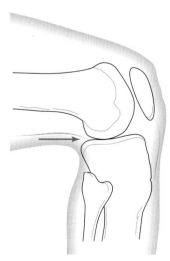

Figure 19-1. The knee joint (lateral view).

All three types of arthrokinematic motion are used during knee flexion and extension. The convex femoral condyles move on the concave tibial condyles or vice versa, depending upon whether it is an open- or closed-chain activity. The articular surface of the femoral condyles is much greater than that of the tibial condyles. If the femur rolled on the tibia from flexion to extension, the femur would roll off the tibia before the motion was complete (Fig. 19-3A). Therefore, the femur must **glide** posteriorly on the tibia as it **rolls** into extension (Fig. 19-3B). It should also be noted that the articular surface of the femoral medial condyle is longer than that of the lateral condyle (Fig. 19-4A). As extension occurs, the articular surface of the femoral lateral condyle is used up while some articular surface remains on the medial condyle (Fig. 19-4B). Therefore, the medial condyle of the femur must also glide posteriorly to use its entire articular surface (Fig. 19-4C). It is this posterior gliding of the medial condyle during the last few degrees of weight-bearing extension (closed-chain action) that causes the femur to **spin** (rotate medially) on the tibia (see Fig. 19-3B).

Looking at the same spin, or rotational, movement during non-weight-bearing extension (open-chain action), note that the tibia rotates laterally on the femur (see Fig. 19-4). These last few degrees of motion lock the knee in extension; this is sometimes called the *screw-home mechanism* of the knee. With the knee fully extended, an individual can stand for a long time without using muscles. For knee flexion to occur, the knee must be "unlocked" by laterally rotating the femur on the tibia. This small amount of rotation of the femur on the tibia, or vice versa, keeps the knee from being a true hinge joint. Because this rotation is not an independent motion, it will not be considered a knee motion.

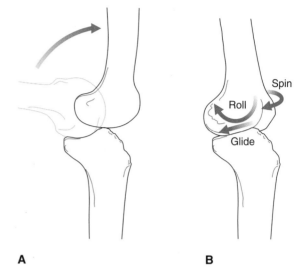

A   **B**

Figure 19-3.   Arthrokinematic movements of the knee joint surfaces in a closed-chain activity of knee extension in which the femur moves on the tibia (medial view). **(A)** Pure rolling of the femur would cause it to roll off the tibia as the knee extends. **(B)** Normal motion of the knee demonstrates a combination of rolling, gliding (posteriorly), and spinning (medially) in the last 20 degrees of extension.

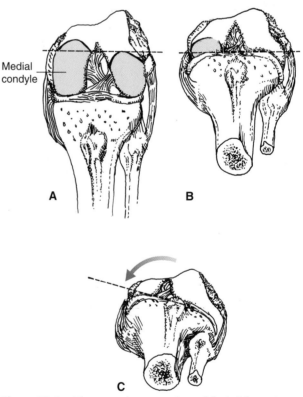

A   **B**

C

Figure 19-4.   The screw-home motion of the left knee. In the weight-bearing position (closed-chain activity), the femur rotates medially on the tibia as the knee moves into the last few degrees of extension.

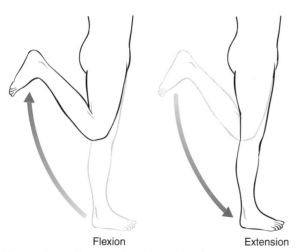

Flexion   Extension

Figure 19-2.   Knee motions (lateral view).

Articulation between the femur and patella is referred to as the **patellofemoral joint** (Fig. 19-5). The smooth, posterior surface of the patella glides over the patellar surface of the femur. The main functions of the patella involve increasing the mechanical advantage of the quadriceps muscle and protecting the knee joint. An increased mechanical advantage is achieved by lengthening the quadricaps moment arm. As discussed in Chapter 8 (in the "Torque" section), moment arm is the perpendicular distance between the muscle's line of action and the center of the joint (axis). By placing the patella between the quadriceps, or patellar tendon, and the femur, the action line of the quadriceps muscles is farther away (Fig. 19-6). Hence, the moment arm lengthens, allowing the muscle to have greater angular force. Without the patella, the moment arm would be shorter and much of the muscle's force would be a stabilizing force directed back into the joint.

The **Q angle,** or *patellofemoral angle,* is the angle between the quadriceps muscle (primarily the rectus femoris muscle) and the patellar tendon. It is determined by drawing a line from the anterior superior iliac spine (ASIS) to the midpoint of the patella, and from the tibial tuberosity to the midpoint of the patella. Although the rectus femoris attaches to the anterior inferior iliac spine (AIIS), the ASIS lies just above the AIIS and is easier to palpate. The angle formed by the intersection of these lines represents the Q angle (Fig. 19-7). In knee extension, this angle ranges from 13 to 19 degrees in normal individuals. The angle tends to be greater in females, because the pelvis is generally wider in women. Many different knee and patellar problems, such as patellofemoral pain syndrome, are associated with Q angles greater or smaller than this range.

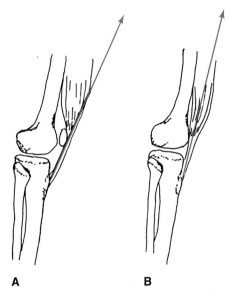

Figure 19-6.   Moment arm of the quadriceps muscles is greater with a patella **(A),** than without a patella **(B)** (side view).

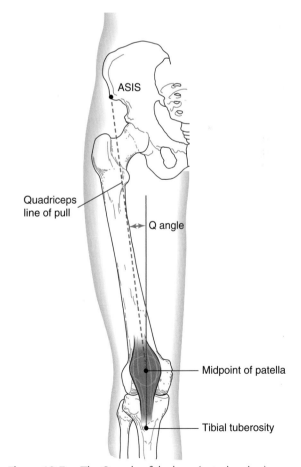

Figure 19-7.   The Q angle of the knee (anterior view).

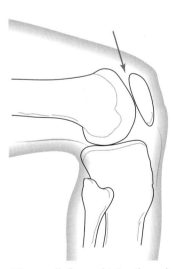

Figure 19-5.   The patellofemoral joint (lateral view).

Bones and Landmarks

The knee is composed of the distal end of the femur articulating with the proximal end of the tibia. The landmarks of the femur significant to the knee are the following (see Figs. 18-7 and 19-8):

Head
The rounded portion covered articulating with the acetabulum.

Neck
The narrower portion located between the head and the trochanters.

Greater Trochanter
Large projection located laterally between the neck and the body of the femur, providing attachment for the gluteus medius and minimus and for most deep rotator muscles.

Lesser Trochanter
A smaller projection located medially and posteriorly, just distal to the greater trochanter; it provides attachment for the iliopsoas muscle.

Body
The long, cylindrical portion between the bone ends; also called the *shaft.* It is bowed slightly anteriorly.

Medial Condyle
Distal medial end.

Lateral Condyle
Distal lateral end.

Lateral Epicondyle
Projection proximal to the lateral condyle.

Medial Epicondyle
Projection proximal to the medial condyle.

Adductor Tubercle
Small projection proximal to the medial epicondyle to which a portion of the adductor magnus muscle attaches.

Linea Aspera
Prominent longitudinal ridge or crest running most of the posterior length.

Pectineal Line
Runs from below the lesser trochanter diagonally toward the linea aspera. It provides attachment for the adductor brevis.

Patellar Surface
Located between the medial and lateral condyle anteriorly. It articulates with the posterior surface of the patella.

The landmarks of the tibia significant to the knee are as follows (Fig. 19-9):

Intercondylar Eminence
A double-pointed prominence on the proximal surface at about the midpoint, which extends up into the intercondylar fossa of the femur.

Medial Condyle
The proximal medial end.

Lateral Condyle
The proximal lateral end.

Plateau
The enlarged proximal end, including the medial and lateral condyles and the intercondylar eminence.

Tibial Tuberosity
Large projection at the proximal end on the anterior surface in the midline.

The **fibula** is lateral to, and smaller than, the tibia. It is set back from the anterior surface of the tibia, allowing a large space for muscle attachment (Fig. 19-10).

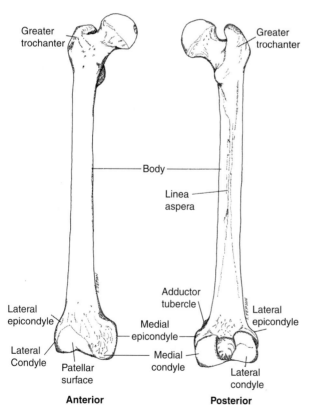

Greater trochanter · Greater trochanter · Body · Linea aspera · Adductor tubercle · Lateral epicondyle · Medial epicondyle · Lateral epicondyle · Lateral Condyle · Patellar surface · Medial condyle · Medial condyle · Lateral condyle

Anterior   **Posterior**

Figure 19-8. Right femur.

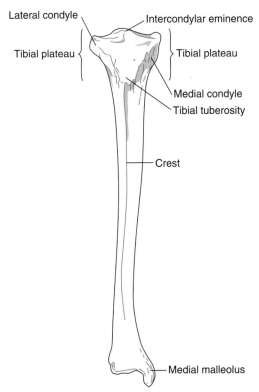

Figure 19-9.   Right tibia (anterior view).

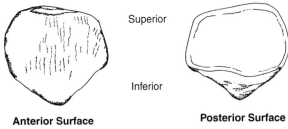

Figure 19-11.   The patella.

This feature gives the lower leg its rounded circumference. The fibula is not part of the knee joint, because it does not articulate with the femur. Although it provides a point of attachment for some of the knee structures, it has a larger role at the ankle.

The **patella** is a triangular sesamoid bone within the quadriceps muscle tendon (Fig. 19-11). It has a broad, superior border and a somewhat pointed distal portion.

The **calcaneus** (see Fig. 19-10) is the most posterior of the tarsal bones and is commonly known as the *heel*. It is identified here because it provides attachment for the gastrocnemius muscle.

Ligaments and Other Structures

As stated earlier, the knee is held together not by its bony structure but by ligaments and muscles. The cruciate and collateral ligaments are the two main sets of ligaments for this task (Fig. 19-12). The cruciates are located within the joint capsule and are therefore called *intracapsular ligaments*. Situated between the

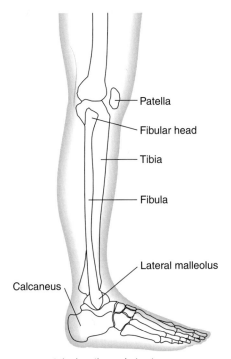

Figure 19-10.   Right leg (lateral view).

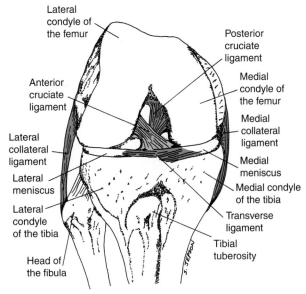

Figure 19-12.   The right knee in flexion (anterior view).

medial and lateral condyles, the cruciates cross each other obliquely (*cruciate* means "resembling a cross" in Latin). They are named for their attachment on the *tibia* (Fig. 19-13). The **anterior cruciate ligament** attaches to the anterior surface of the tibia in the inter-condylar area just medial to the medial meniscus. It spans the knee laterally to the posterior cruciate ligament, and it runs in a superior and posterior direction to attach posteriorly on the lateral condyle of the femur. The **posterior cruciate ligament** attaches to the posterior tibia in the intercondylar area, and it runs in a superior and anterior direction on the medial side of the anterior cruciate ligament. It attaches to the anterior femur on the medial condyle. In summary, the anterior cruciate runs from the anterior tibia to the posterior femur, and the posterior cruciate runs from the posterior tibia to the anterior femur.

The cruciates provide stability in the sagittal plane. The anterior cruciate ligament keeps the femur from being displaced posteriorly on the tibia. Conversely, it keeps the tibia from being displaced anteriorly on the femur. It tightens during extension, preventing excessive hyperextension of the knee. When the knee is partly flexed, the anterior cruciate keeps the tibia from moving anteriorly. Conversely, the posterior cruciate ligament keeps the femur from displacing anteriorly on the tibia or the tibia from displacing posteriorly on the femur. It tightens during flexion and is injured much less frequently than the anterior cruciate ligament.

Located on the sides of the knee are the collateral ligaments (see Fig. 19-12). The **medial collateral ligament,** or tibial collateral ligament is a flat, broad ligament

attaching to the medial condyles of the femur and tibia. Fibers of the medial meniscus are attached to this ligament, which contributes to frequent tearing of the medial meniscus during excessive stress to the medial collateral ligament. On the lateral side is the **lateral collateral ligament,** or fibular collateral ligament. This round, cordlike ligament attaches to the lateral condyle of the femur and runs down to the head of the fibula, independent of any attachment to the lateral meniscus. It protects the joint from stresses to the medial side of the knee. It is quite strong and not commonly injured.

The collateral ligaments supply stability in the frontal plane. The medial collateral ligament provides medial stability and prevents excessive motion if there is a blow to the lateral side of the knee. The lateral collateral ligament provides stability to the medial side. Because their attachments are offset posteriorly and superiorly to the axis of flexion, the collateral ligaments tighten during extension, contributing to the stability of the knee, and slacken during flexion.

Located on the superior surface of the tibia, the **medial** and **lateral menisci** (plural of *meniscus*) are two half-moon, wedge-shaped fibrocartilage disks. They are designed to absorb shock (Fig. 19-14). Because they are thicker laterally than medially and because the proximal surfaces are concave, the menisci deepen the relatively flat joint surface of the tibia. Perhaps because of its attachment to the medial collateral ligament, the medial meniscus is torn more frequently.

There are two types of end feel at the knee joint. With knee flexion, the end feel is soft (soft tissue approximation) due to the contact between the muscle bellies of the thigh and leg. With knee extension, the end feel is firm (soft tissue stretch) due to tension of the joint capsule and ligaments.

The purpose of a bursa is to reduce friction, and approximately 13 of them are located at the knee joint. They are needed because the many tendons located

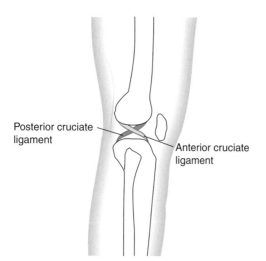

Figure 19-13. Cruciate ligaments are named for their attachment on the tibia (side view).

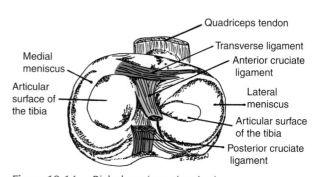

Figure 19-14. Right knee (superior view).

around the knee have a relatively vertical line of pull against bony areas or other tendons. Figure 19-15 illustrates many of the bursae around the knee as viewed from the medial side. Table 19-1 summarizes the most commonly discussed bursae.

The **popliteal space** is the area behind the knee, and it contains important nerves (tibial and common peroneal) and blood vessels (popliteal artery and vein). This diamond-shaped fossa is bound superiorly on the medial side by the semitendinosus and semimembranosus muscles and by the biceps femoris muscle on the lateral side (Fig. 19-16). The inferior boundaries are the medial and lateral heads of the gastrocnemius muscle.

The **pes anserine** (Latin for "goose foot") **muscle group** is made up of the sartorius, gracilis, and semitendinosus (Fig. 19-17) muscles. Each muscle has a different proximal attachment. The sartorius muscle arises anteriorly from the iliac spine, the gracilis muscle arises medially from the pubis, and the semitendinosus muscle arises posteriorly from the ischial tuberosity. They all cross the knee posteriorly and medially, then join together to attach distally on the anterior medial surface of the proximal tibia. This arrangement can also be seen in

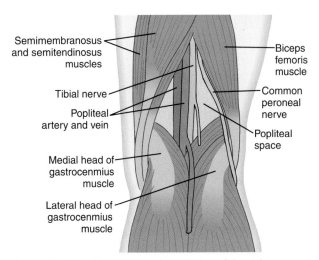

Figure 19-16. The muscular boundaries of the right popliteal space (posterior view).

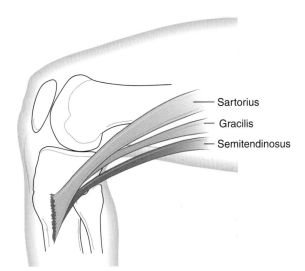

Figure 19-17. The three muscle attachments of pes anserine (medial view).

Figure 18-29. Orthopedic surgeons sometimes alter this common attachment to provide medial stability to the knee.

Muscles of the Knee

Many of the two-joint muscles of the knee were discussed with the hip. However, further clarification of these muscles does need to be made. Table 19-2 shows the muscles that cross the knee, although not all have a major function.

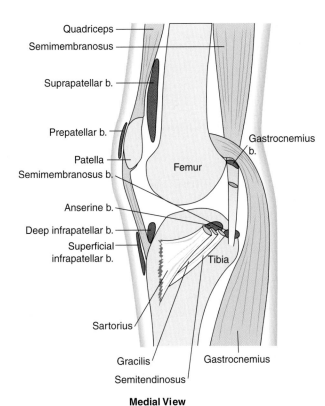

Medial View

Figure 19-15. Bursae around the knee joint (side view).

Table 19-1	Bursae of the Knee
Name	**Location**
Anterior	
Prepatellar	Between the patella and skin
Deep infrapatellar	Between proximal tibia and patellar ligament
Infrapatellar	Between tibial tuberosity and skin
Suprapatellar*	Between distal femur and quadriceps tendon
Posterior	
Gastrocnemius*	Between lateral head of gastrocnemius muscle and capsule
Biceps	Between fibular collateral ligament and biceps tendon
Popliteal*	Between popliteus tendon and lateral femoral condyle
Gastrocnemius*	Between medial head of gastrocnemius muscle and capsule
Semimembranosus	Between tendon of semimembranosus muscle and tibia
Lateral	
Iliotibial	Deep to the iliotibial band at its distal attachment
Fibular collateral ligament	Deep to the fibular collateral ligament next to the bone
Medial	
Anserine	Deep to sartorius, gracilis, and semitendinosus tendons

*Communicates with knee joint.

Anterior Muscles

The quadriceps muscles are comprised of four muscles that cross the anterior surface of the knee (Fig. 19-18). The **rectus femoris muscle** is the only one of this group to cross the hip. Its proximal attachment is on the AIIS. It runs almost straight down the thigh, where it is joined by the three vasti muscles and blends into the quadriceps tendon (also called the *patellar tendon*). This tendon encases the patella, crosses the knee joint, and attaches to the tibial tuberosity. The rectus femoris muscle is a prime mover in hip flexion and knee extension.

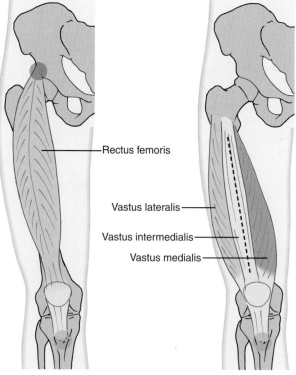

Figure 19-18.   The quadriceps muscle group (anterior view). The three vasti muscles lie deep to the rectus femoris. The vastus medialis and lateralis attach proximally on the posterior femur but join the other two muscles to cross the knee anteriorly.

Table 19-2	Muscles of the Knee	
Area	**One-Joint Muscle**	**Two-Joint Muscle**
Anterior	Vastus lateralis	Rectus femoris
	Vastus medialis	
	Vastus intermedialis	
Posterior	Biceps femoris	Biceps femoris
	(short)	(long)
	Popliteus	Semimembranosus
		Semitendinosus
		Sartorius
		Gracilis
		Gastrocnemius
Lateral		Tensor fascia latae

The **vastus lateralis muscle** is located lateral to the rectus femoris muscle. It originates from the linea aspera of the femur and spans the thigh laterally to join the other quadriceps muscles at the patella. The **vastus medialis muscle** also comes from the linea aspera, but it spans the thigh medially. Located deep to the rectus femoris muscle is the **vastus intermedialis muscle.** It arises from the anterior surface of the femur and spans the thigh anteriorly. It blends together with the other vasti muscles along its length. All four quadriceps muscles attach to the base of the patella and the tibial tuberosity via the patellar tendon. Because all four muscles span the knee anteriorly, they all extend the knee. Because the rectus femoris muscle also spans the hip anteriorly, it flexes the hip.

Rectus Femoris Muscle

O	AIIS
I	Tibial tuberosity via patellar tendon
A	Hip flexion, knee extension
N	Femoral nerve (L2, L3, L4)

Vastus Lateralis Muscle

O	Linea aspera
I	Tibial tuberosity via patellar tendon
A	Knee extension
N	Femoral nerve (L2, L3, L4)

Vastus Medialis Muscle

O	Linea aspera
I	Tibial tuberosity via patellar tendon
A	Knee extension
N	Femoral nerve (L2, L3, L4)

Vastus Intermedialis Muscle

O	Anterior femur
I	Tibial tuberosity via patellar tendon
A	Knee extension
N	Femoral nerve (L2, L3, L4)

Posterior Muscles

Three muscles that are known collectively as the *hamstring muscles* cover the posterior thigh. They consist of the semimembranosus, the semitendinosus, and the biceps femoris muscles (Fig. 19-19). They have a common site of origin on the ischial tuberosity.

The **semimembranosus muscle** runs down the medial side of the thigh deep to the semitendinosus muscle and inserts on the posterior surface of the medial

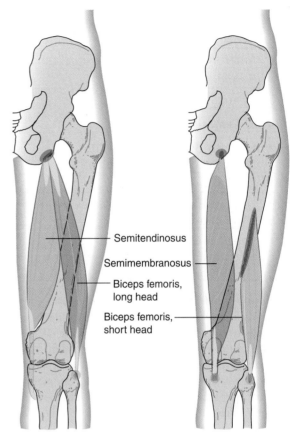

Figure 19-19. The hamstring muscle group (posterior view).

Labels: Semitendinosus; Semimembranosus; Biceps femoris, long head; Biceps femoris, short head

condyle of the tibia. The **semitendinosus muscle** has a much longer and narrower distal tendon that moves anteriorly after spanning the knee joint posteriorly. It attaches to the anteromedial surface of the tibia with the gracilis and sartorius muscles. The **biceps femoris muscle** has two heads and runs laterally down the thigh on the posterior side. The long head arises with the other two muscles on the ischial tuberosity, but the short head arises from the lateral lip of the linea aspera. Both heads join together, spanning the knee posteriorly to attach laterally on the head of the fibula and, by a small slip, to the lateral condyle of the tibia. The short head of the biceps femoris is the only part of the hamstring muscle group that has a function only at the knee. The other parts have a function at both the hip and the knee.

Semimembranosus Muscle

O	Ischial tuberosity
I	Posterior surface of medial condyle of tibia
A	Extend hip and flex knee
N	Sciatic nerve (L5, S1, S2)

Semitendinosus Muscle

O	Ischial tuberosity
I	Anteromedial surface of proximal tibia
A	Extend hip and flex knee
N	Sciatic nerve (L5, S1, S2)

Biceps Femoris Muscle

O	Long head: ischial tuberosity Short head: lateral lip of linea aspera
I	Fibular head
A	Long head: extend hip and flex knee Short head: flex knee
N	Long head: sciatic nerve (S1, S2, S3) Short head: common peroneal nerve (L5, S1, S2)

The **popliteus muscle** is a one-joint muscle located posteriorly at the knee in the popliteal space, deep to the two heads of the gastrocnemius muscles (Fig. 19-20). It originates on the lateral side of the lateral condyle of the femur and crosses the knee posteriorly at an oblique angle to insert medially on the posterior proximal tibia. Because it spans the knee posteriorly, it flexes the knee. It is credited with "unlocking" the knee, as it initiates knee flexion.

Popliteus Muscle

O	Lateral condyle of femur
I	Posterior medial condyle of tibia
A	Initiates knee flexion
N	Tibial nerve (L4, L5, S1)

The **gastrocnemius muscle** is a two-joint muscle that crosses the knee and the ankle (Fig. 19-21). It is an extremely strong ankle plantar flexor but also has a significant role at the knee. It attaches by two heads to the posterior surface of the medial and lateral condyles of the femur. After descending the posterior leg superficially, it forms a common *Achilles tendon* (often called the *heel cord by laymen*) with the soleus muscle and attaches to the posterior surface of the calcaneus. Although its major function is at the ankle, it does span the knee posteriorly, has a good angle of pull, and is a large muscle. Therefore, its contribution as a knee flexor cannot be overlooked. In addition, its unusual contribution to knee *extension* has been demonstrated in individuals with no quadriceps muscle function (Fig. 19-22). In a closed kinetic chain action with the foot planted on the ground so that the distal segment (leg) is stationary, the proximal segment (thigh) becomes the movable part. This is also a reversal of muscle action in which the femur is pulled posteriorly, or into knee extension. This feature of the gastrocnemius muscle makes it possible for a person to stand upright without the use of quadriceps muscles.

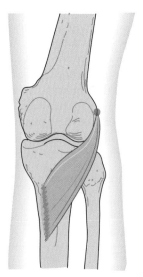

Figure 19-20.   The popliteus muscle (posterior view).

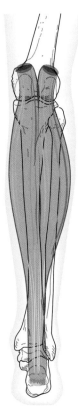

Figure 19-21.   The gastrocnemius muscle (posterior view).

medially, contributing greatly to medial stability. The gastrocnemius and hamstring muscles provide posterior stability both medially and laterally, and the quadriceps muscles provide anterior stability.

Anatomical Relationships

Muscles cross the knee either anteriorly or posteriorly. The rectus femoris is the most superficial muscle of the anterior group. At the mid- and lower thigh, the vastus lateralis and the vastus medialis are superficial on either side of the rectus femoris (Fig. 19-23). Deep to the rectus femoris and between the two vasti muscles is the vastus intermedialis (Fig. 19-24).

The hamstring muscles are on the posterior thigh. Superficially, the biceps femoris (long head) is on the lateral side, and the semitendinosus is on the medial side. Deep to these muscles is the short head of the biceps femoris (laterally) and the semimembranosus (medially). The deepest muscle at the distal end of the thigh is the

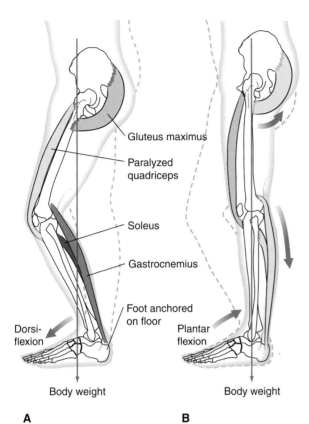

A   **B**

Figure 19-22.   Side view. **(A)** With a paralyzed quadriceps unable to pull the knee into extension, the body weight line falls behind the knee, causing flexion. However, in a combined reversal of muscle action of the gluteus maximus and gastrocnemius muscles, knee extension during stance is possible. **(B)** In the closed-chain position, they pull the knee into extension. The soleus assists by plantar flexing the dorsiflexed ankle into a neutral ankle position. This puts the body weight line in front of the knee and ankle axes and allows the knee to remain extended.

Gastrocnemius Muscle

O	Medial and lateral condyles of femur
I	Posterior calcaneus
A	Knee flexion, ankle plantar flexion
N	Tibial nerve (S1, S2)

The gracilis, sartorius, and tensor fascia latae muscles span the knee joint posteriorly, but because of their angle of pull, their size in relation to other muscles, and other such factors, they do not have a prime mover function. However, they do provide stability to the joint.

The **tensor fascia latae muscle** spans the knee laterally, essentially in the middle of the joint axis for flexion and extension. It contributes greatly to lateral stability. The **gracilis** and **sartorius muscles** span the knee

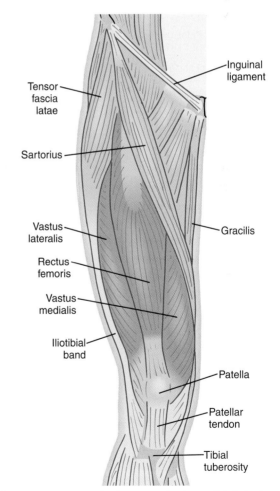

Figure 19-23.   Anterior knee muscles (superficial view).

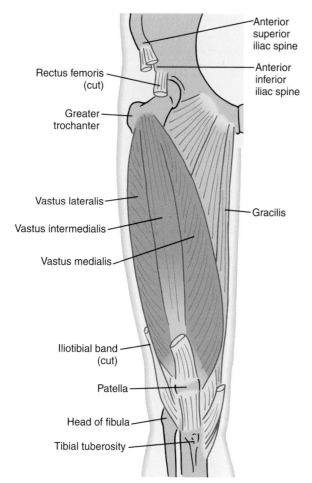

Figure 19-24.   Anterior knee muscles (deep view).

Rectus femoris (cut)
Greater trochanter
Vastus lateralis
Vastus intermedialis
Vastus medialis
Iliotibial band (cut)
Patella
Head of fibula
Tibial tuberosity
Anterior superior iliac spine
Anterior inferior iliac spine
Gracilis

Table 19-3	Prime Movers of the Knee	
Action	**Muscle**
Extension	Quadriceps group
	Rectus femoris
	Vastus medialis
	Vastus intermedialis
	Vastus lateralis
Flexion	Hamstring group
	Semimembranosus
	Semitendinosus
	Biceps femoris
	Popliteus
	Gastrocnemius

popliteus. It lies deep to the proximal heads of the gastrocnemius.

The sartorius crosses the knee on the medial side, anterior to the gracilis, followed more posteriorly by the semitendinosus (pes anserine; see Fig. 18-29). The tensor fascia latae crosses the knee joint laterally by way of the iliotibial band.

Summary of Muscle Action

Table 19-3 summarizes the actions of the prime movers of the knee.

Summary of Muscle Innervation

The femoral and sciatic nerves play a major part in the innervation of the knee joint. The femoral nerve innervates the quadriceps muscle group, and the sciatic nerve innervates the hamstring muscle group.

The other two knee flexors, the popliteus and gastrocnemius muscles, receive innervation from the tibial nerve. (Not included in this discussion or in Table 19-4 are the two-joint hip muscles that span the knee but do not act as prime movers at the knee—the sartorius, gracilis, and tensor fascia latae muscles.) The knee extensors receive innervation from the femoral nerve, which comes off the spinal cord at a higher level than does innervation of the knee flexors. This is significant when dealing with individuals with spinal cord injuries. Tables 19-4 and 19-5 summarize the innervation to the knee. It should be noted that there is some discrepancy among various sources regarding spinal cord level of innervation.

Common Knee Pathologies

Genu valgum, also called "knock knees," is an alignment of the lower extremity in which the distal segments (ankles) are positioned more laterally than normal. The knees tend to touch while the ankles are apart. **Genu varum** (bowlegs) is the opposite alignment problem in which the distal segments are positioned more medially than normal. The ankles tend to touch while the knees are apart. Malalignment at one joint often affects alignment at an adjacent joint. Therefore, coxa varus is seen in conjunction with genu valgus, while coxa valgus may be seen in conjunction with genu varus. **Genu recurvatum,** also called, "back knees" is the positioning of the tibiofemoral joint in which range of motion goes beyond 0 degrees of extension.

Patellar tendonitis, or jumper's knee, is characterized by tenderness at the patellar tendon and results from the overuse stress or sudden impact overloading associated with jumping. It is commonly seen in basketball players, high jumpers, and hurdlers.

Table 19-4	Innervation of the Muscles of the Knee	
Muscle	Nerve	Spinal Segment
Quadriceps		
Rectus femoris	Femoral	L2, L3, L4
Vastus lateralis	Femoral	L2, L3, L4
Vastus intermedialis	Femoral	L2, L3, L4
Vastus medialis	Femoral	L2, L3, L4
Hamstrings		
Semimembranosus	Sciatic	L5, S1, S2
Semitendinosus	Sciatic	L5, S1, S2
Biceps femoris—long head	Sciatic	L5, S1, S2
Biceps femoris—short head	Common peroneal	L5, S1, S2
Others		
Popliteus	Tibial	L4, L5, S1
Gastrocnemius	Tibial	S1, S2

Osgood-Schlatter disease is a common overuse injury among adolescents. It involves the traction-type epiphysis on the tibial tuberosity of growing bone where the tendon of the quadriceps muscle attaches. **Popliteal cyst,** or Baker's cyst, is actually misnamed as a "cyst." This general term refers to any synovial hernia or bursitis involving the posterior aspect of the knee.

Although there is no universal agreement on terminology and causation, **patellofemoral pain syndrome** generally refers to a common problem causing diffuse anterior knee pain. It is generally considered the result of a variety of alignment factors, such as increased Q angle, patella alta (high-riding patella), quadriceps weakness or tightness, weakness of hip lateral rotators, and excessive foot pronation. **Chondromalacia patella** is the softening and degeneration of the cartilage on the posterior aspect of the patella, causing anterior knee pain. Abnormal tracking of the patella within the patellofemoral groove causes the patellar articular cartilage to become inflamed, leading to its degeneration. **Prepatellar bursitis** (housemaid's knee) occurs when there is constant pressure between the skin and the patella. It is commonly seen in carpet layers and is the result of repeated direct blows or sheering stresses on the knee.

Terrible triad is a knee injury caused by a single blow to the knee and involves tears to the anterior

Table 19-5	Segmental Innervation of the Knee					
Spinal Cord Level	L2	L3	L4	L5	S1	S2
Knee Extensors						
Rectus femoris	X	X	X			
Vastus lateralis	X	X	X			
Vastus intermedialis	X	X	X			
Vastus medialis	X	X	X			
Knee Flexors						
Popliteus			X	X	X	
Semitendinosus				X	X	X
Semimembranosus				X	X	X
Biceps femoris				X	X	X
Gastrocnemius					X	X

cruciate ligament, the medial collateral ligament, and the medial meniscus. **Miserable malalignment syndrome** is an alignment problem of the lower extremity involving increased anteversion of the femoral head and is associated with genu valgus, increased tibial torsion, and a pronated flat foot.

Points to Remember

- The body commonly experiences forces such as traction, approximation, shear, bending, and rotation. These forces also have other names.
- The muscle's point of attachment to the bone is used to determine leverage. With a second-class lever, resistance occurs between the axis and the force. With a third-class lever, force is in the middle.
- The longer the force arm, the easier it is to move the part. Conversely, the longer the resistance arm, the harder it is to move the part.

- End feel is the quality of the feel when slight pressure is applied at the end of the joint's passive range.
- An open kinetic chain requires that the distal segment is free to move and the proximal segment(s) remain stationary.
- To stretch a one-joint muscle, it is necessary to put any two-joint muscles on a slack over the joint not crossed by the one-joint muscle.
- To contract a two-joint muscle most effectively, start with it being stretched over both joints.
- A muscle becomes actively insufficient when it contracts over all its joints as the same time.
- When determining whether a concentric or eccentric contraction is occurring, decide
  - if the activity is accelerating against gravity or slowing down gravity, or
  - if a weight greater than the pull of gravity is affecting the activity.
- Reversal of muscle action occurs when the origin moves toward the insertion.

Review Questions

General Anatomy Questions

1. Describe the knee joints:
   a. Number of axes:
      Knee _____
      Patellofemoral _____
   b. Shape of joint:
      Knee _____
      Patellofemoral _____
   c. Type of motion allowed:
      Knee _____
      Patellofemoral _____
2. Describe knee joint motion in terms of planes and axes.
3. What is the "Q angle"? Why is it important?
4. Which bones make up the knee joint?
5. Why is the action of the popliteus muscle often described as "unlocking" the joint?
6. What is the pes anserine?
7. An individual with a spinal cord injury at L3 would be expected to have what knee motion?

8. In Figure 19-22:
   a. What type of kinetic chain activity is demonstrated?
   b. Is it possible for the muscles to perform this function in either an open or closed kinetic chain?
   c. Is either the gastrocnemius or gluteus maximus muscle working in a reversal of muscle action role?
9. A snowboarder catches an edge and falls. His board twists in one direction as his body twists in the opposite direction. What is the most likely type of force experienced at the knee?
10. When assessing the knee collateral ligaments, the examiner pulls laterally on your ankle while pushing medially on your knee.
    a. What type of load is placed on your lower extremity?
    b. Which side of your knee undergoes a tensile stress?
    c. Which side of your knee undergoes a compressive stress?

Review Questions—cont'd

Functional Activity Questions

1. Analyze the person's position lying on the two benches illustrated in Figure 19-25 to determine if one is more advantageous than the other for strengthening the hamstrings by doing leg curls. Note that the knees remain extended in both positions.
   a. What is the hamstring action at the hip and at the knee?
   b. What is the position of the hips in Figure 19-25A?
   c. What is the position of the hips in Figure 19-25B?
   d. In what position would the hamstrings be actively insufficient?
   e. Which person's position on the bench will more effectively work the hamstrings?
   f. Why?

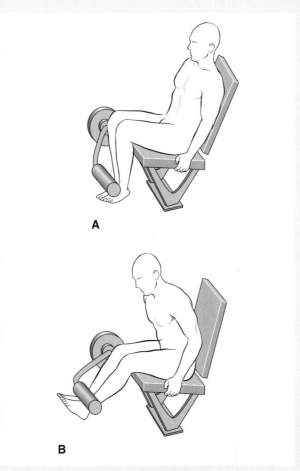

Figure 19-26.   Starting positions for knee extension exercise.

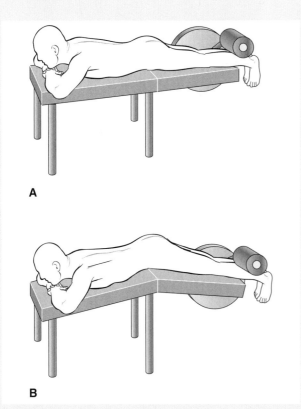

Figure 19-25.   Bench positions for hamstring curl exercise.

2. Analyze the person's sitting positions illustrated in Figure 19-26 to determine if one is more advantageous than the other for strengthening the knee extensors. Knee extension is the motion being performed.
   a. What are the hip positions in Figures 19-26A and 19-26B?
   b. What are the names of the one-joint muscles performing the knee extension?
   c. What is the name of the two-joint muscle, and what hip and knee motions does it perform?
   d. Describe the length-tension effect on these muscles in each position.
   e. Which person's position will more effectively work the rectus femoris?
   f. Which person's position will more effectively work the vasti muscles?

(continued on next page)

Review Questions—cont'd

3. What is the sequence of right-knee motions when stepping up onto a curb leading with the right foot, starting with the right knee extended?
   a. Placing right foot up on curb:
   b. Bringing left foot up on curb:

4. Identify the sequence of knee motions (starting with the knee in extension) for kicking a ball and identify the activity of the rectus femoris during each phase.
   a. What is the knee motion when preparing to kick?
   b. Over what joints is the rectus femoris being elongated?
   c. What is the knee motion when making ball contact?
   d. What is happening to the rectus femoris at the knee during ball contact?
   e. What is the knee motion during follow-through?
   f. What is happening to the rectus femoris during follow-through?

5. What compensatory motions may occur when stepping up onto a curb if your right leg were in a long leg cast?
   a. Which would be the leading leg?
   b. What pelvic motion would assist in getting the right leg up on the curb?

Clinical Exercise Questions

1. What types of exercises are occurring during a "wall sit"? Keeping the head, shoulders, and back against the wall with your feet shoulder-width apart, slowly slide down the wall until the thighs are almost parallel to the floor. Hold that position for the count of five. Return to the starting position.
   During the slide-down phase:
   a. What is the knee motion?
   b. What type of contraction (isometric, concentric, or eccentric) is occurring?
   c. What muscles are performing this action?
   d. Is this an open- or closed-chain activity?
   During the holding phase:
   a. What type of contraction (isometric, concentric, or eccentric) is occurring?
   b. What muscles are performing this action?
   During the return phase:
   a. What is the knee motion?
   b. What type of contraction (isometric, concentric, or eccentric) is occurring?
   c. What muscles are performing this action?

2. Sit on the edge of a table with your right leg resting on the table and your left leg over the side with your left foot on the floor. Keeping the back and right leg straight, lean forward at the right hip. See Figure 19-27 for the starting position.
   a. What are the right hip and knee motions?
   b. Is stretching or strengthening occurring?
   c. What muscles are involved?

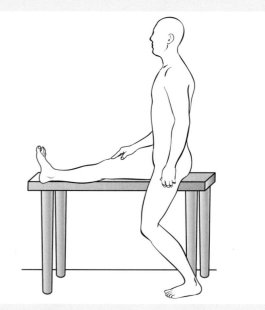

Figure 19-27. Starting position.

3. Lying supine, raise your right leg up toward the ceiling about 24 inches, keeping your right knee straight.
   a. What are the right hip and knee motions?
   b. Is stretching or strengthening occurring?
   c. What muscles are involved?
   d. Is this an open- or closed-chain activity?

4. Standing on your left leg and holding on to something for balance, bend your right knee and grasp your right foot. Slowly pull your right heel toward your right buttock.
   a. What are the right hip and knee motions?
   b. Is stretching or strengthening occurring?
   c. What muscles are involved?

5. When performing passive range of motion (PROM) on an individual's knee, the end feel for flexion should be _____ and _____ for extension.

Review Questions—cont'd

6. Sit on the edge of a table with a 10-pound weight on your ankle. Hold each of the following positions for 30 seconds:
   - Knee fully extended (position A)
   - Knee flexed 30 degrees (position B)
   - Knee flexed 60 degrees (position C)
   a. Which position is easier to hold? Which is more difficult?
   b. Identify the force, resistance, axis, and lever class.
   c. How does the resistance arm length change as you move from position A to position C?
   d. How does the force arm length change as you switch positions?

7. In a standing position, loop an elastic band around the back of your knee and anchor the other end around a heavy table leg or in a doorjamb. You may want to pad the back of the knee with a small towel. Face the anchor point and be far enough away so that there is sufficient tension in the elastic band (Fig. 19-28). From a partly flexed position, slowly straighten the knee, and keep the foot on the floor. Hold for the count of five, and then bend it (returning to starting position).
   Straighten phase:
   a. What knee motion is occurring?
   b. What type of contraction is occurring?
   c. What muscles are involved?
   d. Is this an open- or closed-chain activity?
   Holding phase:
   a. What is the position of the knee?
   b. What type of contraction is occurring?
   c. What muscles are involved?

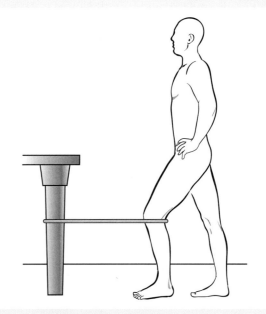

Figure 19-28.   Starting position.

   Bending phase:
   a. What knee motion is occurring?
   b. What type of contraction is occurring?
   c. What muscles are involved?

8. A clinician is applying force to the lower leg of a patient who is trying to extend the knee (Fig. 19-29). Can the clinician apply more force to the patient's leg by pushing down just below the knee (A) or just above the ankle (B)? Why?

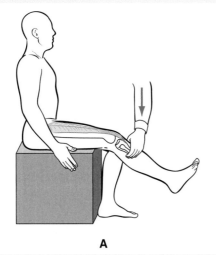

A

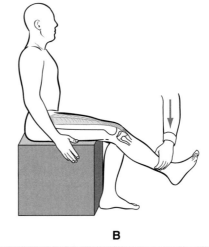

B

Figure 19-29.   Point of force application.

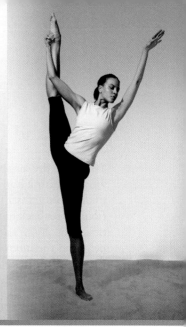

CHAPTER 20
Ankle Joint and Foot

Bones and Landmarks

  Functional Aspects of the Foot

Joints and Motions

  Ankle Motions

  Ankle Joints

  Foot Joints

Ligaments and Other Structures

  Arches

Muscles of the Ankle and Foot

  Extrinsic Muscles

  Intrinsic Muscles

  Anatomical Relationships

  Summary of Muscle Innervation

  Common Ankle Pathologies

Points to Remember

Review Questions

  General Anatomy Questions

  Functional Activity Questions

  Clinical Exercise Questions

The leg (the portion of the lower extremity extending from the knee to the ankle) consists of the tibia and fibula. A strong interosseous membrane keeps the two bones together and provides a greater surface area for muscle attachment (Fig. 20-1).

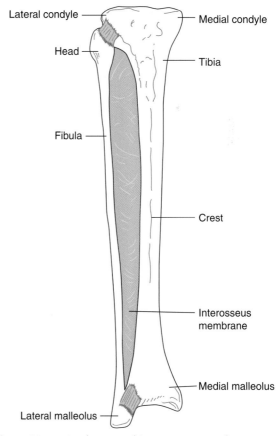

Figure 20-1. Leg bones and interosseous membrane (anterior view).

Bones and Landmarks

The tibia, the larger of the two bones, is the only true weight-bearing bone of the leg. Triangular in shape, the tibia's apex (crest) is located anteriorly. The long, thin fibula is set back in line with the posterior surface of the tibia (Fig. 20-2). Lateral to the tibia, this forms a channel, with the interosseous membrane as the floor; this permits attachment of several muscles without distorting the shape of the leg. Landmarks of the **tibia** pertaining to the ankle are as follows (see Fig. 20-1):

Medial Condyle
The proximal medial end.

Lateral Condyle
The proximal lateral end.

Crest
Anterior and most prominent of the three borders.

Medial Malleolus
The enlarged distal medial surface.

The landmarks of the **fibula** are as follows:

Head
Enlarged proximal end.

Lateral Malleolus
Enlarged distal end.

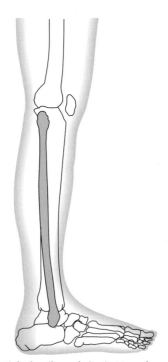

Figure 20-2.   Right leg (lateral view). Note the posterior position of the fibula.

The bones of the foot include the tarsals, metatarsals, and phalanges. The seven **tarsal bones** and their landmarks consist of the following (Fig. 20-3):

Calcaneus
Largest and most posterior tarsal bone.

Calcaneal Tuberosity
Projection on the posterior inferior surface of the calcaneus.

Sustentaculum Tali
Medial superior part projecting out from the rest of the calcaneus, supporting the medial side of the talus. Three tendons loop around this projection, changing directions from the posterior leg to the plantar foot.

Talus
Sitting on the calcaneus, it is the second largest tarsal.

Navicular
On the medial side in front of the talus and proximal to the three cuneiforms.

Tuberosity of Navicular
Projection on the medial side of the navicular; easily seen on the medial border of the foot

Cuboid
On the lateral side of the foot proximal (superior) to the fourth and fifth metatarsals and distal (inferior) to the calcaneus.

Cuneiforms
Three in number and named the first through third, going from the medial toward the lateral side in line with the metatarsals. The first is the largest of the three.

The **metatarsals** are numbered one through five, starting medially (see Fig. 20-3). Normally, the first and fifth metatarsals are weight-bearing bones, and the second, third, and fourth are not. We tend to stand on a triangle. Weight is borne from the base of the calcaneus to the heads of the first and fifth metatarsals. The significant features and landmarks of the metatarsals are as follows:

Base
Proximal end of each metatarsal.

Head
Distal end of each bone.

First
Thickest and shortest metatarsal; located on the medial side of the foot. Articulates with the first cuneiform

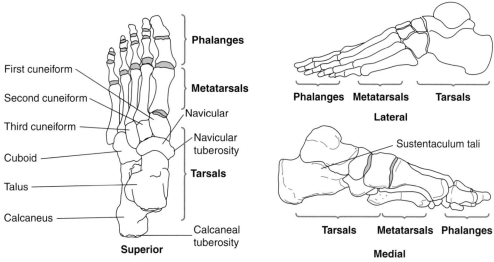

Figure 20-3.   Bones of the left foot (superior, lateral, and medial views).

Second
The longest; articulates with the second cuneiform.

Third
Articulates with the third cuneiform.

Fourth
Together with the fifth metatarsal, articulates with the cuboid.

Fifth
Has prominent tuberosity located on the lateral side of its base.

The **phalanges** of the foot have the same composition as those of the hand (see Fig. 20-3). The first digit, the **great toe,** has a proximal and distal phalanx but no middle phalanx. The second through fifth digits, also called the four **lesser toes,** each have a proximal, middle, and distal phalanx.

Functional Aspects of the Foot

The foot can be divided into three parts (Fig. 20-4). The hindfoot is made up of the talus and calcaneus. In the gait cycle, the hindfoot is the first part of the foot that makes contact with the ground, thus influencing the function and movement of the other two parts. The midfoot is made up of the navicular, the cuboid, and the three cuneiform bones. The mechanics of this part of the foot provide stability and mobility as it transmits movement from the hindfoot to the forefoot. The forefoot is made up of the five metatarsals and all of the phalanges. This part of the foot adapts to the level of the ground. It is also the last part of the foot to make contact with the ground during stance phase.

The ankle joint and foot perform three main functions: acting as a shock absorber as the heel strikes the ground at the beginning of stance phase, adapting to the level (or unevenness) of the ground, and providing a stable base of support from which to propel the body forward.

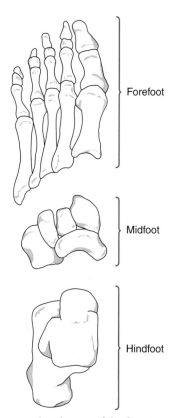

Figure 20-4.   Functional areas of the foot (superior view).

Joints and Motions

Ankle Motions

Motions of the ankle joint and foot need to be defined, because there is not uniform agreement among authors (Fig. 20-5). **Plantar flexion** is movement toward the plantar surface of the foot, whereas **dorsiflexion** occurs when the dorsal surface of the foot moves toward the anterior surface of the leg. These motions occur in the *sagittal plane around the frontal axis.* Due to conflicting definitions, the terms **flexion** and **extension** should not be used. As a case in point, functionally speaking, plantar flexion is the same as extension in that it is part of the general extension movement of the hip, knee, and ankle. However, anatomically speaking, plantar flexion is not a true flexion because there is no approximation of two segments.

Movement in the *frontal plane around the sagittal axis* is called *inversion* and *eversion.* **Inversion** is the raising of the medial border of the foot, turning the forefoot inward. **Eversion,** the opposite motion, is the raising of the lateral border of the foot, turning the forefoot outward. Movement in the transverse plane is called **adduction** and **abduction.** These motions occur primarily in the forefoot and accompany inversion and eversion, respectively.

In recent years, clinicians have begun using *supination* and *pronation* to describe ankle joint and foot motion. **Supination** describes a combination of plantar flexion, inversion, and adduction, and **pronation** describes a combination of dorsiflexion, eversion, and abduction. To avoid further confusion of terms, *valgus* and *varus* must be defined. These terms are more commonly used to describe a *position,* usually an abnormal one. **Valgus** refers to a position in which the distal segment is situated away from the midline. Conversely, **varus** refers to a position in which the distal segment is located toward the midline. Therefore, a calcaneal valgus is a position in which the distal (inferior) part of the calcaneus is angled away from the midline (Fig. 20-6). These terms will not be used here because *motion,* not *position,* is the emphasis.

In summary, the terminology commonly used by clinicians to describe ankle and foot motions are *dorsiflexion, plantar flexion, supination* (a combination of plantar flexion, inversion, and forefoot adduction), and *pronation* (a combination of dorsiflexion, eversion, and forefoot abduction). These motions are illustrated in Figure 20-5. However, when describing muscle action, *inversion* and *eversion* are used in place of *supination* and *pronation,* respectively.

Two joints with little motion that are not part of the true ankle joint but that play a small role in the proper

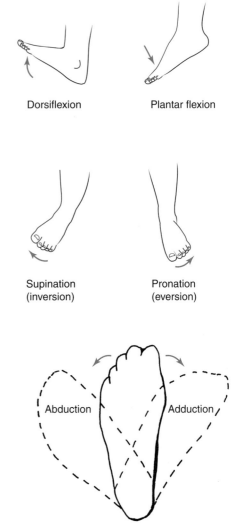

Figure 20-5.   Ankle joint and foot motions.

function of the ankle are the tibiofibular joints (Fig. 20-7). The **superior tibiofibular joint** is the articulation between the head of the fibula and the posterior lateral aspect of the proximal tibia. It is a plane joint that allows a relatively small amount of gliding and rotation of the fibula on the tibia. Being a synovial joint, it has a joint capsule. Ligaments reinforce the capsule, and the joint functions to dissipate the torsional stresses applied at the ankle joint. The **inferior tibiofibular joint** is a syndesmosis (fibrous union) between the concave distal tibia and the convex distal fibula. Because it is not a synovial joint, there is no joint capsule. However, fibrous tissue separates the bones and several ligaments that hold the joint together. Much of the ankle joint's strength depends upon a strong union at this joint. The ligaments holding the inferior tibiofibular joint together allow slight movement to accommodate the motion of the talus.

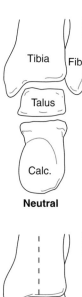

Neutral

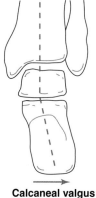

Calcaneal valgus

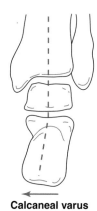

Calcaneal varus

Posterior View

Figure 20-6. Calcaneal positions.

Ankle Joints

The true **ankle joint** (*talocrural joint* or *talotibial joint*) is made up of the distal tibia, which sits on the talus with the medial malleolus of the tibia fitting down around the medial aspect of the talus, and the lateral malleolus of the fibula, which fits down around the lateral aspect. This type of joint often is described using a carpentry term: *tenon and mortise joint*. A mortise is a notch that is

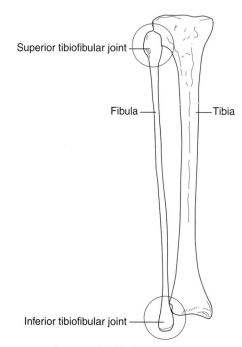

Figure 20-7. The two tibiofibular joints (anterior view).

cut in a piece of wood to receive a projecting piece (tenon) shaped to fit. Therefore, the malleoli of the tibia and fibula would be the mortise, and the talus would be the tenon (Fig. 20-8). This joint connects the leg and foot and is responsible for controlling the majority of foot motion relative to the leg.

In summary, the ankle is a uniaxial hinge joint consisting of articulation between the distal end and medial malleolus of the tibia and the lateral malleolus of the fibula with the talus. The ankle joint allows approximately 30 to 50 degrees of plantar flexion and 20 degrees of dorsiflexion. In the anatomical position, the ankle is in a neutral position. Because the axis of rotation is at an angle, it is considered **triplanar,** a term used to describe

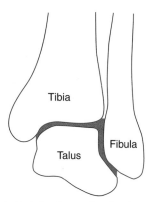

Figure 20-8. Ankle joint (posterior view).

motion around an obliquely oriented axis that passes through all three planes.

At this axis, the lateral malleolus extends more distally and lies more posteriorly than the medial malleolus. To visualize this positioning, place the ends of your index fingers at the distal ends of the malleoli on your left ankle (Fig. 20-9). Notice that when viewed from above, the finger on the lateral malleolus side is more posterior. When viewed from the front, the finger is more distal. Imagine the fingers as a straight rod passing through the joint. Notice that the fingers do not line up in a pure side-to-side direction. The left finger is slightly posterior and inferior, while the right finger is slightly anterior and superior. This is essentially the axis of the ankle joint. It tips approximately 8 degrees from the transverse plane, 82 degrees from sagittal plane, and 20 to 30 degrees from the frontal plane. During ankle

dorsiflexion, the foot not only comes up but also moves out slightly (abduction). During ankle plantar flexion, the foot moves down and in (adduction).

Motion at the Ankle Joint

In an open kinetic chain, with the leg fixed and the foot free to move, the angle of the joint axis causes the foot to abduct during dorsiflexion and adduct during plantar flexion. The opposite action occurs with closed chain: The foot is fixed on the ground, and the leg moves over it. During dorsiflexion, the leg medially rotates on the foot. With the foot fixed and the leg moving over it, the angle of the joint axis causes the leg to medially rotate on the foot. During ankle plantar flexion, the leg laterally rotates on the foot. This rotation is allowed because of the slight movement that is possible at the tibiofibular joints. It is an accessory movement much like the rotation of the CMC joint of the thumb. This movement is not possible to do in an open chain. Table 20-1 summarizes the motions of the ankle and foot.

In terms of arthrokinematics, the convex talus glides posteriorly on the concave tibia during ankle dorsiflexion and glides anteriorly during ankle plantar flexion. The end feel of both dorsiflexion and plantar flexion is firm and is classified as soft tissue stretch. This is due to the tension of the joint capsule, ligaments, and tendons.

The **subtalar,** or talocalcaneal, **joint** consists of the inferior surface of the talus articulating with the superior surface of the calcaneus (Fig. 20-10). It is a plane

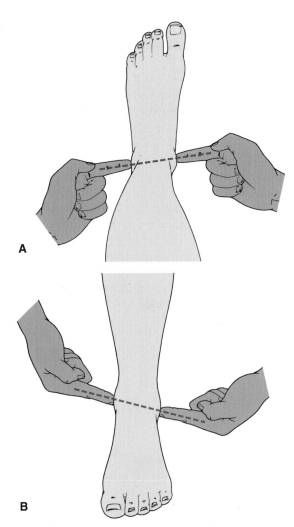

A

B

Figure 20-9.   Axis of motion for the ankle joint. **(A)** Superior view. **(B)** Anterior view.

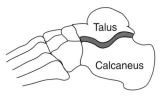

Figure 20-10.   Subtalar joint (lateral view).

Table 20-1	Ankle and Foot Motions	
	Ankle Dorsiflexion	Ankle Plantar Flexion
Open Kinetic Chain		
Leg fixed Foot moves	Foot abducts	Foot adducts
Closed Kinetic Chain		
Foot fixed Leg moves	Leg medially rotates	Leg laterally rotates

synovial joint with 1 degree of freedom. The motions of inversion and eversion occur around an oblique axis.

The **transverse tarsal joint** (midtarsal joint; Fig. 20-11) is made up of the anterior surfaces of the talus and calcaneus articulating with the posterior surfaces of the navicular and the cuboid, respectively. Although they lie next to each other, very little movement occurs between the navicular and the cuboid. The motions of the transverse tarsal joint link the hindfoot and forefoot in inversion and eversion.

Because the motions of these two joints occur on an oblique axis (triplanar), they are combinations of movements. Functionally, the subtalar and transverse tarsal joints cannot be separated. For the sake of simplicity, *inversion/eversion* will be used to describe motions occurring at both the subtalar and transtarsal joints. **Inversion** will include a combination of adduction, supination, and plantar flexion, while **eversion** will include a combination of abduction, pronation, and dorsiflexion. Therefore, when the ankle moves in plantar flexion and dorsiflexion, these motions are occurring primarily at the talocrural joint. When the ankle moves in inversion and eversion, these motions are occurring primarily at the subtalar and transverse tarsal joints. The combined motions of all these joints allow the foot to assume almost any position in space. This is quite useful in allowing the foot to adapt to irregular surfaces such as those found when walking on uneven ground. For example, think about the many foot positions needed when climbing on rocks at the beach or in the mountains.

Foot Joints

The **metatarsophalangeal (MTP)** joints consist of the metatarsal heads articulating with the proximal phalanges (Fig. 20-12). Like the metacarpophalangeal joints of the hand, there are five joints allowing flexion, extension, hyperextension, abduction, and adduction (Fig. 20-13). The first MTP joint is much more mobile. It allows approximately 45 degrees of flexion and extension and 90 degrees of hyperextension. The second through fifth MTP joints allow about 40 degrees of flexion and extension and only about 45 degrees of hyperextension. Hyperextension is very important during the toe-off phase of walking. The point of reference for abduction and adduction is the second toe. Like the middle finger, the second toe abducts in both directions but adducts only as a return motion from abduction.

Also like the hand, each of the lesser toes (two through five) has a **proximal interphalangeal (PIP)** and a **distal interphalangeal (DIP) joint.** Individually, these joints are not as significant as they are in the hand, because the foot requires less dexterity. The great toe has a proximal and distal phalanx but no middle phalange. Therefore, like the thumb, it has only one phalangeal joint, the **interphalangeal (IP) joint** (see Fig. 20-12).

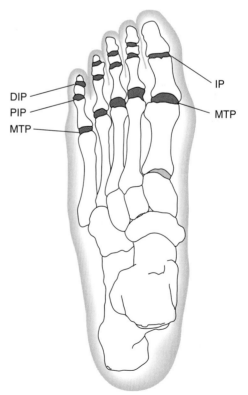

Figure 20-12. Joints of the phalanges of the foot (superior view). Note that the great toe has only two joints whereas the four lesser toes have three.

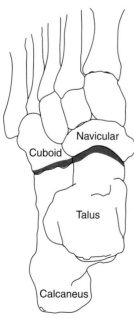

Figure 20-11. Transverse tarsal joint (superior view).

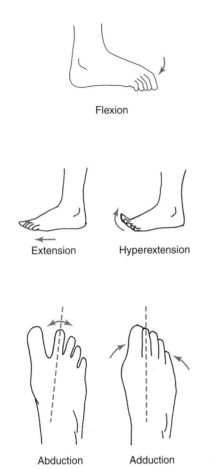

Flexion

Extension   Hyperextension

Abduction   Adduction

Figure 20-13.   Toe motions.

Ligaments and Other Structures

The ankle joint, a synovial joint, has a joint capsule. This **capsul**e is rather thin anteriorly and posteriorly but is reinforced by collateral ligaments on the sides. These collateral ligaments are actually groups of several ligaments. The collateral ligament on the medial side is a triangular **deltoid ligament** whose apex is located along the tip of the medial malleolus. Its broad base spreads out to attach to the talus, navicular, and calcaneus in four parts (Fig. 20-14). The anterior fibers attach to the navicular (tibionavicular ligament). The middle fibers (tibiocalcaneal ligament) descend directly to the sustentaculum tali of the calcaneus. The posterior fibers (posterior tibiotalar ligament) run backward to the talus. The deep fibers (anterior tibiotalar ligament) can barely be seen from the medial side, because they are deep to the tibionavicular portion. The deltoid ligament strengthens the medial side of the ankle joint, holds the calcaneus and navicular against the talus, and helps maintain the medial longitudinal arch.

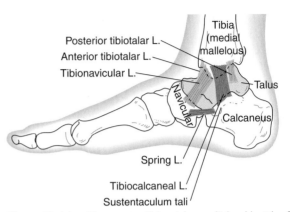

Figure 20-14.   Ligaments of the right medial ankle. The four parts of the deltoid ligament. Note that the dotted lines show the outline of the talus under the ligaments.

On the lateral side of the ankle joint is a group of three ligaments commonly and collectively referred to as the **lateral ligament** (Fig. 20-15). The three parts of this ligament connect the lateral malleolus to the talus and calcaneus. The rather weak anterior talofibular ligament attaches the lateral malleolus to the talus. Posteriorly, the fairly strong posterior talofibular ligament runs almost horizontally to connect the lateral malleolus to the talus. In the middle is the long and fairly vertical calcaneofibular ligament that attaches the malleolus to the calcaneus. Numerous other ligaments attach the various tarsals to each other, to the metatarsals, and so on. They tend to be named for the bones to which they attach. Their individual names and locations will not be discussed here.

Arches

Because the foot is the usual point of impact with the ground, it must be able to absorb a great deal of shock, adjust to changes in terrain, and propel the body forward.

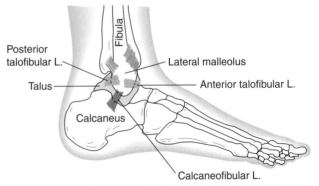

Figure 20-15.   Ligaments of the right lateral ankle. The three parts of the lateral ligament.

To allow these actions to occur, the bones of the foot are arranged in arches. We stand on a triangle that distributes weight-bearing from the base of the calcaneus to the heads of the first and fifth metatarsals (Fig. 20-16). Between these three points are two arches (medial and lateral longitudinal; Fig. 20-17) at right angles to the third (transverse) arch (Fig. 20-18).

The **medial longitudinal arch** makes up the medial border of the foot, running from the calcaneus anteriorly through the talus, navicular, and three cuneiforms

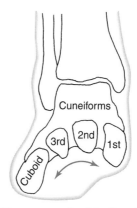

Figure 20-18.   Transverse arch of the foot (frontal view).

anteriorly to the first three metatarsals (Fig. 20-17A). The talus is at the top of the arch; it is often referred to as the *keystone* because it receives the weight of the body. An essential part of an arch, the keystone is usually the central, or topmost, part. The arch depresses somewhat during weight-bearing and then recoils when the weight is removed. Normally, it never flattens or touches the ground.

The **lateral longitudinal arch** runs from the calcaneus anteriorly through the cuboid to the fourth and fifth metatarsals (Fig. 20-17B). It normally rests on the ground during weight-bearing.

The **transverse arch** (see Fig. 20-18) runs from side to side through the three cuneiforms to the cuboid. The second cuneiform is the keystone of this arch.

These three arches are maintained by (1) the shape of the bones and their relation to each other, (2) the plantar ligaments and fascia (Figs. 20-19 and 20-20), and (3) the muscles. The ligaments and fascia are perhaps the most important features. The **spring ligament**

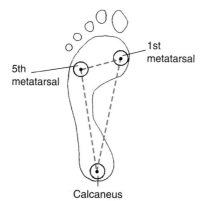

Figure 20-16.   The main weight-bearing surfaces of the right foot (plantar view).

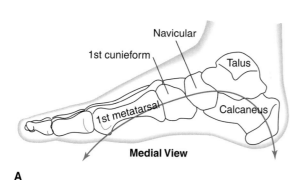

Medial View

A

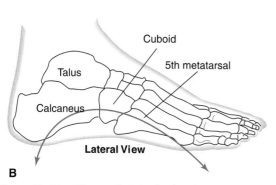

Lateral View

B

Figure 20-17.   The two longitudinal arches of the right foot: **(A)** Medial longitudinal arch. **(B)** Lateral longitudinal arch.

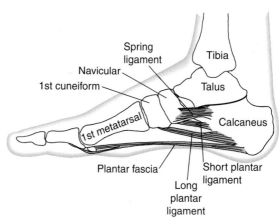

Figure 20-19.   Support structures of the right foot and arches (medial view).

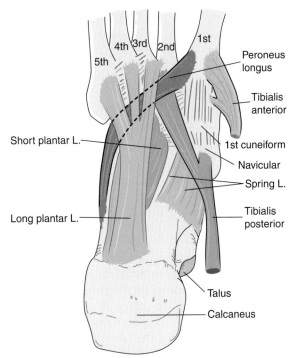

Figure 20-20.   Support structures of the right foot and arches (inferior view).

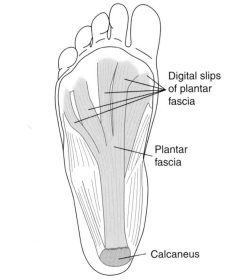

Figure 20-21.   Plantar fascia (plantar view).

(plantar calcaneonavicular ligament) attaches to the calcaneus and runs forward to the navicular. It is short and wide, and it is most important because it supports the medial side of the longitudinal arch.

The **long plantar ligament,** the longest of the tarsal ligaments, is more superficial than the spring ligament. It attaches posteriorly to the calcaneus and runs forward to attach on the cuboid and bases of the third, fourth, and fifth metatarsals. It is the primary support of the lateral longitudinal arch. The long plantar ligament is assisted by the **short plantar ligament,** which also attaches the calcaneus to the cuboid. It mostly lies deep to the long plantar ligament. Both longitudinal arches are supported by the superficially located **plantar fascia,** which runs from the calcaneus forward to the proximal phalanges. It acts as a tie-rod, keeping the posterior segments (calcaneus and talus) from separating from the anterior portion (anterior tarsals and metatarsal heads). This plantar fascia increases the stability of the foot and arches during weight-bearing and walking (Fig. 20-21).

The arches are also supported by muscles, mainly the invertors and evertors of the foot. The tibialis posterior, the flexor hallucis longus, and the flexor digitorum longus muscles all span the ankle posteriorly on the medial side, passing under the sustentaculum tali of the calcaneus. Thus, they give some support to

the medial side of the foot. The flexor hallucis longus and flexor digitorum longus muscles span the medial longitudinal arch and help support it. The peroneus longus muscle spans the foot from the lateral to the medial side, providing support to the transverse and lateral longitudinal arches. The intrinsic muscles provide more support than the extrinsics, because any motion will involve them. However, the total muscular support to the arches has been estimated to bear only about 15% to 20% of the total stress to the arches.

Muscles of the Ankle and Foot

Extrinsic Muscles

As in the wrist and hand, there are extrinsic and intrinsic muscles in the ankle and foot. The extrinsic muscles originate on the leg, and the intrinsic muscles originate on the tarsal bones. The extrinsic muscles of the leg are found in groups of three or combinations of three and are located in four anatomical areas. Those four anatomical areas also represent the four compartments of the leg, separated by heavy fascia. Within each compartment is a group of muscles that have a common function(s). They are the (1) superficial posterior, (2) deep posterior, (3) anterior, and (4) lateral groups/compartments (see Figs. 20-33 through 20-37). All have proximal attachments on the femur, tibia, or fibula, and all cross the ankle joint. Table 20-2 summarizes these muscles. Assistive movers are the muscles

Table 20-2	Extrinsic Muscles of the Ankle and Foot	
Muscle	Joint Crossing	Possible Actions
Posterior Group		
Superficial Posterior Group		
Gastrocnemius	Posterior	Plantar flexion
Soleus	Posterior	Plantar flexion
(Plantaris)	Posterior	Plantar flexion
Deep Posterior Group		
Tibialis posterior	Posterior, medial	Plantar flexion, inversion
Flexor digitorum longus	Posterior, medial	Plantar flexion, inversion, lesser toe flexion
Flexor hallucis longus	Posterior, medial	Plantar flexion, inversion, great toe flexion
Anterior Group		
Tibialis anterior	Anterior, medial	Dorsiflexion, inversion
Extensor hallucis longus	Anterior, medial	Dorsiflexion, inversion, great toe extension
Extensor digitorum longus	Anterior	Dorsiflexion, lesser toe extension
Lateral Group		
Peroneus longus	Posterior, lateral	Eversion, plantar flexion
Peroneus brevis	Posterior, lateral	Eversion, plantar flexion
(Peroneus tertius)	Anterior	Eversion, dorsiflexion

indicated in parentheses. All other muscles listed are prime movers.

Superficial Posterior Group

The superficial posterior group includes the gastrocnemius, soleus, and plantaris muscles. The **gastrocnemius muscle** is a two-joint muscle that crosses the knee and the ankle (Fig. 20-22). It is an extremely strong ankle plantar flexor. It attaches by two heads to the posterior surface of the medial and lateral condyles of the femur. After descending the posterior leg superficially, it forms a common *Achilles tendon* (often called the *heel cord by laymen*) with the soleus muscle and attaches to the posterior surface of the calcaneus. Although its major function is at the ankle, it does span the knee posteriorly and has a significant role at the knee.

Gastrocnemius Muscle

O	Medial and lateral condyles of femur
I	Posterior calcaneus
A	Knee flexion; ankle plantar flexion
N	Tibial nerve (S1, S2)

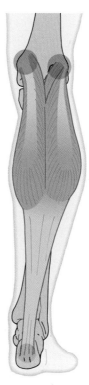

Figure 20-22.   The gastrocnemius muscle (posterior view).

The **soleus muscle** is a large, one-joint muscle located deep to the gastrocnemius muscle (Fig. 20-23). Originating on the posterior tibia and fibula, it spans the posterior leg, blending with the gastrocnemius muscle to form the large, strong Achilles tendon that inserts on the posterior calcaneus. Because the soleus muscle spans the ankle in the midline, its only function is to plantar flex the ankle. The two heads of the gastrocnemius and soleus muscles make up what is sometimes referred to as the **triceps surae muscle,** meaning "three-headed calf" muscle.

Soleus Muscle

O	Posterior tibia and fibula
I	Posterior calcaneus
A	Ankle plantar flexion
N	Tibial nerve (S1, S2)

The **plantaris muscle** is a long, thin, two-joint muscle with no significant function (see Fig. 20-23). It originates on the posterior surface of the lateral epicondyle of the femur, spans the posterior leg medially, and blends with the gastrocnemius and soleus muscles in the Achilles tendon. Theoretically, it should flex the knee and plantar flex the ankle. However, because of its size in relation to the prime movers of those actions, it is assistive at best.

Plantaris Muscle

O	Posterior lateral condyle of femur
I	Posterior calcaneus
A	Very weak assist in knee flexion and ankle plantar flexion
N	Tibial nerve (L4, L5, S1)

Deep Posterior Group

The deep posterior group is made up of the tibialis posterior, the flexor hallucis longus, and the flexor digitorum longus muscles. They all attach to the posterior tibia and/or fibula, and all terminate in the foot. Because they all cross the ankle posteriorly, they can plantar flex it. However, because of their size in relation to the soleus and gastrocnemius muscles, their role is only assistive in ankle plantar flexion.

The **tibialis posterior muscle** is the deepest-lying posterior muscle. Its proximal attachment is on the interosseous membrane and adjacent portions of the tibia and fibula (Fig. 20-24). It descends on the posterior aspect of the leg, looping around the medial malleolus to attach on the navicular with fibrous expansions to the cuboid, the three cuneiforms, the sustentaculum tali of the calcaneus, and the bases of the second

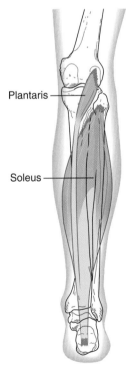

Figure 20-23. The soleus and plantaris muscles (posterior view).

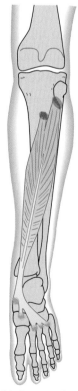

Figure 20-24. The tibialis posterior muscle (posterior view). Note that the foot is in extreme plantar flexion.

through fourth metatarsals. Because the tibialis posterior muscle crosses the ankle medially and posteriorly, it can invert and plantar flex the ankle. As mentioned above, because of its size in relation to the other plantar flexors, it is only assistive in plantar flexion.

Tibialis Posterior Muscle

O	Interosseous membrane, adjacent tibia and fibula
I	Navicular and most tarsals and metatarsals
A	Ankle inversion; assists in plantar flexion
N	Tibial nerve (L5, S1)

Situated mostly on the lateral side of the leg, the **flexor hallucis longus muscle** arises from the posterior fibula and interosseous membrane. It descends the leg posteriorly, loops around the medial malleolus through a groove in the posterior talus, and goes under the sustentaculum tali of the calcaneus. This muscle travels down the foot through the two heads of the flexor hallucis brevis muscle to attach at the base of the distal phalanx of the great toe (Fig. 20-25). This distal attachment is similar to the flexor digitorum profundus and superficialis muscles in the hand. The flexor

hallucis longus muscle flexes the great toe and assists in inversion and, to a lesser degree, assists in plantar flexion of the ankle.

Flexor Hallucis Longus Muscle

O	Posterior fibula and interosseous membrane
I	Distal phalanx of the great toe
A	Flexes great toe; assists in inversion and plantar flexion of the ankle
N	Tibial nerve (L5, S1, S2)

Situated mostly on the medial side of the leg, the **flexor digitorum longus muscle** arises from the posterior tibia (Fig. 20-26). It descends the leg posteriorly, loops around the medial malleolus, and runs down the foot, splitting into four tendons and inserting into the distal phalanx of the second through fifth toes. This muscle passes through the split in the flexor digitorum brevis tendon in a fashion similar to the flexor digitorum profundus muscle, which goes through the split in the flexor digitorum superficialis muscle in the hand. It

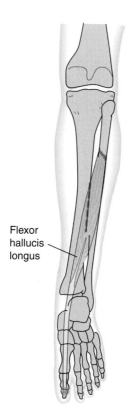

Flexor hallucis longus

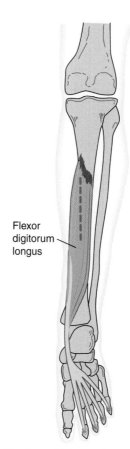

Flexor digitorum longus

Figure 20-25.   The flexor hallucis longus muscle (posterior view). Note that the foot is in extreme plantar flexion.

Figure 20-26.   The flexor digitorum longus muscle (posterior view). Note that the foot is in extreme plantar flexion.

flexes the four lesser toes and assists in inversion and plantar flexion of the ankle.

Flexor Digitorum Longus Muscle

O	Posterior tibia
I	Distal phalanx of four lesser toes
A	Flexes the four lesser toes; assists in ankle inversion and plantar flexion of the ankle
N	Tibial nerve (L5, S1)

The relationships among the deep posterior muscles are interesting, as they cross and intertwine with one another from their proximal to distal attachments (Fig. 20-27). Table 20-3 summarizes this changing relationship. Note that at their origins, the tibialis posterior muscle is in the middle of these three muscles. Where they loop around the medial malleolus, the flexor digitorum longus is in the middle. At their insertions, the flexor hallucis longus is in the middle. The flexor digitorum longus is on the opposite side from where it was at the origin. This feature of changing relationship provides added strength, much like a

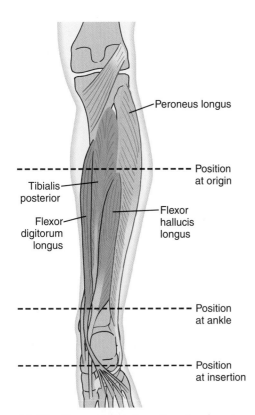

Figure 20-27. From origin to insertion, the changing positions of the flexor digitorum longus (D), the tibialis posterior (T), and the flexor hallucis longus (H) provide added strength (posterior and plantar views of leg and foot).

Table 20-3	Deep Posterior Group		
Location	**Relationship**		
Origin (medial to lateral)	FDL	TP	FHL
Medial malleolus (superior to inferior)	TP	FDL	FHL
Insertion (medial to lateral)	TP	FHL	FDL

braided rope that is stronger than a rope in which the individual fibers run parallel to one another.

Anterior Group

The anterior muscle group is made up of the tibialis anterior, the extensor hallucis longus, and the extensor digitorum longus muscles. They all attach proximally on the anterior lateral leg and cross the ankle anteriorly.

The **tibialis anterior muscle** originates on the lateral side of the tibia and interosseous membrane, then descends the leg to insert medially on the first cuneiform and the base of the first metatarsal (Fig. 20-28). It makes up most of the anterior lateral leg's bulk. Because the tibialis anterior muscle spans the ankle anteriorly and medially, it dorsiflexes and inverts the ankle.

Tibialis Anterior Muscle

O	Lateral tibia and interosseous membrane
I	First cuneiform and first metatarsal
A	Ankle inversion and dorsiflexion
N	Deep peroneal nerve (L4, L5, S1)

The **extensor hallucis longus muscle,** a thin muscle lying deep to and between the tibialis anterior and the extensor digitorum longus muscles, originates on the fibula and interosseous membrane and inserts into the base of the distal phalanx of the great toe (Fig. 20-29). Its primary function is to extend the great toe, but this muscle also assists in dorsiflexing and inverting the ankle.

Extensor Hallucis Longus Muscle

O	Fibula and interosseous membrane
I	Distal phalanx of great toe
A	Extends first toe; assists in ankle inversion and dorsiflexion
N	Deep peroneal nerve (L4, L5, S1)

The **extensor digitorum longus muscle** is the most lateral of the anterior muscles. It attaches to most of the anterior fibula, the interosseous membrane, and the

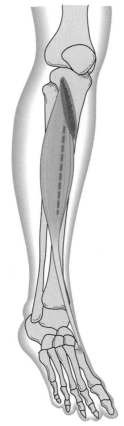

Figure 20-28. The tibialis anterior muscle (anterolateral view).

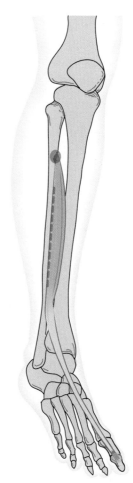

Figure 20-29. The extensor hallucis longus muscle (anterolateral view).

lateral condyle of the tibia. It descends the leg to attach to the distal phalanx of the four lesser toes (Fig. 20-30). The extensor digitorum longus muscle functions primarily to extend the second through fifth toes, but it also assists in dorsiflexing the ankle. It does not have an inversion/eversion role, because it crosses the joint through the middle of that axis.

Extensor Digitorum Longus Muscle

O	Fibula, interosseous membrane, tibia
I	Distal phalanx of four lesser toes
A	Extends four lesser toes, assists in ankle dorsiflexion
N	Deep peroneal nerve (L4, L5, S1)

Lateral Group

The lateral group of muscles consists of the peroneus longus, peroneus brevis, and peroneus tertius muscles. They all originate proximally on the fibula and run distally to the foot. Two cross the ankle joint posteriorly, and one crosses the ankle anteriorly.

The **peroneus longus muscle** is the most superficial of the peroneal muscles. Arising from the proximal end of the fibula and interosseous membrane, it descends the lateral leg and loops behind the lateral malleolus along with the peroneus brevis muscle. At this point, the peroneus longus muscle goes deep, crossing the foot obliquely from the lateral to the medial side and inserting into the plantar surface of the first metatarsal and first cuneiform (Fig. 20-31). This distal attachment is very close to the attachment of the tibialis anterior muscle. Together, the peroneus longus and tibialis anterior muscles are sometimes referred to as the **stirrup of the foot,** because the peroneus longus muscle descends the leg laterally before crossing the foot medially to join the tibialis anterior muscle. The tibialis anterior muscle descends the leg medially to meet the peroneus longus muscle, forming a U, or stirrup (see Fig. 20-20). Crossing the foot as it does, the peroneus longus muscle provides some support to the lateral longitudinal and transverse arches of the foot. Its prime

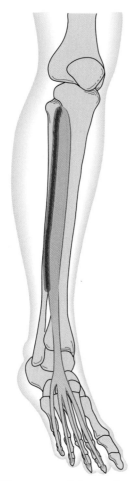

Figure 20-30. The extensor digitorum longus muscle (anterolateral view).

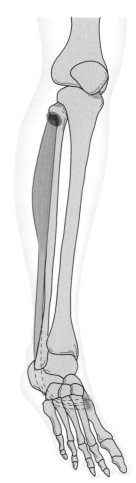

Figure 20-31. The peroneus longus muscle (anterolateral view). Dotted lines indicate location on plantar surface.

function is to evert the ankle, although this muscle can assist somewhat in ankle plantar flexion.

Peroneus Longus Muscle

O	Lateral proximal fibula and interosseous membrane
I	Plantar surface of first cuneiform and metatarsal
A	Ankle eversion; assists in ankle plantar flexion
N	Superficial peroneal nerve (L4, L5, S1)

Deep to the peroneus longus muscle is the smaller, shorter **peroneus brevis muscle.** It attaches laterally on the distal fibula, descends the leg, and loops behind the lateral malleolus before coming forward to attach on the base of the fifth metatarsal (Fig. 20-32). The peroneus brevis muscle is superficial from the lateral malleolus forward. Like the peroneus longus muscle,

the primary function of this muscle is to evert the ankle, although it can assist somewhat in plantar flexion.

Peroneus Brevis Muscle

O	Lateral distal fibula
I	Base of fifth metatarsal
A	Ankle eversion; assists in plantar flexion
N	Superficial peroneal nerve (L4, L5, S1)

The **peroneus tertius muscle,** which is not present in all people, is difficult to identify and often is confused as part of the extensor digitorum longus muscle. This muscle arises from the distal medial fibula and interosseous membrane. It crosses the ankle anteriorly to insert on the dorsal surface of the base of the fifth metatarsal, near the peroneus brevis muscle (see Fig. 20-32). Theoretically, this muscle should dorsiflex and evert the ankle, but due to its size, it is assistive at best.

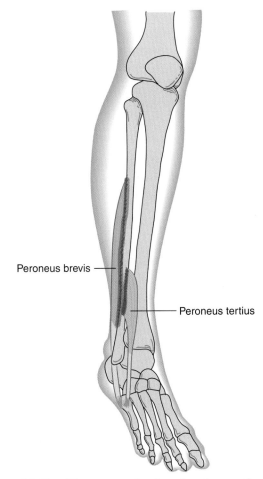

Figure 20-32.   The peroneus brevis and tertius muscles (anterolateral view).

Table 20-4	Actions of Ankle Prime Movers
Action	**Muscle**
Plantar flexion	Gastrocnemius, soleus
Dorsiflexion	Tibialis anterior
Inversion	Tibialis anterior, tibialis posterior
Eversion	Peroneus longus, peroneus brevis
Flexion of second through fifth toes	Flexor digitorum longus
Flexion of first toe	Flexor hallucis longus
Extension of second through fifth toes	Extensor digitorum longus
Extension of first toe	Extensor hallucis longus
No prime mover action	Plantaris, peroneus tertius

the extensor digitorum brevis, the extensor hallucis brevis muscles, and the dorsal interossei, which are between the metatarsals and dorsal to the plantar interossei. Table 20-5 summarizes the intrinsic muscles according to surface location, depth location, function, and similar structure in the hand. Table 20-6 summarizes the innervation of the intrinsic muscles.

Anatomical Relationships

To appreciate the relationships between muscles of the ankle and foot, they should be put into anterior, lateral, and posterior groups, with superficial and deep subgroups. The posterior group has six muscles arranged in three layers. The gastrocnemius is the only superficial muscle that is located posteriorly (Fig. 20-33). Deep to it are the very long, thin plantaris muscle and the large, one-joint soleus muscle (Fig. 20-34). The deepest layer has the flexor digitorum longus, the tibialis posterior, and the flexor hallucis longus arranged from medial to lateral (Fig. 20-35). As noted earlier, the interrelationship of these muscles changes two more times before reaching their insertions (see Table 20-3).

Of the lateral group, the peroneus longus is superficial and the peroneus brevis lies deep to it. Just above the lateral malleolus, the peroneus brevis can be palpated just anterior to the peroneus longus (Fig. 20-36). Below the malleolus, the peroneus longus cannot be seen or palpated, because it goes deep to cross the plantar surface of the foot. However, at the base of the fifth metatarsal, the tendon of the peroneus brevis should be seen coming from behind the malleolus and the tendon

Peroneus Tertius Muscle

O	Distal medial fibula
I	Base of fifth metatarsal
A	Assists somewhat in ankle eversion and dorsiflexion
N	Deep peroneal nerve (L4, L5, S1)

Table 20-4 summarizes the actions of the prime movers of the ankle.

Intrinsic Muscles

Intrinsic muscles have both attachments distal to the ankle joint. Because we do not use these muscles in the foot to perform intricate actions, they tend not to be as well developed as their counterparts in the hand. Their names tell a great deal about their location and action. All intrinsic muscles are located on the plantar surface, essentially in layers; the exceptions to this are

Table 20-5	Intrinsic Muscles of the Foot	
Muscle	Action	Comparable Hand Muscle
Dorsal Surface		
Extensor digitorum brevis	Extends PIP joints of digits 2–4	None
Extensor hallucis brevis	Extends PIP joint of first digit	None
Plantar Surface		
First Layer (most superficial)		
Abductor hallucis	Abducts; flexes IP of first toe	Abductor pollicis brevis
Flexor digitorum brevis	Flexes PIP of digits 2–5	Flexor digitorum superficialis
Abductor digiti minimi	Flexes; abducts fifth digit	Same name
Second Layer		
Quadratus plantae	Straightens diagonal line of pull of flexor digitorum longus	None
Lumbricales	Flexes MPs; extends PIPs and DIPs	Same name
Third Layer		
Flexor hallucis brevis	Flexes MP of first digit	Flexor pollicis brevis
Adductor hallucis	Adducts; flexes first digit	Adductor pollicis
Flexor digiti minimi	Flexes PIP of fifth digit	Same name
Dorsal Surface		
Fourth Layer (deepest)		
Dorsal interossei	Abducts second through fourth digits	Same name
Plantar interossei	Adducts second through fourth digits	Palmar interossei

of the peroneus tertius should be seen coming in front of the malleolus. Do not confuse it as a tendon of the extensor digitorum longus. Note that it does not go to the fifth toe.

The tibialis anterior muscle comes from the proximal lateral tibia and is superficial as it runs the entire

Table 20-6	Innervation of the Intrinsic Foot Muscles
Muscle	Nerve
Dorsal Surface	
Extensor digitorum brevis	Deep peroneal
Extensor hallucis brevis	Deep peroneal
Plantar Surface	
Abductor hallucis	Tibial
Flexor digitorum brevis	Tibial
Abductor digiti minimi	Tibial
Quadratus plantae	Tibial
Lumbricales	Tibial
Flexor hallucis brevis	Tibial
Adductor hallucis	Tibial
Flexor digiti minimi	Tibial
Dorsal interossei	Tibial
Plantar interossei	Tibial

distance to the medial side of the ankle. Just above the ankle, the tendons of the tibialis anterior, the extensor hallucis longus, and the extensor digitorum longus can be seen from medial to lateral (Fig. 20-37). Note that the extensor digitorum longus has a tendon running to the second, third, fourth, and fifth toes. Be sure to note, too, the difference between the tendon of the extensor digitorum longus going to the fifth toe and the tendon of the peroneus tertius going only to the base of the fifth metatarsal.

The intrinsic muscles of the foot are arranged in essentially four layers on the plantar surface. The first muscular layer lies deep to the plantar fascia (see Fig. 20-21). The flexor digitorum brevis lies in the midline, with tendons going to the second through the fifth toes. On the medial side lies the abductor hallucis, and on the lateral side is the abductor digiti minimi (Fig. 20-38). The second layer has two intrinsic muscles and tendons of two extrinsic muscles (flexor digitorum longus and flexor hallucis longus) (Fig. 20-39). The quadratus plantae runs from the calcaneus toward the tendon of the flexor digitorum longus, where it attaches just before the flexor digitorum longus splits into four tendons that go to the second through fifth toes. When it contracts, the quadratus plantae straightens the long toe flexor's line of pull. The tendon of the flexor hallucis longus can also be seen in this layer. The

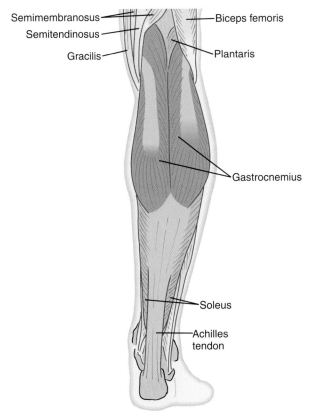

Figure 20-33. Muscles of the posterior leg, superficial layer (posterior view, right leg).

Labels: Semimembranosus, Semitendinosus, Gracilis, Biceps femoris, Plantaris, Gastrocnemius, Soleus, Achilles tendon

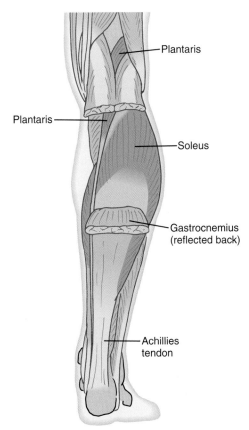

Figure 20-34. Middle layer of the posterior group. The middle section of the gastrocnemius muscle has been removed.

Labels: Plantaris, Plantaris, Soleus, Gastrocnemius (reflected back), Achillies tendon

lumbricales are four intrinsic muscles that arise from the tendons of the flexor digitorum longus, pass on the medial side of the four lesser toes, and attach on the tendons of the extensor digitorum longus on the dorsal surface. The third layer has the two heads of the flexor hallucis brevis medially, the two heads of the adductor hallucis in the middle, and the flexor digiti minimi laterally (Fig. 20-40). The fourth and deepest layer includes the interossei muscles. As their names imply, they lie between the bones (metatarsals) on the palmar and dorsal sides (Fig. 20-41). They have the same function as their counterparts in the hand and have very similar attachments (see Figs. 13-25 and 13-26 for a comparison). Unlike their counterparts in the hand, the second toe is the one from which the other toes either abduct or adduct.

The intrinsic muscles on the dorsum of the foot lie underneath or next to their counterpart extrinsic muscles (Fig. 20-42). The extensor hallucis brevis is just lateral to the extensor hallucis longus. The three tendons of extensor digitorum brevis are deep to the extensor digitorum longus and attach laterally to its distal attachment on the second, third, and fourth toes.

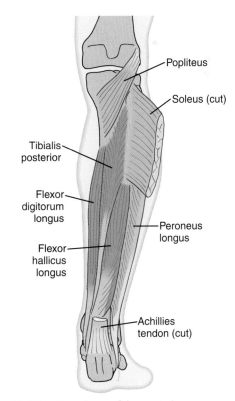

Figure 20-35. Deep layer of the posterior group.

Labels: Popliteus, Soleus (cut), Tibialis posterior, Flexor digitorum longus, Peroneus longus, Flexor hallicus longus, Achillies tendon (cut)

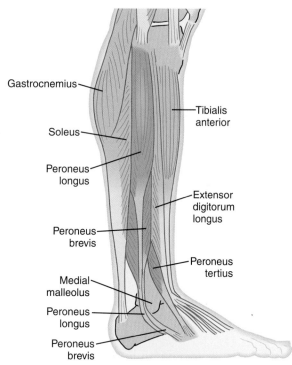

Figure 20-36.   Muscles of the right lateral group (lateral view).

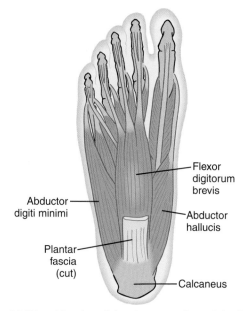

Figure 20-38.   Muscles of the plantar surface of the foot—first (superficial) layer (plantar view).

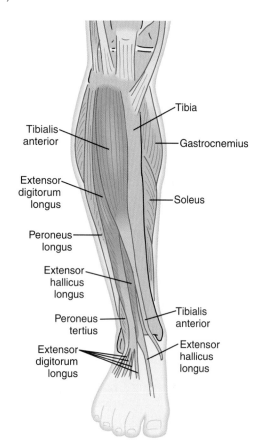

Figure 20-37.   Muscles of the right anterior group (anterior view).

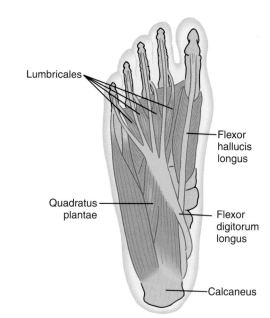

Figure 20-39.   Muscles of the plantar surface of the foot—second layer (plantar view).

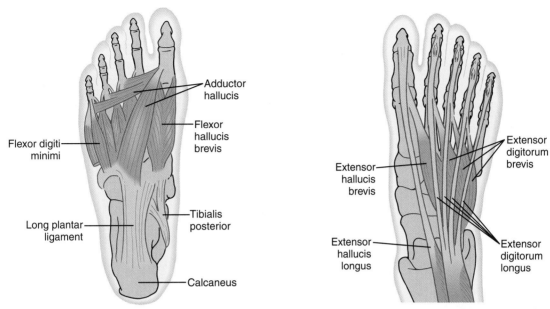

Figure 20-40.   Muscles of the plantar surface of the foot—third layer (plantar view).

Figure 20-42.   Intrinsic muscles of the dorsum of the foot.

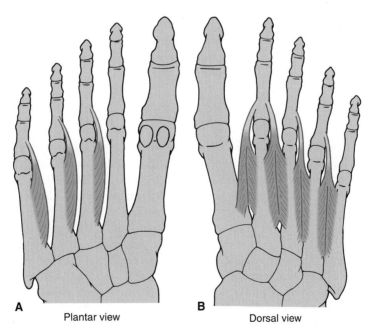

A   Plantar view   **B**   Dorsal view

Figure 20-41.   Muscles of the plantar surface of the right foot—fourth (deepest) layer. **(A)** Plantar interossei. **(B)** Dorsal interossei.

Summary of Muscle Innervation

The ankle and foot muscles fall into relatively tidy groupings according to innervation. Those muscles located on the posterior leg and plantar surface of the foot receive innervation from the **tibial nerve.** Similar to the hand, the plantar foot divides into two groups. The lateral plantar branch of the tibial nerve innervates muscles located on the lateral side, and the medial plantar branch innervates those on the medial side.

The **superficial peroneal nerve** innervates muscles on the lateral side of the leg (peroneals). The peroneus tertius muscle is the exception, because it crosses the ankle anteriorly and receives innervation with the other anterior muscles from the **deep peroneal nerve.**

Tables 20-6, 20-7, and 20-8 summarize ankle and foot innervation according to nerve and spinal

Table 20-7	Innervation of the Muscles of the Leg and Foot	
Muscle	**Nerve**	**Spinal Segment**
Gastrocnemius	Tibial	S1, S2
Soleus	Tibial	S1, S2
Plantaris	Tibial	L4, L5, S1
Tibialis posterior	Tibial	L5, S1
Flexor digitorum longus	Tibial	L5, S1
Flexor hallucis longus	Tibial	L5, S1, S2
Peroneus longus	Superficial peroneal	L4, L5, S1
Peroneus brevis	Superficial peroneal	L4, L5, S1
Peroneus tertius	Deep peroneal	L4, L5, S1
Extensor digitorum longus	Deep peroneal	L4, L5, S1
Extensor digitorum brevis	Deep peroneal	L5, S1
Extensor hallucis longus	Deep peroneal	L4, L5, S1
Tibialis anterior	Deep peroneal	L4, L5, S1
Abductor hallucis	Medial plantar (tibial)	L4, L5
Flexor hallucis brevis	Medial plantar (tibial)	L4, L5, S1
Flexor digitorum brevis	Medial plantar (tibial)	L4, L5
Lumbricales (medial 1)	Medial plantar (tibial)	L4, L5
Lumbricales (lateral 3)	Lateral plantar (tibial)	S1, S2
Abductor digiti minimi	Lateral plantar (tibial)	S1, S2
Quadratus plantae	Lateral plantar (tibial)	S1, S2
Adductor hallucis	Lateral plantar (tibial)	S1, S2
Flexor digiti minimi	Lateral plantar (tibial)	S1, S2
Dorsal interossei	Lateral plantar (tibial)	S1, S2
Plantar interossei	Lateral plantar (tibial)	S1, S2

segment. As has been noted in previous chapters, there is some variation among sources regarding spinal cord level. *Gray's Anatomy* is used as the reference source when discrepancy occurs.

Common Ankle Pathologies

Shin splints is a general term given to exercise-induced pain along the medial edge of the tibia, usually a few inches above the ankle to midway up the tibia. Most commonly, inflammation of the periosteum causes the pain. Shin splints are an overuse injury that can result from running on hard surfaces, running on tiptoes, and playing sports that involve a lot of jumping. **Medial tibial stress syndrome** is a more specific term that includes anterior leg pain not associated with a stress fracture.

Deformities of the foot and toes often affect other joints of the lower extremity and trunk, especially during walking or running. A normal foot is defined as **plantigrade,** in that the sole is at right angles to the leg when a person is standing. **Equinus foot** (horse's foot) means that the hindfoot is fixed in plantar flexion. A **calcaneus foot** is one that is fixed in dorsiflexion. **Pes cavus** refers to an abnormally high arch, while **pes planus** (flat foot) is the loss of the medial longitudinal arch. **Hallux valgus** is caused by pathological changes in which the great toe develops a valgus deformity (distal end pointed laterally). **Hallux rigidus** is a degenerative condition of the first MTP joint associated with pain and diminished range of motion. In the following lesser toe deformities, all MTP joints are hyperextended: In **hammer toe,** the PIP is flexed and the DIP is extended. **Mallet toe** is just the opposite; it has an extended PIP joint and a flexed DIP joint. **Claw toe** has a flexed PIP joint and a flexed DIP joint.

Metatarsalgia is a general term referring to pain around the metatarsal heads. The individual often describes the pain as a bruise, or "like walking on pebbles." The pain usually becomes worse with increased activity. **Morton's neuroma** is caused by abnormal pressure on the plantar digital nerves commonly at the web space between the third and fourth

Table 20-8	Segmental Innervation of the Ankle Joint and Foot			
Spinal Cord Level	L4	L5	S1	S2
Gastrocnemius			X	X
Soleus			X	X
Plantaris	X	X	X	
Tibialis posterior		X	X	
Flexor digitorum longus		X	X	
Flexor hallucis longus		X	X	X
Peroneus longus	X	X	X	
Peroneus brevis	X	X	X	
Peroneus tertius	X	X	X	
Extensor digitorum longus	X	X	X	
Extensor digitorum brevis		X	X	
Extensor hallucis longus	X	X	X	
Tibialis anterior	X	X	X	
Abductor hallucis	X	X		
Flexor hallucis brevis	X	X	X	
Flexor digitorum brevis	X	X		
Lumbricales	X	X	X	X
Abductor digiti minimi			X	X
Quadratus plantae			X	X
Adductor hallucis			X	X
Flexor digiti minimi			X	X
Dorsal interossei			X	X
Plantar interossei			X	X

metatarsals. This pressure can result in pain and numbness in the toe area that gets worse with activity, such as running. **Turf toe** is caused by forced hyperextension of the great toe at the MTP joint. It is commonly seen in football, baseball, or soccer players.

The ankle is considered the most frequently injured joint in the body. **Ankle sprains** are probably the most common injury among recreational and competitive athletes, and the lateral ligament is the most frequently injured ligament in these groups. Lateral or inversion sprains occur when the foot lands in a plantar-flexed and inverted position. One or more of the lateral ligament's three parts may be stretched or torn.

An **ankle fracture** often occurs when a person trips over an unexpected obstacle or falls from a height, and it usually involves a twisting component to the ankle. The lateral malleolus is most commonly involved. A **bimalleolar fracture** involves both malleoli, while a **trimalleolar fractures** involves both malleoli and the posterior lip of the tibia.

Plantar fasciitis is a common overuse injury, resulting in pain in the heel. The plantar fascia helps to maintain the medial longitudinal arch and acts as a shock absorber during weight-bearing. The pain is usually located at the point where the fascia attaches to the calcaneus on the plantar surface. **Achilles tendonitis,** an inflammation of the gastrocnemius-soleus tendon, is sometimes a precursor to a **ruptured Achilles tendon.** With a complete rupture, the individual loses the ability to plantar flex the ankle. To determine if the tendon is intact, have an individual lie prone with the feet off the edge of the table. Squeeze on the muscle belly of the gastrocnemius muscle. If the tendon is intact, slight plantar flexion will occur, but no motion will occur if the tendon is ruptured.

A **triple arthrodesis** is a surgical procedure that fuses the talocalcaneal, calcaneocuboid, and talonavicular joints. It provides medial-lateral stability of the foot and relieves pain at the subtalar joint, but inversion and eversion at the ankle are lost. Ankle dorsiflexion and plantar flexion remain because the talotibial joint has not been involved.

> ## Points to Remember
> - Stretching is performed on *relaxed* muscles and strengthening occurs when muscles contract.
> - To stretch a two-joint muscle, stretch it over both joints at the same time within pain limits of that muscle.
> - To stretch a one-joint muscle when a two-joint muscle crosses the same joint, select a joint position that stretches a two-joint muscle over only one joint.
> - The excursion of a one-joint muscle being stretched will be greater than the range allowed by the joint.
> - The excursion of a two-joint muscle is less than the combined range allowed by both joints.
> - A muscle contraction is strongest if the muscle is stretched before it contracts.
> - A muscle loses power quickly as it shortens.
> - Two-joint muscles maintain their force of contraction for a longer period than a one-joint muscle. This is because they are able to elongate over one joint while shortening over the other joint.

Review Questions

General Anatomy Questions

1. Describe the ankle (talotibial) joint:
   a. Number of axes:
   b. Shape of joint:
   c. Type of action allowed:
   d. Bones involved:

2. What bones are involved in the subtalar joint? What bones are involved in the transverse tarsal joint?

3. What are the functions of the interosseous membrane?

4. What ligaments provide medial stability to the ankle? What is their collective name?

5. What ligaments provide lateral stability to the ankle? What is their collective name?

6. What are the names of the two longitudinal arches?

7. List the bones involved in each longitudinal arch.

8. List the bones involved in the transverse arch.

9. What is the function of the arches?

10. Which muscles pass behind the medial malleolus?

11. Which extrinsic muscles attach on the medial side of the foot?

12. Which muscles pass behind the lateral malleolus?

13. Which extrinsic muscles attach on the lateral side of the foot?

14. Which muscles form the "stirrup" of the foot? Describe how the stirrup is formed.

15. Would an individual with a spinal cord injury at L4 be able to actively do ankle plantar flexion?

Functional Activity Questions

Identify the main ankle joint action or position in the following activities:

1. Pushing your foot down on the accelerator pedal while driving

2. Standing in high heels

3. Walking up a steep slope

4. Walking down a steep slope

5. Foot on floor with the heel as the pivot point, creating a "windshield wiper" motion of the foot

6. Walking on your heels

7. Taking off when jumping, hopping, or skipping

Clinical Exercise Questions

1. Answer the following questions about each muscle:
   Gastrocnemius
   a. Number of joints crossed?
   b. Knee motion?
   c. Ankle motion?
   Soleus
   a. Number of joints crossed?
   b. Knee motion?
   c. Ankle motion?

Review Questions—cont'd

2. Place your hands on the wall at shoulder level. Stand with your left foot 24 inches from the wall and your right foot about 12 inches from the wall (Fig. 20-43). Keeping your left leg straight and your right foot flat on the floor, lean in toward the wall, leading with your pelvis and allowing your right knee to bend. In terms of what is occurring at the left knee and ankle, answer the following questions:

   a. What are the joint positions or motions that are occurring
      at the left knee? _____
      at the left ankle? _____

   b. To be in the above position, is the left gastrocnemius contracting/stretching?

   c. To be in the above position, is the left soleus contracting/stretching?

   d. Which of these two muscles is being stretched more than the other?

   e. Why?

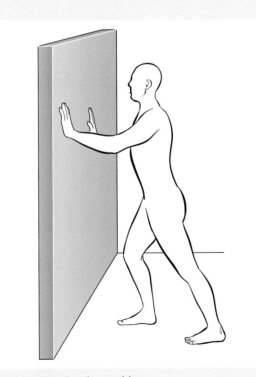

Figure 20-43.   Starting position.

3. Repeat the position of the exercise in question 2, except this time bend your left knee as you lean into the wall.

   a. What are the joint positions or motions that are occurring
      at the left knee? _____
      at the left ankle? _____

   b. In this new position, is the left gastrocnemius stretched or slack at the knee?

   c. In this new position, is the left gastrocnemius stretched or slack at the ankle?

   d. In this new position, is the left soleus stretched at the knee?

   e. In this new position, is the left soleus stretched at the ankle?

   f. Which of these two muscles is stretched more?

   g. Why?

4. Standing upright and holding on to the back of a chair for balance, rise up on your toes as high as possible.

   a. What are the joint positions or motions that are occurring
      at the knee? _____
      at the ankle? _____

   b. Is the gastrocnemius shortening or elongating over the knee?

   c. Is the gastrocnemius shortening or elongating over the ankle?

   d. Does the soleus have an action at the knee?

   e. Is the soleus shortening or elongating over the ankle?

   f. Why is the gastrocnemius stronger than the soleus in this position?

(continued on next page)

Review Questions—cont'd

5. Sitting with your knees bent, roll your feet and legs until the soles of your feet are together (Fig. 20-44).
   a. Is inversion or eversion the joint motion (or attempted joint motion) at the ankle?
   b. What type of muscle contraction (isometric, concentric, or eccentric) is occurring?
   c. What are the prime movers of this action?

6. Sitting on the floor with knee extended, loop an elastic band around the midfoot with the ankle plantar flexed and anchor the other end around a heavy table leg. Be far enough away to create sufficient tension in the elastic band. Bring your toes up toward your knees as much as possible. Hold for the count of five. Return to the starting position.
   a. What motion is occurring in each of the three phases?
   b. What type of contraction is occurring in each phase?
   c. What muscles are involved as prime movers?
   d. Is this an open or closed kinetic chain?

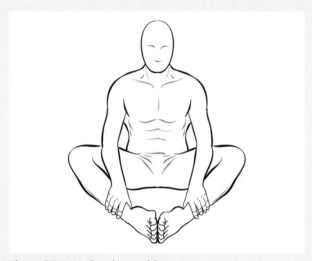

Figure 20-44. Starting position.

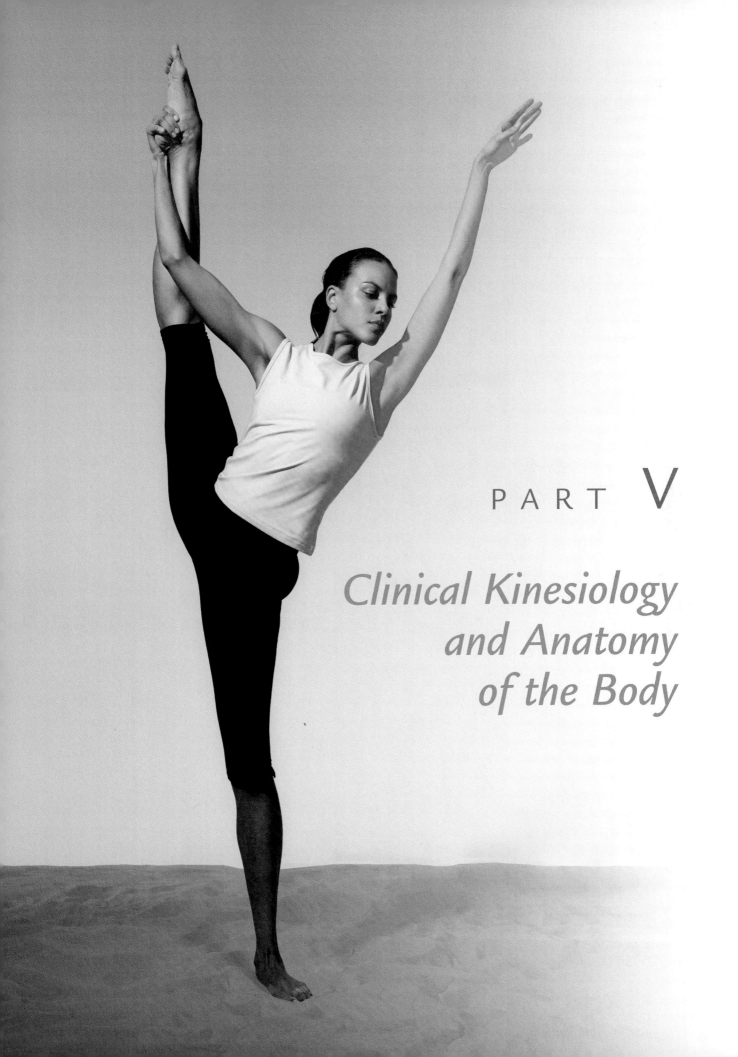

PART V

Clinical Kinesiology
and Anatomy
of the Body

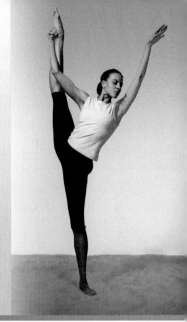

CHAPTER 21
Posture

Vertebral Alignment

Development of Postural Curves

Standing Posture

Lateral View

Anterior View

Posterior View

Sitting Posture

Supine Posture

Common Postural Deviations

Review Questions

General Anatomy Questions

Functional Activity Questions

Clinical Exercise Questions

In general, posture is the position of your body parts in relation to each other at any given time. Posture can be static, as in a stationary position such as standing, sitting, or lying. It can be dynamic as the body moves from one position to another. Posture deals with alignment of the various body segments. These body segments can be compared to blocks. If you start stacking blocks, one directly on top of the other, the column will remain relatively stable. However, if you stack them off center from each other, the column will remain upright only if the block (or blocks) above offsets the block(s) below and remains within the base of support. In the human body, each joint involved with weight-bearing can be considered a postural segment.

Vertebral Alignment

The vertebral column can be compared to the column of blocks. It is not completely straight but has a series of counterbalancing anterior-posterior curves. These curves, which must be maintained during rest and activity, act as shock absorbers and reduce the amount of injury. The thoracic and sacral curves offset the cervical and lumbar curves (Fig. 21-1). The thoracic and sacral curves are concave anteriorly and convex posteriorly, and are seen when viewed in the sagittal plane. Conversely, the lumbar and cervical curves are just the opposite—convex anteriorly and concave posteriorly. Remember that a curve has two sides to it: a concave side and a convex side. Therefore, whether a curve is concave or convex depends on to which side you are referring.

When one or more of these vertebral curves either increases or decreases significantly from what is considered good posture, poor posture results. For example, a "sway back" is an increased lumbar curve, whereas a "flat back" is a decreased thoracic curve. In most cases,

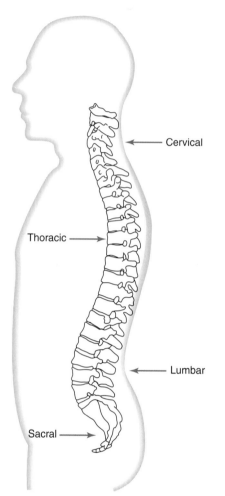

Figure 21-1.   The four major curves of the vertebral column (lateral view).

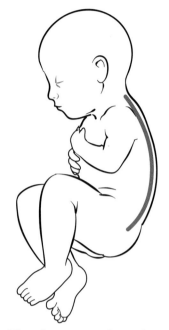

Figure 21-2.   The primary curve of a newborn (lateral view).

if there is an increased lumbar curve, there is also an increased thoracic curve. No lateral curves should exist. Any lateral curvature of the spine is a pathological condition called *scoliosis.*

Development of Postural Curves

At birth, the entire vertebral column is flexed. When viewed from the sagittal plane, it is anteriorly concave. This concave curve is called a **primary curve** (Fig. 21-2). The thoracic and sacral curves are considered primary curves for this reason. When lying in a prone position, a 2- to 4-month-old infant begins to lift its head; at approximately 5 to 6 months of age, an infant begins bilateral lifting of its lower extremities. These two anti-gravity extension actions create the **secondary curves.** These are the anteriorly convex curves of the cervical and lumbar regions.

Think of the pelvis in the upright position as a bowl of water. If the bowl is level, it will hold water. If the bowl is tipped forward or backward, water will spill out. Similarly, the position of the pelvis has great influence on the vertebral column, especially the lumbar region. The pelvis should maintain a neutral position. A position is neutral when (1) the anterior superior iliac spine (ASIS) and the posterior superior iliac spine (PSIS) are level with each other in a transverse plane and (2) the ASIS is in the same vertical plane as the symphysis pubis. When the pelvis is in a neutral position, the lumbar curve has the desired amount of curvature. When the pelvis tilts anteriorly, lumbar curvature increases **(lordosis).** When the pelvis tilts posteriorly, lumbar curvature decreases (flat back). Figure 17-13 illustrates these positions.

With weight evenly distributed on both legs, the pelvis should remain level from side to side, with both ASISs being at the same level. During walking, however, the pelvis dips from side to side as weight shifts from stance to swing phase. This **lateral pelvic tilt** is controlled by the hip abductors, mainly the gluteus medius and gluteus minimus, and by the trunk lateral benders, mainly the erector spinae and quadratus lumborum. If you bend your left knee and lift your foot off the ground, your pelvis on the left side becomes unsupported and will drop. Force couple action of the hip abductors and trunk lateral benders hold the pelvis level. The right hip abductors on the opposite side contract to pull the pelvis down on the right side while trunk lateral benders on the left (same side) contract to pull the pelvis up on the left side. These motions are illustrated in Figure 17-21. An abnormal lateral pelvic tilt can also occur if both legs are not of equal length. This will result in a lateral curvature, or scoliosis.

Muscle contractions are primarily responsible for keeping the body in the upright position in both static and dynamic posture. The muscles most involved are called **antigravity muscles** (Fig. 21-3). These are the hip and knee extensors and the trunk and neck extensors. Other muscles involved (perhaps to a lesser extent but also important in maintaining the upright position) are the trunk and neck flexors and lateral benders, the hip abductors and adductors, and the ankle pronators and supinators. If all of these muscles were to relax, the body would collapse.

The ankle plantar flexors and dorsiflexors are important in controlling postural sway (Fig. 21-4). **Postural sway** is anterior-posterior motion of the upright body caused by motion occurring primarily at the ankles. This sway is the result of constant displacement and correction of the center of gravity within the base of support.

To demonstrate this, stand upright with your feet slightly apart. Lean your entire body slowly forward by bending at the ankles. You will reach a point where you will need to either correct the forward lean or you will lose your balance. Notice that your ankle plantar flexors contract to bring you back to an upright position. Next, lean backward and notice what happens. Again, you will reach a point where you either need to correct the lean

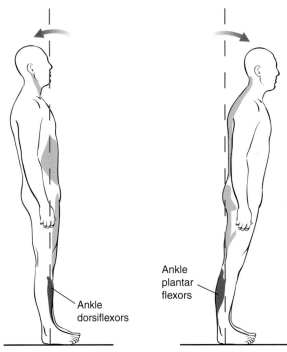

Figure 21-4.   Postural sway.

or lose your balance. Notice that your ankle dorsiflexors contract to bring you back to an upright position.

A high center of gravity and small base of support tend to increase the amount of postural sway. To again demonstrate this, stand upright with your feet slightly apart. Notice how much your body tends to move back and forth. Next, observe the amount of sway when you stand on your toes in the upright position with your feet close together. You should notice much more motion in the latter position, because you have raised your center of gravity higher and made your base of support smaller.

Good posture, which means good alignment, is important because it decreases the amount of stress placed on bones, ligaments, muscles, and tendons. Good alignment also improves function and decreases the amount of muscle energy needed to keep the body upright. For example, if the knee is in full extension, little muscle contraction is needed to keep the knee from buckling. However, when the knee is partially flexed, the muscles at that joint (knee extensors) must contract to keep the knee from collapsing. Because standing is a closed-chain activity, muscles at the hip and ankle must also contract to keep the body's center of gravity over its base of support.

To watch a ballet dancer move is to watch good posture in motion. Ballet aspires to show motion in an aesthetically beautiful manner. What is most beautiful is also most functional. Maintaining good postural alignment and keeping one's center of gravity well within

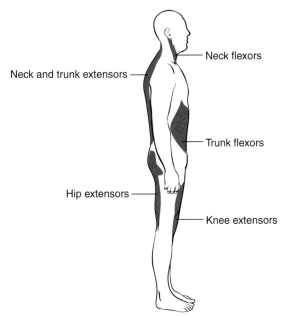

Figure 21-3.   Antigravity muscles (lateral view).

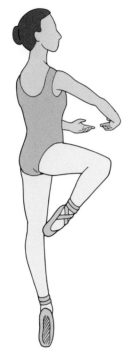

Figure 21-5. A ballet dancer must maintain good posture during motion.

Lateral View

In the standing position and viewed from the **lateral position,** the plumb line should be aligned so that it passes slightly in front of the lateral malleolus (Fig. 21-6). For ideal posture, the body segments should be aligned so that the plumb line passes through the landmarks in the order listed below:

Head
Through the earlobe.

Shoulder
Through the tip of the acromion process.

Thoracic Spine
Anterior to the vertebral bodies.

Lumbar Spine
Through the vertebral bodies.

one's base of support places less stress on body parts and allows for better balance. Ballet dancers learn the basic elements of good posture from the very beginning of their training. They are instructed in various ways to get taller, tighten their knee muscles, tighten their abdominal muscles to flatten the abdomen "like a pancake," and hold their buttocks "like a rock." In other words, dancers assume and maintain good alignment. The dancer in Figure 21-5 is maintaining good body alignment while balancing over a fairly small base of support. She is maintaining this posture dynamically as she turns (pirouette) on pointe (toes extended and ankle in extreme plantar flexion).

Standing Posture

Posture is easier to describe in a static standing position, because, except for a slight amount of sway when standing, the body is not moving. However, many of the guidelines for static posture can be applied to dynamic posture. Assessing a person's posture can be done most accurately with the use of a plumb line suspended from the ceiling or a posture grid behind the person as a point of reference. A plumb line is a string or cord with a weight attached to the lower end. Because the string is weighted, it makes a perfectly straight vertical line of gravity.

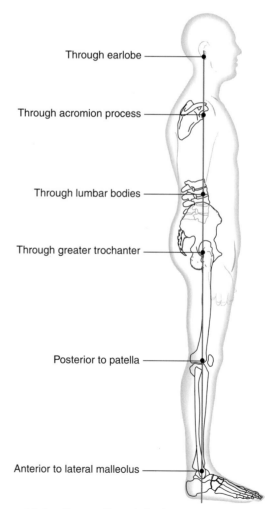

Through earlobe

Through acromion process

Through lumbar bodies

Through greater trochanter

Posterior to patella

Anterior to lateral malleolus

Figure 21-6. Posture (lateral view).

Pelvis
Level.

Hip
Through the greater trochanter (slightly posterior to the hip joint axis).

Knee
Slightly posterior to the patella (slightly anterior to the knee joint axis) with the knees in extension.

Ankle
Slightly anterior to the lateral malleolus, with the ankle joint in a neutral position between dorsiflexion and plantar flexion.

Table 21-1 summarizes common postural deviations that can be detected from the side view. Because standing is a closed kinetic chain activity, the position or motion of one joint will affect the position or motions of other joints.

Anterior View

In the standing position and viewed from the **anterior position,** the plumb line should be aligned to pass through the midsagittal plane of the body, thus dividing the body into two equal halves (Fig. 21-7). The body segments listed below should be aligned in the following order:

Head
Extended and level, not flexed or hyperextended.

Shoulders
Level and not elevated or depressed.

Sternum
Centered in the midline.

Hips
Level, with both ASISs in the same plane.

Legs
Slightly apart.

Knees
Level and not bowed or knock-kneed.

Ankles
Normal arch in feet.

Feet
Slight outward toeing.

Posterior View

In the standing position and viewed from the **posterior position,** the plumb line should also be aligned to pass

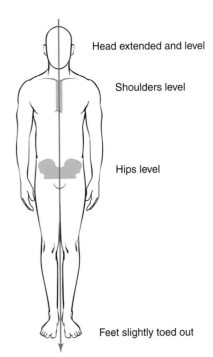

Figure 21-7.   Posture (anterior view).

Head extended and level

Shoulders level

Hips level

Feet slightly toed out

through the midsagittal plane of the body, dividing the body into two equal halves (Fig. 21-8). The following body segments should be aligned in the order listed below:

Head
Extended, not flexed or hyperextended.

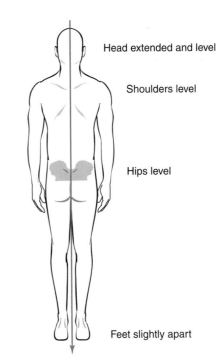

Figure 21-8.   Posture (posterior view).

Head extended and level

Shoulders level

Hips level

Feet slightly apart

Table 21-1	Summary of Common Postural Deviations		
	Lateral View	**Posterior View**	**Anterior View**
Head	Forward	Tilted Rotated	Tilted Rotated Mandible asymmetrical
Cervical spine	Exaggerated curve Flattened curve		
Shoulders	Rounded	Elevated Depressed	Elevated Depressed
Scapulae		Abducted Adducted Winged	
Thoracic spine	Exaggerated curve	Lateral deviation	
Lumbar spine	Exaggerated curve Flattened curve	Lateral deviation	
Pelvis	Anterior pelvic tilt Posterior pelvic tilt	Lateral pelvic tilt Pelvis rotated	
Hip			Medially rotated Laterally rotated
Knee	Genu recurvatum Flexed knee	Genu varum Genu valgum	External tibial torsion Internal tibial torsion
Ankle/foot	Forward posture Flattened longitudinal arch Exaggerated longitudinal arch	Pes planus Pes cavus	Hallux valgus Claw toe Hammertoe Mallet toe

Shoulders
Level and not elevated or depressed.

Spinous Processes
Centered in the midline.

Hips
Level, with both PSISs in the same plane.

Legs
Slightly apart.

Knees
Level and not bowed or knock-kneed.

Ankles
Calcaneus should be straight.

Sitting Posture

Good postural alignment while sitting is important, because sitting can place a great deal of pressure on the intervertebral disk. Studies have shown that disk pressure in the sitting position increases by slightly less than half of the amount of disk pressure in the standing position. To state the obvious, shifting weight onto the front part of the vertebrae will increase the amount of pressure placed on the intervertebral disks. As the person leans forward, disk pressure increases. As a person reaches forward or picks up a weight, disk pressure further increases as the weight or length of the lever arm increases. Figure 21-9 illustrates disk pressure in various positions. Disk pressure is least when you are lying supine. It increases as you stand and increases more as you sit. Leaning forward in these positions increases the disk pressure, and leaning forward with an object in your hand obviously increases it even more.

If the lumbar curve decreases, as often happens when sitting with the back unsupported (Fig. 21-10), the pressure on the intervertebral disks and posterior structures increases. A chair with the seat inclined anteriorly, such as the kneeling stool (Fig. 21-11), can decrease disk pressure by tilting the pelvis forward slightly. This helps to maintain the lumbar curve. However, because the back is unsupported, increased and sustained muscle contraction is required to keep the body upright.

Shifting weight onto the front part of the vertebra is not always a problem. Although disk pressure increases in this position, the stresses placed on the posterior part of the vertebra (the facet joints) decreases. Therefore, if a person has a facet joint problem, a flexed position is

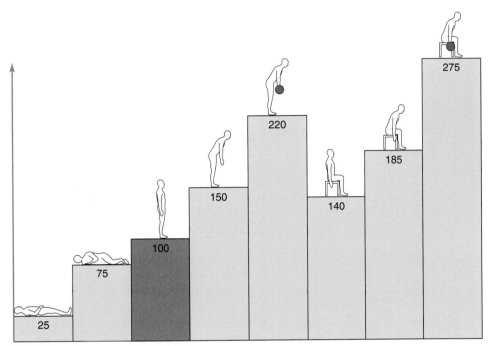

Figure 21-9.   Disk pressures in various positions.

generally more desirable. Conversely, if a person has a disk problem, an extended position is usually more desirable.

In sitting postures, a chair with lumbar support that maintains lumbar lordosis places the least amount of pressure on the disks. Maintaining the vertebral curves, keeping the feet flat on the floor, having the low back supported, and keeping the upper body in good alignment are key elements of good sitting posture. Figure 21-12 demonstrates the best posture while working at a computer. The neck and trunk are upright, the trunk is supported, and the lumbar spine has a support. The top of the monitor is at eye level. A person should not have to hyperextend the head to view the screen. The shoulders are relaxed. The elbows are flexed and close to the body. The hands, wrists, and forearms are straight and parallel to the ground. The chair should allow the hips and knees to be flexed. The thighs are parallel to the ground and the lower legs are vertical, allowing the feet to be flat on the floor or on a footrest.

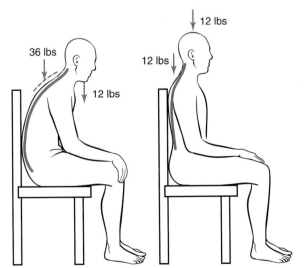

Figure 21-10.   Slouched posture increases disk pressure.

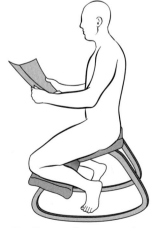

Figure 21-11.   Kneeling stool posture reduces disk pressure.

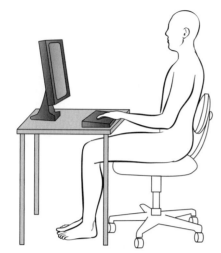

Figure 21-12.   Sitting posture at computer.

Supine Posture

Lying down is considered a resting position (Fig. 21-13). The least amount of intervertebral disk pressure occurs while lying supine (see Fig. 21-9). If you could run a plumb line horizontally, it would intersect many of the same landmarks as in the standing position. Good alignment in this position is also important. A good resting surface should be firm enough to avoid loss of the lumbar curve, yet soft enough to conform and give support to the normal curves of the body. In the side-lying position, the bottom leg is extended and the top leg is flexed. Placing a pillow between the legs can increase comfort by keeping the hips in good alignment. Lying prone is usually not recommended because of the increased pressure placed on the neck. In this position, using a pillow only increases the stresses on the neck.

When actively moving about and changing positions, whether vacuuming the rug, picking up a box from the floor, or raking leaves, keeping the body (especially the trunk) in good postural alignment is important. Most principles of good body mechanics involve avoiding stress to the trunk and maintaining the spinal curves, which involve maintaining good posture.

Common Postural Deviations

Table 21-1 summarizes the common postural deviations seen when assessing posture. It is not within the scope of this book to describe the individual causes and effects of postural problems. However, some general statements regarding cause and effect should be made.

Deviation from "good" posture is considered "poor" or "bad" posture. Causes of poor posture can be the result of structural problems. These structural problems may result from a congenital malformation such as a hemivertebra. The deviation may be an acquired deformity caused by trauma such as a compression fracture. Postural deviations also may result from neurological conditions that cause paralysis or spasticity. In addition, postural problems may be functional, or nonstructural, in nature. A person who sits or stands for long periods of time will tend to slouch. This can result in a muscle imbalance.

Generally, if a person tends to maintain a posture in which a curve is increased, the muscles on the concave side will tend to tighten while the muscles on the convex side tend to weaken. For example, you would expect a person with a lumbar lordosis to have tight back extensors and weak abdominal muscles. Also, postures that tend to increase the lordotic curves (cervical and lumbar) will increase pressure on the more posterior facet joints and decrease pressure on the more anterior intervertebral disks. Conversely, an increase in the kyphotic curves (thoracic and sacral) will increase the pressure on the intervertebral disks while decreasing the pressure on the facet joints.

It should be noted that the terms *kyphotic* and *lordotic* can lead to confusion. They are used to describe both the normal amount of curvature and the abnormal or excessive. *Scoliosis* is a term that refers to a lateral curvature. However, any amount of scoliosis is considered abnormal.

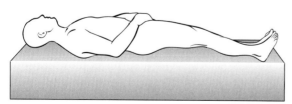

Figure 21-13.   Lying posture.

Review Questions

General Anatomy Questions

1. If a person had an excessive cervical lordosis, would you expect the cervical extensors or flexors to be tight?

2. Which position—side, front, or back—would be best to assess the condition in question 1?

3. If a person had an anterior tilt of the pelvis, would you expect the hip flexors or hip extensors to be tight?

4. To assess the condition in question 3, which position—the side, front, or back—would be best?

5. What position should the shoulders be in relation to each other?

6. Which position—side, front, or back—would be best to assess the position of the shoulders in relation to each other?

7. When using a plumb line to assess a person's posture in the lateral standing position, you should begin by lining up the plumb line with what body structure?

8. For ideal posture (when viewed laterally), where should the plumb line pass on the following structures:
   a. Knee
   b. Hip
   c. Shoulder
   d. Head

Functional Activity Questions

1. Sitting in a chair with a back and armrests, put your hands together, resting them between your thighs near your knees. Your shoulder girdles are in what position?

2. Sitting in the same position as in question 1, move from that position to one with your forearms resting on the arms of the chair. How does the position of your shoulder girdles change from their position in question 1?

3. Sitting slouched down in the chair, keep your back in contact with the back of the chair and slide your buttocks forward. What position does your head assume?

4. Carry a heavy book bag on your right shoulder. By changing posture, how do you keep the strap from sliding off your shoulder?

During Pregnancy:

5. In what direction does the woman's center of gravity shift?

6. There is a tendency for the pelvis to tilt in which direction in the sagittal plane?

7. What type of change would occur in the lumbar spine?

8. Those changes in the pelvic and lumbar positions could lead to
   a. which trunk muscle group becoming tight?
   b. which trunk muscle group becoming stretched?

9. As compensatory posture, would you expect the hip flexors or extensors to become tight?

Clinical Exercise Questions

1. Sit in front of a computer. Pretend (if necessary) that you are wearing bifocals that require you to look through the bottom of the lenses for close-up work. This can be simulated by wrapping plastic wrap on the top half of a pair of eyeglasses or sunglasses. To read the screen, what position does the head and neck assume?

2. If the position in the exercise in question 1 became a chronic posture,
   a. muscle groups on which side of the neck would become tighter?
   b. muscle groups on which side of the neck would become stretched?

3. Stand upright with equal weight on both feet and a 1- to 3-inch block under your left foot (depending on your height). Does your pelvis remain level? If not, which side of the pelvis is higher?

(continued on next page)

Review Questions—cont'd

4. If the posture in the exercise in question 3 became a permanent condition,
   a. muscle groups on which side of the trunk would become tighter?
   b. muscle groups on which side of the trunk would become stretched?

5. Continuing with the exercise in question 3:
   a. Which side of the intervertebral disk would be compressed? Distracted?
   b. Which side of the intervertebral disk would be distracted?
   c. The intervertebral foramen on which side would be opened more?
   d. The intervertebral foramen on which side would be made smaller?

6. Lie supine, hug your knees to your chest, and bring your knees and forehead together. Hug the knees close to your chest (Fig. 21-14).
   a. What trunk muscle group is being stretched?
   b. Which part of the intervertebral disk is being compressed?

7. Lie prone with your hips and knees extended. Rise up and rest on your elbows (Fig. 21-15).
   a. What trunk muscles are being stretched?
   b. Which part of the intervertebral disk is being compressed?

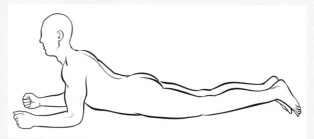

Figure 21-15.   Exercise position. Lie prone, resting on elbows.

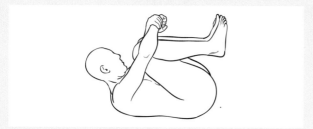

Figure 21-14.   Exercise position. Lie supine, hugging knees to chest.

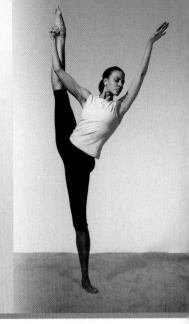

CHAPTER 22
Gait

Definitions

Analysis of Stance Phase

Analysis of Swing Phase

Additional Determinants of Gait

Age-Related Gait Patterns

Abnormal (Atypical) Gait

Muscular Weakness/Paralysis

Joint/Muscle Range-of-Motion Limitation

Neurological Involvement

Pain

Leg Length Discrepancy

Points to Remember

Review Questions

General Anatomy Questions

Functional Activity Questions

Clinical Exercise Questions

Walking is the manner or way in which you move from place to place with your feet. *Gait* is the process or components of walking. Each person has a unique style, and this style may change slightly with mood. When you are happy, your step is lighter, and there may be a "bounce" in your walk. Conversely, when you are sad or depressed, your step may be heavy. For some people, their walking pattern is so unique that they can be identified from a distance even before their face can clearly be seen. Regardless of the numerous different styles, the components of normal gait are the same.

In the most basic sense, walking requires balancing on one leg while the other leg moves forward. This requires movement not only of the legs but also of the trunk and arms. To analyze gait, you must first determine what joint motions occur. Then, based upon that information, you must decide which muscles or muscle groups are acting.

Definitions

Certain definitions must be made to describe gait. **Gait cycle,** also called **stride,** is the activity that occurs between the time one foot touches the floor and the time the same foot touches the floor again (Fig. 22-1). A **stride length** is the distance traveled during the gait cycle.

A **step** is basically one-half of a stride. It takes two steps (a right one and a left one) to complete a stride or gait cycle. These steps should be equal. A **step length** is that distance between the heel strike of one foot and the heel strike of the other foot (see Fig. 22-1). With an increased or decreased walking speed, the step length will increase or decrease, respectively. Regardless of speed, the step length of each leg should remain equal.

Walking speed, or **cadence,** is the number of steps taken per minute. It can vary greatly. Slow walking may be as slow as 70 steps per minute. However, students on

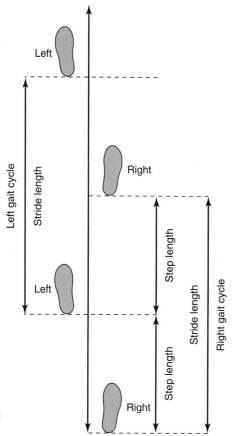

Figure 22-1.   Gait cycle terminology. A right and left step make up a gait cycle (also called *stride*).

their way to an examination have been clocked at much slower speeds. Fast walking may be as fast as 130 steps per minute, although racewalkers will walk much faster. Regardless of speed, the gait cycle is the same; all parts occur in their proper place at the proper time.

There are two phases of the gait cycle (Fig. 22-2). **Stance phase** is the activity that occurs when the foot is in contact with the ground. It begins with the heel strike of one foot and ends when that foot leaves the ground. This phase accounts for about 60% of the gait cycle. **Swing phase** occurs when the foot is not in contact with the ground. It begins as soon as the foot leaves the floor and ends when the heel of the same foot touches the floor again. The swing phase makes up about 40% of the gait cycle.

Perry (1992) identifies three tasks that need to be accomplished during these phases of the gait cycle: (1) weight acceptance, (2) single leg support, and (3) leg advancement. Figure 22-2 shows the phases of the gait cycle. **Weight acceptance** occurs at the very beginning of stance phase, when the foot touches the ground and the body weight begins to shift onto that leg. **Single leg support** occurs next, as the body weight shifts completely onto the stance leg so that the opposite leg can swing forward. The task of **leg advancement** occurs during swing phase.

The gait cycle has two periods of double support and two periods of single support (see Fig. 22-2). When both feet are in contact with the ground at the same time, this is a period of **double support.** This occurs as one leg is beginning its stance phase and the other leg is ending its stance phase. For example, the first period of double support occurs as the right leg is beginning

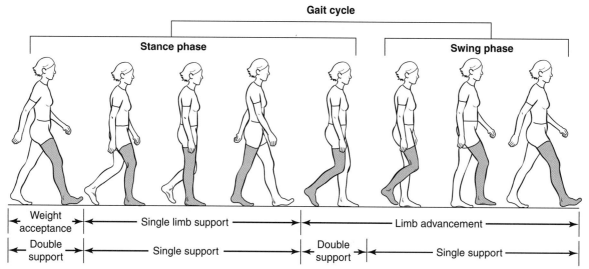

Figure 22-2.   Phases of the gait cycle.

stance phase and the left leg is ending stance phase. The second period of double support occurs as the right leg is ending its stance phase and the left leg is beginning its stance phase. Each period of double support takes up about 10 percent of the gait cycle at an average walking speed. If you increase your walking speed, you spend less time with both feet on the ground. Conversely, when you walk slowly, you spend more time in double support.

A period of **nonsupport**—that is, a time during which neither foot is in contact with the ground—does not occur during walking. However, nonsupport does occur during running. Other than speed, this may be the biggest difference between running and walking. Other activities, such as hopping, skipping, and jumping, have a period of nonsupport but lose the order of progression that walking and running have. In other words, these activities do not include all the parts of stance and swing phase that walking and running have.

The period of **single support** occurs when only one foot is in contact with the ground (see Fig. 22-2). Thus, two periods of single support occur in a gait cycle: once when the right foot is on the ground as the left foot is swinging forward, then again when the left foot bears weight and the right leg swings forward. Each single-support period takes up about 40 percent of the gait cycle.

Many sets of terms have been developed from the original, or traditional, terminology to describe the components of walking. In many cases, although the terminology may be accurate, it is often cumbersome. However, terminology developed by the Gait Laboratory at Rancho Los Amigos (RLA) Medical Center has been gaining acceptance. Perhaps the biggest difference between the two sets of terms is that the traditional terms refer to *points in time*, whereas RLA terms refer to *periods of time*. Traditional terminology accurately reflects key points within the gait cycle, whereas RLA periods accurately reflect the moving or dynamic nature of gait. It is best to be familiar with both sets of terms, because both terminologies will be seen in the literature. Table 22-1 compares traditional terminology with the RLA terms. One can see that they are similar with a few exceptions. Table 22-2, on pages 344 and 345, describes the activities of each phase and the key points to observe. The table reiterates the slight differences between the two sets of terms. However,

Table 22-1　Comparison of Gait Terminology

Traditional		Rancho Los Amigos	
Term	**Definition**	**Term**	**Definition**
Stance Phase			
Heel strike	Heel contacts the ground	Initial contact	Same
Foot flat	Plantar surface of the foot in contact with ground	Loading response	Beginning: Just after initial contact when body weight is being transferred onto leg and entire foot makes contact with the ground Ending: Opposite foot leaves the ground
Midstance	Point at which the body passes over the weight-bearing leg	Midstance	Beginning: Opposite foot leaves the ground Ending: Body is directly over the weight-bearing limb
Heel-off	Heel leaves the ground, while ball of the foot and toes remain in contact with the ground	Terminal stance	Beginning: As the heel of weight-bearing leg rises Ending: Initial contact of the opposite foot; the body has moved in front of the weight-bearing leg
Toe-off	Toes leave the ground, ending stance phase	Preswing	Beginning: Initial contact and weight shifted onto the opposite leg Ending: Just before toes of weight-bearing leg leave the ground

(Continued)

Table 22-1	Comparison of Gait Terminology—cont'd			
	Traditional		**Rancho Los Amigos**	
Term	**Definition**	**Term**	**Definition**	
Swing Phase				
Acceleration	The swing leg begins to move forward	Initial swing	Beginning: The toes leave the ground	
			Ending: The swing foot is opposite the weight-bearing foot, and the knee is in maximum flexion	
Midswing	The swing (non-weight-bearing) leg is directly under the body	Midswing	Beginning: The swing foot is opposite the weight-bearing foot	
			Ending: The swing leg has moved in front of the body and the tibia is in a vertical position	
Deceleration	The leg is slowing down in preparation for heel strike	Terminal swing	Beginning: The tibia is in a vertical position	
			Ending: Just prior to initial contact	

the key points are in the same sequence of the gait cycle, regardless of which terminology is used.

Analysis of Stance Phase

As defined earlier, *stance* is that period in which the foot is in contact with the floor. Traditionally, the stance phase has been broken down into five components: (1) heel strike, (2) foot flat, (3) midstance, (4) heel-off, and (5) toe-off (Fig. 22-3). Some sources give stance phase only four components by combining heel-off and toe-off into one and calling it *push-off*. Because significantly different activities occur during these two periods, it is best to keep them separated.

Heel strike signals the beginning of stance phase, the moment the heel comes in contact with the ground (Fig. 22-4). At this point, the ankle is in a neutral position between dorsiflexion and plantar flexion, and the knee begins to flex. This slight knee flexion provides some shock absorption as the foot hits the ground. The hip is in about 25 degrees of flexion. The trunk is erect and remains so throughout the entire gait cycle. The trunk is rotated toward the opposite (contralateral) side, the opposite arm is forward, and the same-side (ipsilateral) arm is back in shoulder hyperextension. At this point, body weight begins to shift onto the stance leg. In RLA, this is the period of *initial contact*.

The ankle dorsiflexors are active in putting the ankle in its neutral position. The quadriceps, which have been contracting concentrically, switch to contracting eccentrically to minimize the amount of knee flexion. The hip flexors have been active. However, the hip extensors are beginning to contract, keeping the hip

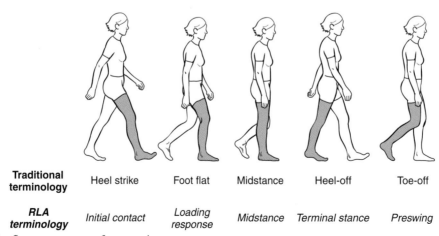

Traditional terminology	Heel strike	Foot flat	Midstance	Heel-off	Toe-off
RLA terminology	*Initial contact*	*Loading response*	*Midstance*	*Terminal stance*	*Preswing*

Figure 22-3. The five components of stance phase.

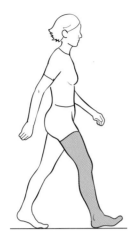

Figure 22-4.   Heel strike (*Initial Contact – RLA*).

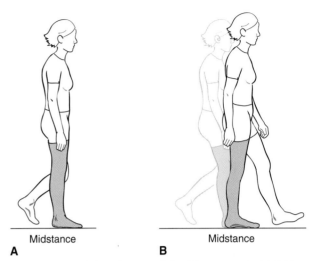

Midstance   Midstance

A   **B**

Figure 22-6.   **(A)** Midstance. **(B)** Midstance period (RLA). The lighter tone shows the beginning of the loading response, and the darker tone shows the ending of this period.

from flexing more. The erector spinae are active in keeping the trunk from flexing. The force of the foot hitting the ground transmits up through the ankle, knee, and hip to the trunk. This would cause the pelvis to rotate anteriorly, flexing the trunk somewhat, if it were not for the erector spinae counteracting this force.

Foot flat, when the entire foot is in contact with the ground, occurs shortly after heel strike (Fig. 22-5). The ankle moves into about 15 degrees of plantar flexion with the dorsiflexors contracting eccentrically to keep the foot from "slapping" down on the floor. The knee moves into about 20 degrees of flexion. The hip is moving into extension, allowing the rest of the body to begin catching up with the leg. Weight shift onto the stance leg continues. Foot flat is roughly comparable to the RLA period called *loading response,* which is that period between the end of heel strike and the end of foot flat.

The point at which the body passes over the weight-bearing foot is called **midstance** (Fig. 22-6). In this phase, the ankle moves into slight dorsiflexion. However, the dorsiflexors become inactive. The plantar flexors begin to contract, controlling the rate at which the leg moves over the ankle. The knee and hip continue to extend; both arms are in shoulder extension, essentially parallel with the body; and the trunk is in a neutral position of rotation. In RLA, *midstance* is the period between the end of foot flat and the end of midstance.

Following midstance is **heel-off,** in which the heel rises off the floor (Fig. 22-7). The ankle will dorsiflex slightly (approximately 15 degrees) and then begin to plantar flex. This is the beginning of the **push-off**

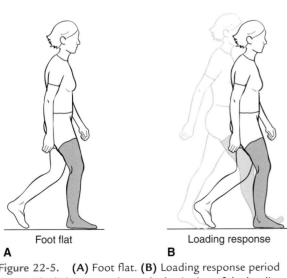

Foot flat   Loading response

A   **B**

Figure 22-5.   **(A)** Foot flat. **(B)** Loading response period (RLA). The lighter tone shows the beginning of the loading response, and the darker tone shows the ending of this period.

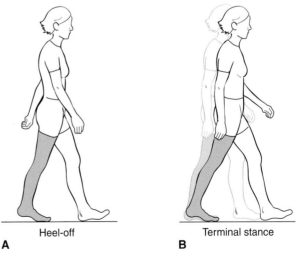

Heel-off   Terminal stance

A   **B**

Figure 22-7.   **(A)** Heel-off. **(B)** Terminal stance period (RLA). The lighter tone shows the beginning and the darker tone shows the ending of this period.

Table 22-2	Key Events of Normal Gait Cycle		
Traditional Terminology	**RLA Terminology**	**Activity**	**Key Points to Observe**
Stance Phase			
Heel strike* Foot touches the floor	*Initial contact* Foot touches the floor	• Stance phase begins • Task of weight acceptance begins • Double leg support begins • Body at lowest point in cycle	• Head and trunk are upright throughout cycle • Ankle dorsiflexed to neutral • Knee extended • Hip flexed • Leg in front of body • Pelvis rotated forward–ipsilateral side • Ipsilateral arm back, contralateral arm forward
Foot flat Entire foot in contact with ground	*Loading response* Begins with foot touching floor, continues until opposite foot leaves the floor	• Weight shift onto stance leg continues • Double leg support ends	• Ankle plantar flexes putting foot on ground • Knee partially flexed, absorbing shock • Hip moving into extension • Body catching up with leg • Ipsilateral arm swinging forward
Midstance Body passes over stance leg	*Midstance* Begins with other leg leaving floor, continues until body is over stance leg	• Body at highest point in cycle • Single leg support begins	• Ankle slightly dorsiflexed • Knee and hip continue extending • Body passes over right foot • Pelvis in neutral position • Both arms parallel with body
Heel-off Heel rises off floor, beginning of push-off	*Terminal stance* Begins with heel rising, continues until other foot touches floor	• Body moves ahead of foot • Single leg support ends	• Ankle slightly dorsiflexed, then begins plantar flexion • Knee extending, then beginning slight flexion • Hip hyperextending • Body ahead of stance leg • Pelvis rotating back—ipsilateral side • Ipsilateral arm swinging forward

Table 22-2	Key Events of Normal Gait Cycle—cont'd		
Traditional Terminology	**RLA Terminology**	**Activity**	**Key Points to Observe**
Toe-off Toe leaves the floor	*Preswing* Begins with other foot touching floor, continues until toes leave floor	• Task of leg advancement begins • Double leg support begins and ends	• Ankle plantar flexed • Knee and hip are flexing • Lateral pelvic tilt on right side • Ipsilateral arm forward
Swing Phase **Acceleration** Leg is behind body, moving forward to catch up	*Initial swing* Begins with foot leaving floor, ends with swinging foot opposite stance foot	• Swing phase (non-weight-bearing) begins • Single leg support begins on contralateral side	• Ankle beginning to dorsiflex • Knee and hip continue flexing • Leg is behind body but moving forward • Pelvis beginning to rotate forward • Ipsilateral arm swinging backward
Midswing Foot swings under and past body	*Midswing* Begins with foot opposite stance foot, ends with tibia in vertical position	• Leg shortens to clear floor • Single leg support on contralateral side continues	• Ankle dorsiflexed • Knee at maximum flexion and begins to extend • Hip at maximum flexion • Leg passing under and moving in front of body • Pelvis in neutral position • Arms parallel with body and moving in opposite directions
Deceleration Leg slowing down, preparing to touch floor	*Terminal swing* Begins with vertical tibia, ends when foot touches floor	• Leg advancement task ends • Single support ends	• Ankle continuing in dorsiflexion • Knee extended • Hip flexed • Leg ahead of body • Pelvis rotated forward–ipsilateral side • Ipsilateral arm back, contralateral arm forward

*__Bold__ indicates traditional terminology. *Italics* indicates Rancho Los Amigos (RLA) terminology.

phase, sometimes called the *propulsion phase,* because the ankle plantar flexors are actively pushing the body forward. The knee is in nearly full extension, and the hip has moved into hyperextension. The leg is now behind the body. The trunk has begun to rotate to the same side, and the arm is swinging forward into shoulder flexion. In RLA, *terminal stance* is that period between the end of midstance and the end of heel-off.

The end of the push-off portion of stance is **toe-off** (Fig. 22-8). The toes are in extreme hyperextension at the MP joints. The ankle moves into about 10 degrees of plantar flexion, and the knee and hip are flexing. The thigh is perpendicular to the ground. In RLA, *preswing* is the period just before and including when the toes leave the ground, signaling the end of stance phase and the beginning of swing phase.

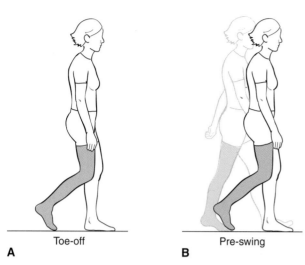

Toe-off

Pre-swing

A   **B**

Figure 22-8. **(A)** Toe-off. **(B)** Preswing period (RLA). The lighter tone shows the beginning and the darker tone shows the ending of this period.

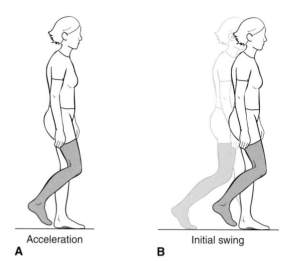

Acceleration

Initial swing

A   **B**

Figure 22-10. **(A)** Acceleration. **(B)** Initial swing period (RLA). The lighter tone shows the beginning and the darker tone shows the ending of this period.

Analysis of Swing Phase

The swing phase consists of three components: acceleration, midswing, and deceleration (Fig. 22-9). These components are all non-weight-bearing activities. The first part is **acceleration** (Fig. 22-10). The leg is behind the body and moving to catch up. The ankle is dorsiflexing, and the knee and hip continue to flex, which is moving the leg forward. In RLA, *initial swing* is that period between the end of toe-off and the end of acceleration.

At **midswing,** the ankle dorsiflexors have brought the ankle to a neutral position. The knee is at its maximum flexion (approximately 65 degrees), as is the hip (at about 25 degrees of flexion). These motions act to shorten the leg, allowing the foot to clear the ground as it swings

through (Fig. 22-11). Further hip flexion moves the leg in front of the body and puts the lower leg in a vertical position. In RLA, *midswing* is that period between the end of acceleration and the end of midswing.

In **deceleration,** the ankle dorsiflexors are active to keep the ankle in a neutral position in preparation for heel strike (Fig. 22-12). The knee is extending, and the hamstring muscles are contracting eccentrically to slow down the leg, keeping it from snapping into extension. The leg has swung as far forward as it is going to. The hip remains in flexion. In RLA, *terminal swing* is that period between the end of midswing and the end of deceleration.

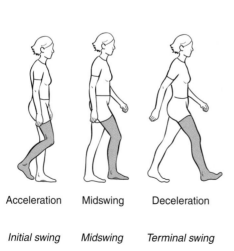

Traditional terminology	Acceleration	Midswing	Deceleration
RLA terminology	*Initial swing*	*Midswing*	*Terminal swing*

Figure 22-9.   Swing phase.

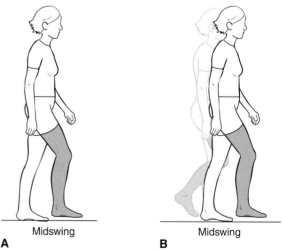

Midswing

Midswing

A   **B**

Figure 22-11. **(A)** Midswing. **(B)** Midswing period (RLA). The lighter tone shows the beginning and the darker tone shows the ending of this period.

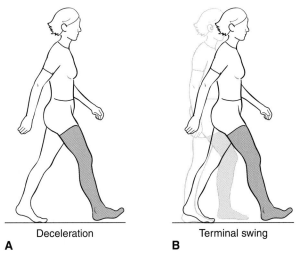

A Deceleration

B Terminal swing

Figure 22-12. **(A)** Deceleration. **(B)** Terminal swing (RLA). The lighter tone shows the beginning and the darker tone shows the ending of this period.

Additional Determinants of Gait

To this point, the description of gait has centered mostly on the lower legs. However, other events are occurring in the rest of the body that must also be considered.

If you held a piece of chalk against the blackboard and walked the board's length, you would see that the line drawn bobs up and down in wavelike fashion. This is described as the **vertical displacement** of the center of gravity (Fig. 22-13). The normal amount of this displacement is approximately 2 inches, being highest at mid-stance and lowest at heel strike *(initial contact)*. There is also an equal amount of **horizontal displacement** of the center of gravity as the body weight shifts from side to side. This displacement is greatest during the single support phase at midstance. In other words, this represents the distance the body's center of gravity must shift horizontally onto one foot so that the other foot can swing forward. This side-to-side displacement is usually about 2 inches.

When you walk, you do not place your feet one step in front of the other but slightly apart. If lines were drawn through the successive midpoints of heel contact *(initial contact)* on each foot, this distance would range from 2 to 4 inches. This is described as the **width of walking base** (Fig. 22-14).

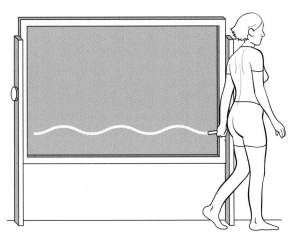

Figure 22-13. Vertical displacement of the body's center of gravity during the gait cycle.

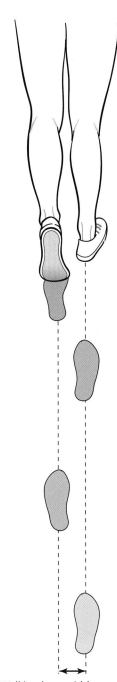

Figure 22-14. Walking base width.

If you walked across the room with your hands on your hips, you would notice that they move up and down as your pelvis on each side drops down slightly. As shown in Figure 22-15, this **lateral pelvic tilt** occurs when weight is removed from the leg at toe-off *(preswing)*. This slight drop is sometimes referred to as the *Trendelenburg sign.* The dip would be greater if it were not for the hip abductors on the opposite side (weight-bearing) and the erector spinae on the same side working together, keeping the pelvis essentially level. When the pelvis drops on the right side (the non-weight-bearing side), the left hip (the weight-bearing side) is forced into adduction. To keep the pelvis level, although it actually dips slightly, the left hip abductors contract to prevent hip adduction. At the same time, the right erector spinae muscle, which has attachment on the pelvis, contracts and "pulls up" on the side of the pelvis that wants to drop (Fig. 22-16).

In addition, step length should normally be equal in both distance and time. The arms should swing with the opposite leg. The trunk rotates forward as the leg progresses through the swing phase. Arms swinging in opposition to trunk rotation controls the amount of trunk rotation by providing counterrotation. The head should be erect, shoulders level, and trunk in extension.

When analyzing someone's gait, it is best to view the person from both the side and the front (and sometimes the back). Step length, arm swing, position of head and trunk, and the activities of the lower

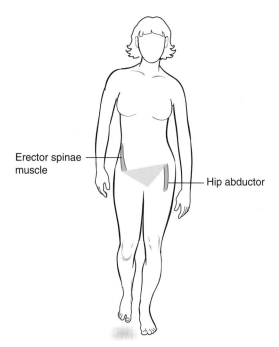

Erector spinae muscle

Hip abductor

Figure 22-16.   Muscles working to minimize lateral pelvic tilt. **(A)** Hip abductors. **(B)** Erector spinae muscles.

leg are usually best viewed from the side. Width of walking base, dip of the pelvis, and position of the shoulders and head should be viewed from the front or back.

Age-Related Gait Patterns

Not all gait patterns that don't comply with "normal" gait characteristics are the result of pathology. The walking patterns of young children and elderly adults have characteristic differences from the walking pattern of younger adults. These are considered age-related, not pathological, changes. The differences seen in young children tend to disappear as they get older. Young children tend to walk with a wider walking base, their cadence is faster, and their stride length is shorter. Initial contact with the floor is with a flat foot, as opposed to heel strike. Their knees remain mostly extended during stance phase. In other words, they tend to take more steps that are short and choppy in a faster period of time. They also have little or no reciprocal arm swing. This is easy to observe as a child walks with an adult.

Even in the absence of pathology, an elderly adult's walking pattern undergoes change. Although there is not universal agreement on the reasons for these changes, it is generally felt that security and fear of falling are major contributors. Typically, older adults

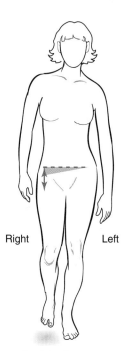

Right   Left

Figure 22-15.   Lateral pelvic tilt.

lose muscle mass, are less active, and often have poorer hearing and vision. It should be recognized that the effects of age are relative to many factors such as health, activity level, and even attitude. Some 70-year-old people may appear "older" than others who are 10 or more years their senior. Given all of these qualifiers, some general statements can be made regarding the changes in the walking pattern of elderly individuals. They tend to walk slower, spending more time in stance phase. Therefore, there are longer periods of double support. Because they take shorter steps, vertical displacement is less. They walk with a wider base, and so have greater horizontal displacement. There are fewer and slower automatic movements, which may increase the chance of stumbling or falling. In turn, this may contribute to increased toe-floor clearance.

Abnormal (Atypical) Gait

The causes of an abnormal gait are numerous. It may be temporary, such as a sprained ankle, or it may be permanent, such as following a stroke. There can be great variation, depending on the severity of the problem. If a muscle is weak, how weak is it? If joint motion is limited, how limited is it? As with all causes of abnormal motion, severity or degree of involvement will always result in a range of variations from minor ones to major ones. There are many methods of classifying abnormal gait. The following is a listing of abnormal gaits based on general cause or basis for the abnormality:

Muscular weakness/paralysis
Joint/muscle range-of-motion (ROM) limitation
Neurological involvement
Pain
Leg length discrepancy

Muscular Weakness/Paralysis

Depending on the cause or severity of the condition, muscle weakness can range from slight weakness to complete paralysis, in which there is no strength at all. Generally speaking, with muscle weakness, the body tends to compensate by shifting the center of gravity over, or toward, the part that is involved. Basically, this reduces the moment of force (torque) on the joint, lessening the muscle strength required. Obviously, the portion of the gait cycle affected will be that portion in which the muscles or joints have a major role. Traditional terminology will be used with RLA terms in italics when there is a difference in terms.

In the case of the **gluteus maximus gait,** the trunk quickly shifts posteriorly at heel strike *(initial contact).* This will shift the body's center of gravity posteriorly over the gluteus maximus, moving the line of force posterior to the hip joints (Fig. 22-17). With the foot in contact with the floor, this requires less muscle strength to maintain the hip in extension during stance phase. This shifting is sometimes referred to as a *rocking horse gait* because of the extreme backward-forward movement of the trunk.

With a **gluteus medius gait,** the individual shifts the trunk over the affected side during stance phase. In Figure 22-18, the left gluteus medius, or hip abductor, is weak, causing two things to happen: (1) the body leans over the left leg during that leg's stance phase, and (2) the right side of the pelvis drops when the right leg leaves the ground and begins swing phase. This gait is also referred to as a

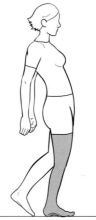

Figure 22-17. Gluteus maximus gait due to muscle weakness/paralysis on right side.

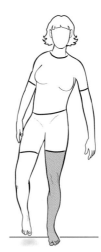

Figure 22-18. Gluteus medius gait.

Trendelenburg gait. Do not confuse it with the normal amount of dipping of the pelvis. Shifting the trunk over the affected side is an attempt to reduce the amount of strength required by the gluteus medius to stabilize the pelvis.

When there is weakness in the **quadriceps** muscle group, several different compensatory mechanisms may be used. Depending on whether only the quadriceps muscles are weak or if there are additional weaknesses in the extremity, various compensatory maneuvers may be used. With quadriceps weakness, the individual may lean the body forward over the quadriceps muscles at the early part of stance phase, as weight is being shifted onto the stance leg. Normally at this time, the line of force falls behind the knee, requiring quadriceps action to keep the knee from buckling. By leaning forward at the hip, the center of gravity is shifted forward and the line of force now falls in front of the knee. This will force the knee backward into extension. Another compensatory maneuver is using the hip extensors and ankle plantar flexors in a closed-chain action to pull the knee into extension at heel strike *(initial contact)*. This reversal of muscle action can be seen in Figure 19-22. In addition, the person may physically push on the anterior thigh during stance phase, holding the knee in extension (Fig. 22-19).

If the **hamstrings** are weak, two things may happen. During stance phase, the knee will go into excessive hyperextension, sometimes referred to as *genu recurvatum gait* (Fig. 22-20). Without the hamstrings to slow the forward swing of the lower leg during the deceleration *(terminal swing)* part of swing phase, the knee will snap into extension.

The amount of weakness of the **ankle dorsiflexors** will determine how an individual may compensate. If there is insufficient strength to move the ankle into

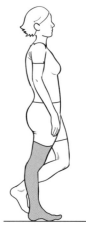

Figure 22-20.   Genu recurvatum gait.

dorsiflexion at the beginning of stance phase, the foot will land with a fairly flat foot. However, if there is no ankle dorsiflexion, the toes will strike first, which is commonly referred to as an **equinus gait** (Fig. 22-21A). Next, weak ankle dorsiflexors may not be able to support the body weight after heel strike and will thus move toward foot flat *(loading response)* as they eccentrically contract. The result is **foot slap.** With the dorsiflexors not being able to slow the descent of the foot, the foot slaps into plantar flexion as more weight is put on the leg. During swing phase, they may not be able to dorsiflex the ankle. Gravity will cause the foot to fall into plantar flexion when it is off the ground. This is called **drop foot.** As a result, the knee will need to be lifted higher for the dropped foot to clear the floor and **steppage gait** will result (Fig. 22-21B). The drum major

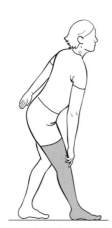

Figure 22-19.   Gait resulting from quadriceps weakness/paralysis.

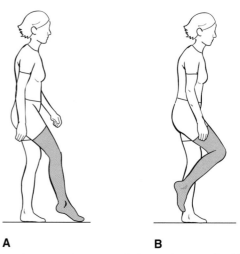

A   **B**

Figure 22-21.   Weakness, paralysis, or absence of ankle dorsiflexors results in **(A)** equinus gait at heel strike *(initial contact—RLA),* and **(B)** steppage gait during swing phase.

in a marching band will utilize the elements of this gait when performing.

When the **triceps surae group** (the gastrocnemius and soleus) is weak, there is no heel rise at push-off *(terminal stance)*, resulting in a shortened step length on the unaffected side. This is sometimes referred to as a *sore foot limp*. Although this gait is noticeable on level ground, it becomes most pronounced when walking up an incline.

A **waddling gait** is commonly seen with muscular and other types of dystrophies, because there is diffuse weakness of many muscle groups. The person stands with the shoulders behind the hips, much like a person with paraplegia would balance resting on the iliofemoral ligament of the hips (Fig. 22-22). There is an increased lumbar lordosis, pelvic instability, and Trendelenburg gait. Little or no reciprocal pelvis and trunk rotation occur. To swing the leg forward, the entire side of the body must swing forward. For example, normally, as the right leg swings forward, the right arm swings backward. In this case, the right arm and leg swing forward together. Add this to the excessive trunk lean of Trendelenburg gait bilaterally, and one can see the waddling nature of the gait. A steppage gait is often present.

Joint/Muscle Range-of-Motion Limitation

In this grouping, the joint is unable to go through its normal range of motion because there is either bony fusion or soft tissue limitation. This limitation can be the result of contractures of muscle, capsule, or skin.

When a person has a **hip flexion contracture,** the involved hip is unable to go into hip extension and

hyperextension during the midstance and push-off phases *(terminal stance)*. To compensate, the person will commonly assume the salutation or greeting position in which the hip is flexed and the person's trunk leans forward as if bowing (Fig. 22-23). The involved leg may also simultaneously flex the knee when it normally would be extended.

With a **fused hip,** increased motion of the lumbar spine and pelvis can greatly compensate for hip motion. A decreased lordosis and posterior pelvic tilt will allow the leg to swing forward (Fig. 22-24A), whereas an increased lordosis and anterior pelvic tilt will swing the leg posteriorly (Fig. 22-24B). This is sometimes referred to as a *bell-clapper gait*. A bell swings

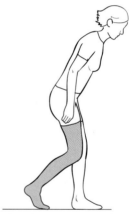

Figure 22-23. Salutation greeting resulting from hip flexion contracture.

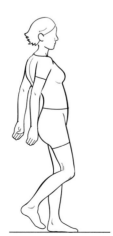

Figure 22-22. Waddling gait.

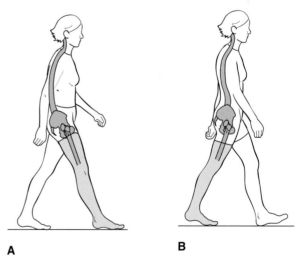

A   **B**

Figure 22-24. Bell-clapper gait resulting from a fused hip. In **(A)** the leg swings forward by flattening the lumbar lordosis and tilting the pelvis posteriorly. In **(B)** the leg swings backward by increasing the lumbar lordosis and tilting the pelvis anteriorly.

back and forth, causing the clapper inside to also move back and forth.

A **knee flexion contracture** will result in excessive dorsiflexion during midstance and an early heel rise during push-off *(terminal stance)*. There is also a shortened step length of the unaffected side. If a **knee fusion** is present, the lower leg will be at a fixed length. That length will depend on the position of the joint. If the knee is in extension, the leg will be unable to shorten during swing phase. To compensate, the person must (1) rise up on the toes of the uninvolved leg in a **vaulting gait** (Fig. 22-25), (2) hike the hip of the involved side, (3) swing the leg out to the side, or (4) do some variation of the three methods. With a **circumducted gait,** the leg begins near the midline at push-off *(terminal stance),* swings out to the side during swing phase, then returns to the midline for heel strike (Fig. 22-26). It is called an **abducted gait** if the leg remains in an abducted position throughout the gait cycle.

Depending on the severity of a **triceps surae contracture,** several things may result. The knee can be forced into excessive extension during midstance, because there is insufficient length of the plantar flexors to allow dorsiflexion. If the gastrocnemius does not have enough extensibility to be stretched over both the ankle and knee, something must give. There will be either limited ankle dorsiflexion or the knee will be pulled into extreme extension. Remember that the gastrocnemius is a two-joint muscle that plantar flexes the ankle and flexes the knee. In weight-bearing, body weight may force a certain amount of dorsiflexion, thus forcing a tight gastrocnemius to pull the knee into extension. In addition, an early heel rise will occur during push-off *(terminal stance),* the knee will be lifted higher during swing phase,

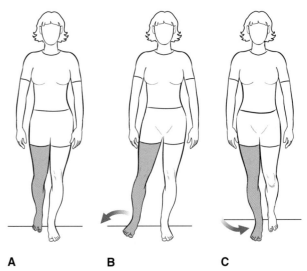

Figure 22-26.   Circumducted gait. **(A)** The leg is in the normal position at the end of stance phase. The leg then swings out and around during swing phase **(B)**, returning to the normal position for the beginning of stance phase **(C)**.

and the toes will land first during heel strike *(initial contact).* The latter is called a *steppage gait.*

An **ankle fusion** is commonly called a *triple arthrodesis* because of fusion of the subtalar joint and the two articulations making up the transtarsal joint. This will result in loss of ankle pronation and supination. Plantar flexion and dorsiflexion will remain but will be limited. Usually, there is a shortened stride length. The person will have more difficulty walking on uneven ground, because the ability to pronate and supinate the foot has been lost.

Neurological Involvement

The amount of gait disturbance depends on the amount and severity of neurological involvement. For example, spasticity of the hip flexors affects moving the leg forward in midstance and terminal stance. Hamstring spasticity can keep the knee in a flexed position, which can interfere with moving the leg forward during stance phase and limit the effectiveness of straightening the leg at the end of the swing. Spasticity of the triceps surae can keep the ankle plantar flexed, creating problems during both stance and swing phase. Spasticity tends to put the foot in a varus position, and flaccidity tends to put the foot in a valgus position.

A **hemiplegic gait** will vary depending on the severity of neurological involvement and the presence and amount of spasticity. Generally speaking, with spasticity there is an extension synergy in the involved lower extremity. The hip goes into extension, adduction, and

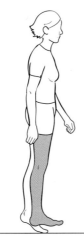

Figure 22-25.   Vaulting gait resulting from a right knee fused in extension. The person must rise up on her toes on the left side to allow the involved right leg to swing through.

medial rotation. The knee is in extension, though often unstable. The ankle demonstrates a drop foot with ankle plantar flexion and inversion (equinovarus), which is present during both stance phase and swing phase. The involved upper extremity may typically be in a flexion synergy (Fig. 22-27). Usually, there will be no reciprocal arm swing. Step length tends to be lengthened on the involved side and shortened on the uninvolved side.

Cerebellar involvement often results in an **ataxic gait.** Lack of coordination leads to jerky uneven movements. Balance tends to be poor, and the person walks with a wide base of support (abducted gait). The person usually has difficulty walking in a straight line and tends to stagger. Reciprocal arm motion also appears to be jerky and uneven. All movements appear exaggerated.

A **parkinsonian gait,** in which one has tremors, demonstrates diminished movement. The posture of the lower extremities and trunk tends to be flexed. The elbows are partially flexed, and there is little or no reciprocal arm swing. Stride length is greatly diminished, and the forward heel does not swing beyond the rear foot. The person walks with a shuffling gait, with the feet flat and weight mostly forward on the toes (Fig. 22-28). The person has difficulty initiating movements. This shuffling gait tends to start slowly and increase in speed, and the person often has difficulty in stopping. It gives the appearance that the person's feet are trying to catch up to the forward-leaning trunk. This is called a **festinating gait.**

Spasticity in the hip adductors results in a **scissors gait.** This gait is most evident during the swing phase, when the unsupported leg swings against or across the stance leg. Needless to say, the walking base is narrowed. The trunk may lean over the stance leg as the swing phase leg attempts to swing past it (Fig. 22-29).

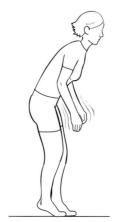

Figure 22-28. Parkinsonian gait.

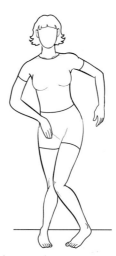

Figure 22-29. Scissors gait.

A **crouch gait** describes the bilateral lower extremity involvement seen in the spastic diplegia associated with cerebral palsy. There is often great variation in the gait from what is considered "typical." There is excessive flexion, adduction, and medial rotation at the hips and flexion at the knees. The ankles are plantar flexed. The pelvis maintains an anterior pelvic tilt, and there is an increased lumbar lordosis. To compensate, the reciprocal arm swing and horizontal displacement are exaggerated.

Pain

When a person has pain in any of the lower extremity's joints, the tendency is to shorten the stance phase. In other words, if it hurts to stand on it, do not stand on it. A shortened, often abducted, stance phase on the involved side results in a rapid and shortened step length on the uninvolved side. Compensation in the reciprocal arm swing also is evident. Reciprocal arm swinging shortens as the step length is shortened, exaggerated, and

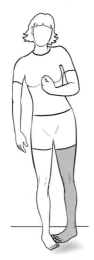

Figure 22-27. Hemiplegic gait.

often abducted. This gait is often referred to as **antalgic gait.** If the pain is caused by a hip problem, the person will lean over that hip during weight-bearing. This will decrease the torque placed on the joint and the amount of pressure placed on the femoral head. Magee (1987) stated that the amount of pressure will be decreased from more than twice the body weight to approximately that of the person's body weight.

Leg Length Discrepancy

We all have legs of unequal length. Often the discrepancy is as much as approximately one- quarter inch between the right and left legs. Because both feet need to be in contact with the ground while in standing posture, how does the body adjust to the difference in leg length? Clinically, these smaller discrepancies are often corrected by inserting heel lifts of various thicknesses into the shoe. Without any other correction, dropping the pelvis on the shorter leg side (affected side) can compensate for a minimal leg length discrepancy. Although this may not look abnormal, it does place added stress on the lower back, hips, and knees. In addition to increased lateral pelvic tilt, the person may compensate by leaning over the shorter leg. This would result in greater lateral leaning of the upper body. These techniques can accommodate leg length discrepancies of up to approximately 3 inches.

When there is **moderate discrepancy,** approximately between 3 and 5 inches (depending on one's height), dropping the pelvis on the affected side will no longer be effective. The person needs to either shorten the uninvolved leg or make the involved leg functionally longer. A longer leg is needed, so the person usually walks on the ball of the foot on the involved (shorter) side. This is called an **equinus gait.** The most obvious change in the gait pattern would be loss of heel strike *(initial contact)* and foot flat *(loading response).*

A person can compensate for severe leg length discrepancy (e.g., any discrepancy more than 5 inches, again, depending on one's height) by using a variety of techniques. In addition to dropping the pelvis and walking in an equinus gait, the person could flex the knee on the uninvolved side. In this case, stance phase would tend to begin with flat foot rather than with the heel strike. The knee would remain in a flexed position for the entire gait cycle. To gain an appreciation for how this may feel or look, walk down the street with one leg in the street and the other on the sidewalk.

When a person has a leg length discrepancy beyond what can be accommodated with heel lifts, it is usually the result of some sort of pathology. For example, a person with a fractured femur that healed in an overriding position would have a shorter leg. If a child who is still growing sustains damage to the epiphyseal plate of one or more long bones of the leg, it could result in arrested growth in that leg. Premature growth stoppage would result in a significant leg length discrepancy if the child had not nearly finished growing. These pathologies are not common, but they can result in significant changes in gait.

Points to Remember

- Stance and swing are the two phases of the gait cycle.
- Using traditional terminology, there are five periods in stance phase: heel strike, foot flat, midstance, heel-off, and toe-off.
- In swing phase, there is acceleration, midswing, and deceleration.
- Using RLA terminology, stance phase also has five periods: initial contact, loading response, midstance, terminal stance, and preswing.
- RLA terms for the swing phase periods are *initial swing, midswing,* and *terminal swing.*
- Additional determinants of gait are vertical and horizontal displacement, walking base width, lateral pelvic tilt, equal step length, and opposite and equal arm swing.

Review Questions

General Anatomy Questions

1. Compare and contrast walking and running.
2. What are the main differences between the traditional terminology and terminology developed by Rancho Los Amigos?
3. What is the phase used for the period that occurs between heel strike and toe-off?
4. What is the time period called when both feet are in contact with the ground? What part of stance phase is each foot in during this period?
5. At what period of stance phase is a person's overall vertical height the greatest?
6. During which phase is the person's foot *not* in contact with the ground?
7. What will happen to the step length and cadence when a person increases his or her walking speed?
8. If unsteady, how does a person tend to adjust his or her walking?
9. If "foot drop" is present, which parts of the swing and stance phases of the person's gait will be altered?
10. If a person has an unrepaired ruptured Achilles tendon, which phase of the gait will be altered?

Functional Activity Questions

Identify the parts of gait that will change during the following:

1. Walking across the ice
2. Walking on a beam that is 4 inches wide
3. Walking down a railroad track with one foot on each side of the track (no train is coming!)
4. Walking in soft, dry sand (similar to running hard uphill)
5. Walking by taking long steps
6. Walking with a long leg brace (also known as a knee-ankle-foot orthosis, or KAFO)
7. The vertical displacement that occurs during walking demonstrates what type of motion?

Clinical Exercise Questions

1. Stand upright as though you had bilateral knee flexion contractures of approximately 45 degrees. Identify how positions of other joints must change to maintain an upright posture.
   a. Ankle
   b. Hip
   c. Pelvis
   d. Lumbar spine

2. Identify the type of muscle contraction and muscle group involved during the following phases of walking:
   a. At the knee going into heel strike
      Type of contraction _____
      Muscle group involved _____
   b. At the ankle during foot flat
      Type of contraction _____
      Muscle group involved _____
   c. At the hip as the leg is moving into midstance
      Type of contraction _____
      Muscle group involved _____
   d. At the hip (in the frontal plane) during toe-off
      Type of contraction _____
      Muscle group involved _____
   e. At the knee during deceleration
      Type of contraction _____
      Muscle group involved _____

3. List the functional changes in gait that a person may use to compensate for a leg length discrepancy. Start with a minimal discrepancy and end with a severe discrepancy.

Bibliography

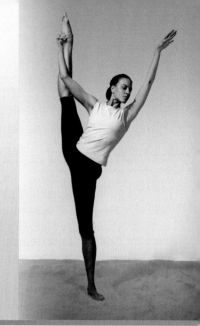

Anderson, MK: Fundamentals of Sports Injury Management. Lippincott Williams & Wilkins, Philadelphia, 2002.

Anderson, MK and Hall, SJ: Fundamentals of Sports Injury Management, ed 2. Lippincott Williams & Wilkins, Philadelphia, 1997.

Anderson, MK, Hall, SJ, and Martin, M: Sports Injury Management, ed 2. Lippincott Williams & Wilkins, Philadelphia, 2002.

Basmajian, J and Blonecker, CE: Grant's Method of Anatomy. Williams & Wilkins, Baltimore, 1989.

Basmajian, J and DeLuca, C: Muscles Alive: Their Functions Revealed by Electromyography, ed 5. Williams & Wilkins, Baltimore, 1985.

Beachey, W: Respiratory Care Anatomy and Physiology: Foundations for Clinical Practice. Mosby, St. Louis, MO, 1998.

Bertoti, DB: Functional Neurorehabilitation Through the Life Span. FA Davis, Philadelphia, 2004.

Brunnstrom, S: Clinical Kinesiology, ed 3. FA Davis, Philadelphia, 1972.

Burt, J and White, G: Lymphedema. Hunter House, Berkeley, 2005.

Cailliet, R: Hand Pain and Impairment, ed 3. FA Davis, Philadelphia, 1982.

Cailliet, R: Hand Pain and Impairment, ed 4. FA Davis, Philadelphia, 1994.

Cailliet, R: Knee Pain and Disability, ed 3. FA Davis, Philadelphia, 1992.

Cailliet, R: Low Back Pain Syndrome, ed 4. FA Davis, Philadelphia, 1988.

Cailliet, R: Neck and Arm Pain, ed 3. FA Davis, Philadelphia, 1991.

Cailliet, R: Shoulder Pain, ed 3. FA Davis, Philadelphia, 1991.

Cailliet, R: Soft Tissue Pain and Disability, ed 3. FA Davis, Philadelphia, 1996.

Calais-Germain, B: Anatomy of Movement. Eastland Press, Seattle, 1993.

Carlin, E: Human Anatomy and Biomechanics: Tapes 1–10 [audio tape]. Audio-Learning, Norristown, PA, 1975.

Cooper, J and Glassow, R: Kinesiology, ed 3. CV Mosby, St. Louis, MO, 1972.

Curtis, BA: Neurosciences: The Basics. Lea & Febiger, Malvern, PA, 1990.

Cyriax, J and Cyriax, P: Illustrated Manual of Orthopaedic Medicine. Butterworth-Heinemann, London, 1983.

Daniels, L and Worthingham, C: Muscle Testing: Techniques of Manual Examination, ed 5. WB Saunders, Philadelphia, 1986.

DesJardins, T: Cardiopulmonary Anatomy and Physiology, ed 4. Thomson Delmar Learning, Clifton Park, NY, 2002.

Donatelli, RA: The Biomechanics of the Foot and Ankle, ed 2. FA Davis, Philadelphia, 1996.

Dufort, A: Ballet Steps: Practice for Performance. Hodder Arnold, London, 1993.

Ellis, H: Clinical Anatomy: A Revision and Applied Anatomy for Clinical Students, ed 10. Blackwell, Malden, MA, 2002.

Evjenth, O and Hamberg, J: Muscle Stretching in Manual Therapy: A Clinical Manual, vol. 1: The Extremities. Alfta Rehab, Alfta, Sweden, 1984.

Gilman, S and Newman, SW: Essentials of Clinical Neuroanatomy and Neurophysiology, ed 10. FA Davis, Philadelphia, 2003.

Goldberg, S: Clinical Anatomy Made Ridiculously Simple. MedMaster, Miami, 1990.

Goodman, CC and Fuller, KS: Pathology: Implications for the Physical Therapist, ed 3. Saunders-Elsevier, St. Louis, MO, 2009.

Goss, CM (ed): Gray's Anatomy of the Human Body, American, ed 29. Lea & Febiger, Philadelphia, 1973.

Gould, J and Davies, G (eds): Orthopaedic and Sports Physical Therapy, ed 2. CV Mosby, St. Louis, MO, 1985.

Hall, SJ: Basic Biomechanics, ed 3. McGraw-Hill, Boston, 1999.

Hamill, J and Knutzen, KM: Biomechanical Basis of Human Movement, ed 2. Lippincott Williams & Wilkins, Philadelphia, 2003.

Hay, J: Biomechanics of Sports Techniques, ed 1. Prentice-Hall, Englewood Cliffs, NJ, 1973.

Hinson, M: Kinesiology, ed 2. WC Brown, Dubuque, Iowa, 1981.

Hole, Jr., JW: Human Anatomy and Physiology, ed 5. WC Brown, Dubuque, IA, 1990.

Hoppenfeld, S: Physical Examination of the Spine and Extremities. Appleton-Century-Crofts, NY, 1976.

Jacob, S and Francone, C: Elements of Anatomy and Physiology, ed 3. WB Saunders, Philadelphia, 1989.

Jenkins, DB: Hollinshead's Functional Anatomy of the Limbs and Back, ed 7. WB Saunders, Philadelphia, 1998.

Jenkins, DB: Hollinshead's Functional Anatomy of the Limbs and Back, ed 8. WB Saunders, Philadelphia, 2002.

Jones, K and Barker, K: Human Movement Explained. Butterworth–Heinemann, Oxford, 1996.

Kapandji, I: Physiology of the Joints: Upper Limbs, vol. 1, ed 2. Livingstone, Edinburgh, 1970.

Kendall, FP and McCreary, EK: Muscles: Testing and Function, ed 3. Williams & Wilkins, Baltimore, 1983.

Kessler, R and Hertling, D: Management of Common Musculoskeletal Disorders: Physical Therapy Principles and Methods. Harper & Row, Philadelphia, 1983.

King, B and Showers, M: Human Anatomy and Physiology, ed 6. WB Saunders, Philadelphia, 1969.

Kingston, B: Understanding Joints: A Practical Guide to Their Structure and Function. Stanley Thornes Ltd, Cheltenham, UK, 2000.

Kisner, C and Colby, LA: Therapeutic Exercise: Foundations and Techniques, ed 4. FA Davis, Philadelphia, 2002.

Lamport, NK, Coffey, MS, and Hersch, GI: Activity Analysis and Application, ed 4. Slack, Thorofare, NJ, 2001.

Landau, BR: Essential Human Anatomy and Physiology, ed 2. Scott, Foresman, Glenview, IL, 1980.

Leeson, C and Leeson, T: Human Structure: A Companion to Anatomical Studies. WB Saunders, Philadelphia, 1972.

Lehmkuhl, LD and Smith, LK: Brunnestrom's Clinical Kinesiology, ed 4. FA Davis, Philadelphia, 1983.

Lesh, SG: Clinical Orthopedics for the Physical Therapist Assistant, ed 1. FA Davis, Philadelphia, 2000.

Levangie, PK and Norkin, CC: Joint Structure and Function, ed 3. FA Davis, Philadelphia, 2001.

Levangie, PK and Norkin, CC: Joint Structure and Function, ed 4. FA Davis, Philadelphia, 2005.

Low, J and Reed A: Basic Biomechanics Explained. Butterworth–Heinemann, Oxford, 1996.

MacConaill, M and Basmajian, J: Muscles and Movements: A Basis for Human Kinesiology. Williams & Wilkins, Baltimore, 1969.

MacLeod, D, Jacobs, P, and Larson, N: The Ergonomics Manual. The Saunders Group, Minneapolis, MN, 1990.

Magee, D: Orthopedic Physical Assessment. WB Saunders, Philadelphia, 1987.

Magee, KR and Saper, JR: Clinical and Basic Neurology for Health Professionals. Year Book Medical, Chicago, 1981.

Manter, JT and Gatz, AJ: Essentials of Clinical Neuroanatomy and Neurophysiology, ed 8. FA Davis, Philadelphia, 1993.

Marieb, EN and Mitchell, SJ: Human Anatomy and Physiology Laboratory Manual, ed 9. Pearson Benjamin Cummings, San Francisco, 2008.

Martini, FH: Fundamentals of Anatomy and Physiology, ed 7. Pearson Benjamin Cummings, San Francisco, 2006.

McGinnis, PM: Biomechanics of Sport and Exercise. Human Kinetics, Champaign, IL, 1999.

McKinnis, LN: Fundamentals of Musculoskeletal Imaging, ed 2. FA Davis, Philadelphia, 2005.

McMillan, B: The Illustrated Atlas of the Human Body, Weldon Owen Pty Ltd, Sydney, 2008.

Melloni, J, et al: Melloni's Illustrated Review of Human Anatomy. JB Lippincott, Philadelphia, 1988.

Miller, B and Keane, C: Encyclopedia and Dictionary of Medicine, Nursing, and Allied Health, ed 4. WB Saunders, Philadelphia, 1989.

Minor, MA and Lippert, LS: Kinesiology Laboratory Manual for Physical Therapist Assistants. FA Davis, Philadelphia, 1998.

Minor, M and Minor, S: Patient Evaluation Methods for the Health Professional. Reston Publishing, Reston, VA, 1985.

Moore, K: Clinically Oriented Anatomy, ed 2. Williams & Wilkins, Baltimore, 1985.

Moore, K: Clinically Oriented Anatomy, ed 3. Williams & Wilkins, Baltimore, 1992.

Moore, K: Clinically Oriented Anatomy, ed 4. Williams & Wilkins, Baltimore, 2004.

Moore, K and Agur, A: Essential Clinical Anatomy, ed 2. Lippincott Williams & Wilkins, Philadelphia, 2002.

Netter, FH: Ciba Collection of Medical Illustrations: Musculoskeletal System: Part I, Anatomy, Physiology, and Metabolic Diseases, vol. 8, ed 1. Ciba-Geigy, Summit, NJ, 1987.

Netter, FH: Ciba Collection of Medical Illustrations: Nervous System, Part I, Anatomy and Physiology, ed 1. Ciba Pharmaceutical, West Caldwell, NJ, 1983.

Neumann, DA: Kinesiology of the Musculoskeletal System: Foundations for Physical Rehabilitation, ed 1. Mosby, St. Louis, MO, 2002.

Nolan, MF: Clinical Applications of Human Anatomy: A Laboratory Guide, ed l. Slack, Thorofare, 2003.

Nordin, M and Frankel, VH: Basic Biomechanics of the Musculoskeletal System, ed 3. Lippincott Williams & Wilkins, Baltimore, 2001.

Norkin, C and Levangie, P: Joint Structure and Function: A Comprehensive Analysis. FA Davis, Philadelphia, 1983.

Norkin, C and Levangie, P: Joint Structure and Function: A Comprehensive Analysis, ed 2. FA Davis, Philadelphia, 1992.

Norkin, C and White, D: Measurement of Joint Motion: A Guide of Goniometry. FA Davis, Philadelphia, 1985.

Oatis, CA: Kinesiology: The Mechanics and Pathomechanics of Human Movement. Lippincott Williams & Wilkins, Philadelphia, 2004.

Oliver, J: Back Care: An Illustrated Guide. Butterworth-Heinemann, Oxford, 1994.

Olson, TR: ADAM: Student Atlas of Anatomy. Williams & Wilkins, Baltimore, 1996.

Palastanga, N, Field, D, and Soames, R: Anatomy and Human Movement: Structure and Function, ed 2. Butterworth-Heinemann, Oxford, 1994.

Palmer, M and Epler, M: Clinical Assessment Procedures in Physical Therapy. JB Lippincott, Philadelphia, 1990.

Palmer, M and Epler, M: Clinical Assessment Procedures in Physical Therapy, ed 2. JB Lippincott, Philadelphia, 1998.

Paris, SV and Patla, C: E-1 Course Notes: Introduction to Extremity Dysfunction and Manipulation. Institute Press, Atlanta, 1986.

Pedretti, LW: Occupational Therapy: Practice Skills for Physical Dysfunction, ed 4. CV Mosby, St. Louis, MO, 1996.

Pedretti, LW and Early, MB: Occupational Therapy: Practice Skills for Physical Dysfunction, ed 5. CV Mosby, St. Louis, MO, 2001.

Perry J: Gait Analysis: Normal and Pathological Function. Slack, Thorofare, NJ, 1992.

Perry, JF, Rohe, DA, and Garcia, AO: The Kinesiology Workbook, ed 2. FA Davis, Philadelphia, 1996.

Pratt, NE: Clinical Musculoskeletal Anatomy. JB Lippincott, Philadelphia, 1991.

Rasch, P: Kinesiology and Applied Anatomy, ed 7. Lea & Febiger, Philadelphia, 1989.

Richardson, JK and Iglarsh, ZA: Clinical Orthopaedic Physical Therapy. WB Saunders, 1994.

Rolak, LA: Neurology Secrets, ed 4. Elsevier Mosby, St. Louis, MO, 2005.

Romanes, G (ed): Cunningham's Textbook of Anatomy, ed 10. Oxford University Press, New York, 1964.

Rothstein, JM, Roy, SH, and Wolf, SL: The Rehabilitation Specialist's Handbook. FA Davis, Philadelphia, 1991.

Rothstein, JM, Roy, SH, and Wolf, SL: The Rehabilitation Specialist's Handbook, ed 2. FA Davis, Philadelphia, 1998.

Rothstein, JM, Roy, SH, and Wolf, SL: The Rehabilitation Specialist's Handbook, ed 3. FA Davis, Philadelphia, 2005.

Roy, S and Irvin, R: Sports Medicine: Prevention, Evaluation, Management, and Rehabilitation. Prentice-Hall, Englewood Cliffs, NJ, 1983.

Rybski, M: Kinesiology for Occupational Therapy. Slack, Thorofare, NJ, 2004.

Scanlon, VC and Sanders, T: Essentials of Anatomy and Physiology, ed 3. FA Davis, Philadelphia, 1999.

Scanlon, VC and Sanders, T: Essentials of Anatomy and Physiology, ed 4. FA Davis, Philadelphia, 2003.

Shumway-Cook, A and Woollacott, M: Motor Control: Theory and Practical Applications. Williams & Wilkins, Baltimore, 1995.

Sieg, K and Adams, S: Illustrated Essentials of Musculoskeletal Anatomy, ed 2. Megabooks, Gainesville, FL, 1985.

Smith, LK, Weiss, EL, and Lehmkuhl, LD: Brunnstrom's Clinical Kinesiology, ed 5. FA Davis, Philadelphia, 1996.

Soderberg, G: Kinesiology: Application of Pathological Motion. Williams & Wilkins, Baltimore, 1986.

Somers, MF: Spinal Cord Injury—Functional Rehabilitation. Appleton & Lange, Norwalk, CT, 1992.

Stanley, BG and Tribuzi, SM: Concepts in Hand Rehabilitation. FA Davis, Philadelphia, 1992.

Starkey, C and Ryan, J: Evaluation of Orthopedic and Athletic Injuries, ed 2. FA Davis, Philadelphia, 2002.

Steindler, A: Kinesiology of the Human Body: Under Normal and Pathological Conditions. Charles C. Thomas, Springfield, IL, 1955.

Thibodeau, G: Anatomy and Physiology. Times Mirror/Mosby College Publishing, St. Louis, MO, 1986.

Tomberlin, JP and Saunders, HD: Evaluation, Treatment and Prevention of Musculoskeletal Disorders, vol 2: Extremities, ed 3. The Saunders Group, Minneapolis, 1994.

Tortora, G: Principles of Human Anatomy, ed 5. Canfield Press, San Francisco, 1990.

Tortora, G and Anagnostakos, N: Principles of Anatomy and Physiology, ed 3. Harper & Row, New York, 1981.

Tovin, BJ and Greenfield, BH: Evaluation and Treatment of the Shoulder: An Integration of the Guide to Physical Therapist Practice. FA Davis, Philadelphia, 2001.

Tyldesley, B and Grieve, JI: Muscles, Nerves and Movement: Kinesiology in Daily Living. Blackwell Scientific, Oxford, 1989.

Venes, D: Taber's Cyclopedic Medical Dictionary, ed 20. FA Davis, Philadelphia, 2005.

Vidic, B and Suarez, F: Photographic Atlas of the Human Body. CV Mosby, St. Louis, MO, 1984.

Warwick, R and Williams, P (eds): Gray's Anatomy, British ed 35. WB Saunders, Philadelphia, 1973.

Wells, K and Luttgens, K: Kinesiology: Scientific Basis of Human Motion, ed 7. WB Saunders, Philadelphia, 1982.

Whittle, MW: Gait Analysis: An Introduction, ed 4. Butterworth-Heinemann, Oxford, 1996.

Williams, M and Lissner, H: Biomechanics of Human Motion. WB Saunders, Philadelphia, 1962.

Yokochi, C: Photographic Anatomy of the Human Body. University Park Press, Baltimore, 1971.

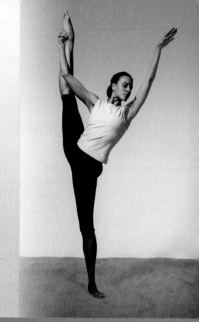

Answers to Review Questions

Chapter 1 Basic Information

1. a. Anterior
   b. Posterior
   c. Inferior
   d. Proximal
   e. Lateral
2. The football is demonstrating curvilinear motion, while the kicker's leg is demonstrating angular motion.
3. Neck hyperextension
4. Shoulder medial rotation
5. Trunk lateral bending
6. Hip lateral rotation
7. Anatomical position and fundamental position are the same except for the forearms, which are supinated in anatomical position and in neutral position (between supination and pronation) in the fundamental position.
8. Dorsal surface of dog, posterior surface of person
9. Angular motion is being used by upper extremity joints—shoulders, elbows, wrists—to propel the wheelchair. Linear motion occurs as the person moves across the room in the wheelchair.
10. Supine
11. Ipsilateral
12. Left hip flexion (slight), adduction, lateral rotation
13. Left knee extension
14. Right forearm supination
15. Neck extension, rotation to the left

Chapter 2 Skeletal System

1. The axial skeleton contains no long or short bones, whereas the appendicular skeleton contains no irregular bones. The bones of the axial skeleton are particularly important in providing support and protection; the appendicular skeleton provides the framework for movement.
2. Compact bone is found in the diaphysis of long bones, and cancellous bone is found in the metaphysis and epiphysis. In other types of bone, cancellous bone is found sandwiched between layers of compact bone.
3. Compact bone is heavier than cancellous bone because it is less porous.
4. An individual's height growth occurs mainly in long bones. The growth occurs at the epiphysis of long bones.
5. Sesamoid bones protect tendons from excess wear. The patella has the additional function of increasing the angle of pull of the quadriceps muscle.
6. a. Foramen, fossa, groove, meatus, sinus
   b. Condyle, eminence, facet, head
   c. Crest, epicondyle, line, spine, trochanter, tuberosity, tubercle
7. Bicipital groove: ditchlike depression
8. Humeral head: rounded articular projection that fits into a joint
9. Acetabulum: deep depression
10. Endosteum
11. Diaphysis
12. Pressure epiphysis
13. Appendicular skeleton
14. Appendicular skeleton
15. Axial skeleton

Chapter 3 Articular System

1. A joint that allows very little or no motion is referred to as a *fibrous joint*. The three types of fibrous joints are synarthrosis, syndesmosis, and gomphosis.

2. A joint that allows a great deal of motion is called a *synovial joint* or *diarthrosis*.

3. Diarthrodial joints can be described by
   a. the number of axes.
   b. the shape of the joint.
   c. the joint motion involved.

4. Tendon

5. Bursa

6. Hyaline cartilage is located on the bone ends of synovial joints and provides a smooth articulating surface. Fibrocartilage is thicker and is located between bones. Fibrocartilage provides shock absorption and spacing. Examples of fibrocartilage are the menisci of the knee and the disks of the vertebrae.

7. The joint motion involved is elbow flexion; it occurs in the sagittal plane around the frontal axis.

8. The joint involved is forearm pronation; it occurs in the transverse plane around the vertical axis.

9. The joint motion involved is finger (MP) adduction; it occurs in the frontal plane around the sagittal axis.

10. Shoulder = 3, elbow = 1, radioulnar = 1, wrist = 2, MCP = 2, PIP = 1, DIP = 1

11. Bones in the skull

12. Shoulder joint; yes; hip joint

13. CMC joint of thumb

14. Amphiarthrosis and cartilaginous

15. Joint capsule

Chapter 4 Arthrokinematics

1. a. Osteokinematic
   b. Arthrokinematic

2. Soft tissue approximation

3. a. Humerus is moving on scapula.
   b. Proximal end of humerus is convex.
   c. Glenoid fossa of scapula is concave.
   d. Convex surface is moving on a fixed concave surface.
   e. Opposite direction

4. a. Compression or approximation
   b. Shear
   c. Traction or distraction
   d. Torsional
   e. Traction or distraction

5. Close-packed position of TMJ is when teeth are clenched.

6. a. Convex
   b. Concave
   c. Concave
   d. Convex
   e. Sellar

7. Roll

8. Glide (slide)

9. a. Yes
   b. Glide (slide)

10. Spin

11. Soft tissue stretch

12. a. Compression
    b. Distraction

13. Torsional

14. Ovoid

15. Accessory; rotation cannot be done alone. It occurs when that joint abducts and flexes, thereby accomplishing opposition.

Chapter 5 Muscular System

1. a. Insertion
   b. Origin

2. Reversal of muscle action

3. a. Agonists in wrist flexion
   b. Antagonists in ulnar/radial deviation

4. a. Gluteus maximus and hamstrings
   b. Hip lateral rotation
   c. Gluteus minimus

5. Active insufficiency

6. Eccentric

7. a. Shoulder abduction
   b. Concentric
   c. Shoulder abductors
   d. Isometric
   e. Elbow extensors

8. a. Shoulder flexion
   b. Concentric
   c. Shoulder flexors during first 90 degrees
   d. Eccentric
   e. Shoulder extensors during second 90 degrees

9. a. Wheelchair push-ups: closed-chain activity
   b. Exercises with weight cuffs: open-chain activity
   c. Overhead wall pulleys: open-chain activity

10. Supine (or prone) lying

11. Anterior surface

12. The hip must be flexed to place the rectus femoris on a slack and the knee is flexed.

13. Oblique

14. Parallel

15. a. Contract
    b. Elasticity

Chapter 6 Nervous System

1. L2

2. Gray matter is unmyelinated tissue, and white matter is myelinated tissue.

3. The brain is protected from trauma by (1) the bony outer layer called the *skull*, (2) three layers of membrane called the *meninges*, and (3) shock absorption provided by cerebrospinal fluid.

4. Motor neurons that synapse above the level of the spinal cord's anterior horn are upper motor neurons. Those synapsing at the cell bodies or axons are lower motor neurons. Pathological conditions occurring to either upper or lower motor neurons have quite different clinical signs.

5. Thoracic nerves directly innervate the muscles near where they arise from the spinal cord. Cervical or lumbar nerves branch or divide, forming a plexus and innervating muscle quite distal from the level of the cord from which they originate.

6. Afferent nerve fibers transmit sensory impulses from the periphery toward the brain. Efferent fibers transmit motor impulses from the brain or spinal cord toward the periphery.

7. The involved nerve is the median nerve. The condition is referred to as *ape hand*.

8. The involved nerve is the peroneal nerve. The condition is referred to as *foot drop*.

9. The muscle group involved with claw hand is the intrinsics, which is mostly innervated by the ulnar nerve.

10. The hematoma would be deep to the dura, the outermost covering of the brain.

11. The intervertebral foramen made up of the inferior vertebral notch of the vertebra above and the superior vertebral notch of the vertebra below

12. Lower motor neuron lesion

13. More like a peripheral nerve lesion because the spinal cord ends at L2. Below that, the cord is made up of a collection of nerve roots.

14. From the spinal cord to the periphery

Chapter 7 Circulatory System

Cardiovascular System

1. Tricuspid valve

2. a. Bicuspid valve
   b. Mitral valve

3. Pulmonic valve, aortic valve

4. Pulmonary arteries, pulmonary veins

5. a. Deoxygenated
   b. Pulmonary veins
   c. Oxygenated
   d. Pulmonary arteries

6. a. AV valves
   b. SL valves

7. It will end up distal to its origin in a leg artery or an arteriole small enough in diameter to prevent its passage.

8. It will end up in one of the pulmonary arteries (or arterioles) in the lung, because it will travel until reaching a vessel with a small enough diameter to prevent further passage.

9. External iliac artery and vein to femoral artery and vein

10. External and internal jugular

11. Common carotid artery

12. Major structures from left femoral vein to lung: (1) left femoral vein, (2) left external iliac vein, (3) left common iliac vein, (4) inferior vena cava, (5) right atrium, (6) right AV valve, (7) right ventricle, (8) pulmonic valve, (9) pulmonary arteries, and (10) lungs

13. a. Diastolic pressure (lowest) occurs when the heart relaxes between beats.
    b. Systolic pressure (highest) occurs while the heart contracts.

Lymphatic System

1. Afferent lymph vessel

2. Subclavian vein

3. (c) Muscle

4. Valves, lymph angion, squeezing action of muscles, movement of diaphragm, and good posture

5. Cervical, axillary, and inguinal regional nodes

6. Thoracic duct

7. Collect, filter, and return lymph to the bloodstream

Chapter 8 Basic Biomechanics

1. a. The wrist, because there is a longer resistance arm when the weight is around the wrist than when it is around the elbow.

2. b. The shorter person, who is not on stilts, has a lower COG.

3. a.

   b.

4. a. Scalar = 5 miles (magnitude only)
   b. Vector = 30 feet to the north (magnitude and direction)

5. More force is required when the hand truck is more horizontal. The force arm remains constant, while changing the angle of the hand truck lengthens or shortens the resistance arm. Lowering the load (angle becomes more horizontal) in effect lengthens the resistance arm and requires the person to exert more force. Raising the load (angle becomes more vertical) shortens the resistance arm and allows the person to use less force to move the hand truck.

6. This demonstrates the concept of the wheel and axle. The smaller push rim will require more force, but the distance the wheelchair will travel with a single push is greater.

7.

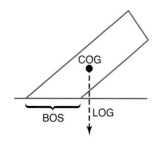

No, the object will fall because the LOG (and COG) is outside the BOS.

8. The BOS of a wheelchair during a "wheelie" is very narrow. To maintain balance, the person must keep the body's COG within that BOS. However, the BOS is very wide when the wheelchair is resting on all four wheels, and it is easy to keep the body's COG within it.

9. Linear force

10. People need to get as close to the bed as possible as it shortens their lever arms; they need to move their legs apart, especially in the A/P direction as it increases their BOS; they need to bend their knees slightly as it lowers their COG.

11. Putting the nut closer to the axis makes the resistance arm shorter, thus easier to crack the nut.

12. Parallel forces; the two people exert an upward force on the mats while the mats (and gravity) exert a downward force. The upward and downward forces are parallel.

13. The medial condyles of the tibia and femur increase the angle of pull of the gracilis. The patella and femoral condyles increase the angle of pull for the quadriceps.

14. Holding the suitcase on the left shifts her COG to the left. By leaning to the right, she is bringing her COG back over the BOS. With a very heavy suitcase, the person's COG shifts farther to the left, so besides leaning to the right, she might raise her right arm out to the side in an attempt to shift the COG more to the right.

15. To increase the amount of friction between the crutch tip and the ground to prevent slippage

Chapter 9 Shoulder Girdle

General Anatomy Questions

1. The shoulder girdle includes the articulations between the scapula and clavicle. The shoulder joint includes the scapula and humerus. The shoulder complex includes the scapula, clavicle, humerus, sternum, and rib cage.

2. a. Use the inferior angle as a point of reference.
   b. When it moves away from the vertebral column, the motion is scapular upward rotation. When it moves back toward the vertebral column to the starting position, the motion is scapular downward rotation.

3. Elevation/depression and protraction/retraction are more linear.

4. Upward and downward rotation are more angular.

5. Scapulohumeral rhythm is the movement relationship between the shoulder girdle and the shoulder joint. After the first 30 degrees, for every 2 degrees of shoulder joint flexion or abduction, the shoulder girdle rotates upwardly 1 degree.

6. Without this shoulder girdle movement, one cannot normally and completely raise the arm above the head.

7. a. Because the three different attachments of the trapezius muscle produce three different lines of pull, the three parts have different muscle actions.
   b. The rhomboid muscles, however, have the same line of pull and thus the same muscle action. There is no functional difference between the rhomboid muscles.

8. The serratus anterior plus the upper and lower trapezius muscles

9. Force couple: a situation in which two or more muscles pull in different, often opposite, directions to accomplish the same motion

10. The rhomboid muscles, the lower and middle trapezius muscles, the levator scapula muscle, and the upper trapezius muscle

11. Pectoralis major

12. a. Pectoralis major
    b. Latissimus dorsi

Functional Activity Questions

1. Downward rotation

2. Upward rotation

3. Elevation

4. Upward rotation and retraction

5. Protraction

6. (1) Concentric, (2) concentric, (3) isometric, (4) isometric, (5) concentric

Clinical Exercise Questions

1. a. Scapular retraction
   b. Middle trapezius, rhomboids
   c. Open

2. a. Scapular retraction
   b. Middle trapezius and rhomboids.
   c. Concentric

3. a. Scapular depression; technically, there is a small amount of upward rotation due to the shoulder flexion from a hyperextended to extended position. This would result in some upward rotation of the scapula.
   b. Lower trapezius, pectoralis minor; upper trapezius, serratus anterior
   c. Concentric

4. a. Scapular protraction and upward rotation
   b. Serratus anterior, pectoralis minor, upper and lower trapezius
   c. Closed

5. a. Scapular retraction and downward rotation
   b. Middle trapezius, rhomboids, levator scapula, pectoralis minor
   c. Concentric contraction; the external weight is greater than the pull of gravity. Therefore, it is an accelerating force, not a decelerating one.

Chapter 10 Shoulder Joint

General Anatomy Questions

1. a. In the frontal plane around the sagittal axis: shoulder abduction/adduction
   b. In the transverse plane around the vertical axis: shoulder medial/lateral rotation, horizontal abduction/adduction
   c. In the sagittal plane around the frontal axis: shoulder flexion/extension

2. The circular arc of the upper extremity formed by a combination of the shoulder motions—flexion, abduction, extension, and adduction

3. Subscapular fossa

4. The supraspinous and infraspinous fossas

5. With the humerus in the vertical position, the bicipital groove facing anteriorly, and the head facing medially, the right humeral head faces toward the left.

6. The **s**upraspinatus, **i**nfraspinatus, **t**eres minor, and **s**ubscapularis muscles; they hold the head of the humerus in toward the glenoid fossa as it moves within the socket.

7. The subscapularis and coracobrachialis muscles and the short head of the biceps brachii muscle

8. The teres major, teres minor, infraspinatus, supraspinatus, and posterior deltoid muscles

9. The anterior deltoid, pectoralis major, and latissimus dorsi muscles

10. a. Clavicular portion
    b. First part of range—to approximately 60 degrees
    c. Its vertical line of pull makes it more effective in the early part of the range and less so as it approaches a more horizontal line of pull.

Functional Activity Questions

1. a. Shoulder hyperextension and medial rotation
   b. Scapular tilt and protraction
2. a. Shoulder abduction and lateral rotation
   b. Scapular upward rotation and retraction
3. a. Shoulder adduction and medial rotation
   b. Scapular downward rotation and protraction
4. a. Shoulder flexion
   b. Scapular upward rotation and protraction
5. a. Shoulder adduction
   b. Scapular downward rotation

Clinical Exercise Questions

1. a. Shoulder horizontal abduction
   b. Concentric contraction of shoulder horizontal abductors
   c. Posterior deltoid, infraspinatus, teres minor
2. a. No
   b. Yes
   c. With a shortened resistance arm, there is less resistance that the force needs to move.
3. a. Shoulder hyperextension
   b. Concentric contraction of shoulder hyperextensors
   c. Latissimus dorsi, posterior deltoid
4. a. Shoulder flexion
   b. Eccentric contraction of shoulder hyperextensors
   c. Latissimus dorsi, posterior deltoid
5. a. Shoulder flexion
   b. Shoulder abduction
   c. Scaption
6. First part:
   a. Shoulder lateral rotation
   b. Concentric
   c. Shoulder lateral rotators: infraspinatus, teres minor, posterior deltoid
   Second part:
   a. Shoulder lateral rotation
   b. Isometric
   c. Shoulder lateral rotators
   Third part:
   a. Shoulder medial rotation
   b. Eccentric
   c. Shoulder lateral rotators
7. Shoulder adductors

Chapter 11 Elbow Joint

General Anatomy Questions

1. a. *Bones in joint:*
      Forearm: radius, ulna
      Elbow: humerus, radius, ulna
   b. *Number of axes:*
      Forearm: 1
      Elbow: 1
   c. *Shape of joint:*
      Forearm: pivot
      Elbow: hinge
   d. *Joint motion allowed:*
      Forearm: supination/pronation
      Elbow: flexion/extension
2. The trochlear notch at the superior end faces anteriorly, the radial notch at the same end faces laterally, and the styloid process at the inferior end is on the medial side.
3. a. Lateral, or radial, collateral ligament
   b. Medial, or ulnar, collateral ligament
   c. Annular ligament
4. The biceps and long head of the triceps muscles
5. Radius, because it is the radius moving around the ulna that produces these motions
6. The pronator quadratus, biceps, and long head of the triceps muscles.
7. The biceps (to radius) and long head of the triceps (to ulna) muscles
8. Anconeus, triceps, and brachialis muscles
9. Long head of triceps
10. a. Shoulder flexion, elbow flexion, forearm supination
    b. Shoulder hyperextension, elbow extension, forearm pronation
11. Same direction
12. a. Biceps
    b. Triceps
    c. Brachioradialis

Functional Activity Questions

1. a. Elbow motion: extension
   b. Forearm motion: supination
2. a. Elbow motion: flexion
   b. Forearm motion: supination (or possibly midposition)
3. a. Elbow motion: extension
   b. Forearm motion: pronation
4. a. Elbow motion: flexion
   b. Forearm motion: supination

5. a. Elbow motion: extension
   b. Forearm motion: midposition

Clinical Exercise Questions

1. a. Forearm supination
   b. Pronator teres, pronator quadratus
2. a. Elbow extension
   b. Concentric
   c. Triceps
   d. Closed chain
3. a. Elbow flexion
   b. Triceps
4. a. Elbow extension
   b. Isometric
   c. Triceps
5. a. Elbow extension
   b. Eccentric
   c. Biceps, brachialis, brachioradialis
   d. Open chain

Chapter 12 Wrist Joint

General Anatomy Questions

1. Proximal row lateral to medial: scaphoid, lunate, triquetrum, pisiform
   Distal row lateral to medial: trapezium, trapezoid, capitate, hamate
2. a. Wrist flexion and extension
   b. Wrist radial and ulnar deviation
   c. No wrist motions occur in the transverse plane around the vertical axis
3. a. *Number of axes:*
      Radiocarpal joint: 2
      Intercarpal joint: 0
   b. *Shape of joint:*
      Radiocarpal joint: condyloid
      Intercarpal joint: plane or irregular
   c. *Joint motion allowed:*
      Radiocarpal joint: flexion/extension, radial/ulnar deviation
      Intercarpal joint: gliding
4. Flexor carpi ulnaris, flexor carpi radialis, palmaris longus
5. Extensor carpi radialis longus and brevis, extension carpi ulnaris
6. If the pisiform bone and "hook" of the hamate bone are visible, it would be the anterior side.
7. Extensor carpi radialis longus and flexor carpi radialis

8. Extensor carpi ulnaris and flexor carpi ulnaris
9. The palmaris longus located on the anterior surface in the middle of the wrist
10. Flexor carpi ulnaris, palmaris longus (with flexor digitorum superficialis and profundus deep to it), flexor carpi radialis (abductor pollicis longus, extensor pollicis long and brevis, which are primarily thumb muscles but also cross the wrist), extensor carpi radialis longus and brevis (extensor digitorum, a finger extensor), and extensor carpi ulnaris
11. Because an articular disk is located between the ulna and the proximal row of carpals
12. You are using a longer lever arm and larger muscles.
13. You are working against gravity when hammering overhead and with gravity when hammering at waist level.
14. For wrist flexion, extension, and ulnar deviation, the end feel is soft tissue stretch. For wrist radial deviation, the end feel is bony.
15. Lateral supracondylar ridge

Functional Activity Questions

1. a. Wrist position: neutral or slight extension
   b. Wrist muscle group: radial deviators
2. a. Wrist position: neutral or slight extension
   b. Wrist muscle group: extensors
3. a. Wrist position: neutral/extension
   b. Wrist muscle group: flexors
4. a. Wrist position: neutral or slight flexion
   b. Wrist muscle group: flexors
5. a. Wrist position: neutral
   b. Wrist muscle group: flexors

Clinical Exercise Questions

1. a. Wrist flexion
   b. Concentric
   c. Wrist flexors
2. a. Wrist extension
   b. Eccentric
   c. Wrist flexors
3. a. Wrist extension
   b. Concentric
   c. Wrist extensors
   d. Elbow flexors
   e. Isometric
4. a. Wrist flexion
   b. Eccentric
   c. Wrist extensors

5. a. Wrist ulnar deviation
   b. Concentric
   c. Wrist ulnar deviators
6. a. Wrist radial deviation
   b. Eccentric
   c. Elasticity of tubing would bring wrist back to neutral if ulnar deviators were not slowing down the motion.
   d. Wrist ulnar deviators

Chapter 13 Hand

General Anatomy Questions

1. a. Finger: MCP abduction/adduction
      Thumb: CMC flexion/extension, MCP and IP flexion/extension
   b. Finger: MCP, PIP, DIP flexion/extension
      Thumb: CMC abduction/adduction
   c. Thumb: CMC opposition/reposition
2. Compare the thumb and fingers:
   a. *Number of bones:*
      Thumb: 4
      Finger: 5
   b. *Number of joints:*
      Thumb: 3
      Finger: 4
   c. *Names of the joints:*
      Thumb: CMC, MCP, IP
      Finger: CMC, MCP, PIP, DIP
3. CMC flexion, abduction, and rotation
4. Rotation
5. It holds the extrinsic tendons close to the wrist.
6. The floor of the carpal tunnel is made up of the carpal bones, and the ceiling is the transverse carpal ligament portion of the flexor retinaculum. The flexor digitorum superficialis and profundus and the flexor pollicis longus muscles and the median nerve run through the carpal tunnel.
7. An extrinsic muscle has its proximal attachment above the wrist and its distal attachment below the wrist. The extrinsic muscles include the flexor digitorum superficialis and profundus, extensor digitorum, extensor digiti minimi, and extensor indicis muscles of the fingers. Extrinsic muscles of the thumb are the flexor pollicis longus, abductor pollicis longus, and extensor pollicis longus and brevis.
8. An intrinsic muscle has both attachments below the wrist; the nine intrinsic muscles include the flexor and abductor pollicis brevis, the opponens and adductor pollicis, the flexor/abductor/opponens digiti minimi, the interossei, and the lumbricales.
9. Thenar muscles are intrinsic muscles on the thumb side (lateral) of the hand; hypothenar muscles are on the little finger side (medial). Any intrinsic muscle with *pollicis* in its name is a thenar muscle, whereas one with *digiti minimi* is a hypothenar muscle.
10. The indentation formed between the tendons of the abductor pollicis longus and extensor pollicis brevis laterally and extensor pollicis longus medially is referred to as the *anatomical snuffbox.*
11. The lumbricales; they attach proximally to the tendons of the flexor digitorum profundus muscle and distally to the tendons of the extensor digitorum muscle.
12. a. Concave
    b. Convex
    c. Same

Functional Activity Questions

1. Holding the handle of a skillet: cylindrical grip
2. Pulling a little red wagon: hook grip
3. Turning pages of a book: pad-to-pad or pad-to-side prehension
4. Fastening snaps or buttons: tip-to-tip prehension
5. Carrying a coffee mug by its handle: lateral prehension
6. Holding a hand of playing cards: lumbrical grip
7. Holding an apple: spherical grip
8. Holding on to a barbell: cylindrical grip
9. Picking up a CD: pad-to-pad or pad-to-side prehension
10. a. Combination of cylindrical and lumbrical grip
    b. Held in neutral position by wrist flexors and radial deviators
    c. Flexor carpi ulnaris and radialis, extensor carpi radialis longus
    d. Elbow flexors in midposition
    e. Biceps, brachialis, and especially brachioradialis
    f. Shoulder flexors and adductors
    g. Anterior deltoid, pectoralis major, teres major, and latissimus dorsi
    h. Shoulder girdle upward rotation and protraction
    i. Upper and lower trapezius, serratus anterior, pectoralis minor

Clinical Exercise Questions

1. Joint motion: finger MCP abduction followed by MCP adduction
Prime movers: dorsal interossei and abductor digiti minimi followed by palmar interossei

2. Joint motion: thumb abduction
Prime movers: abductor pollicis brevis and longus

3. Joint motion: thumb and little finger opposition
Prime movers: opponens pollicis, opponens digiti minimi

4. Joint motion: finger MP flexion and IP extension
Prime movers: lumbricales

5. Joint motion: thumb CMC, MCP, and IP flexion
Prime movers: flexor pollicis longus and brevis

Chapter 14 Temporomandibular Joint

General Anatomy Questions

1. Zygomatic and temporal bones

2. Synonymous terms are mandibular
   a. depression.
   b. elevation.
   c. retraction or retrusion.
   d. protraction or protrusion.
   e. lateral deviation.

3. Mandible and temporal bones

4. Temporalis

5. Masseter

6. Digastric and omohyoid

7. Fifth cranial (trigeminal) nerve

8. Anterior rotation of the mandibular condyle on the disk

9. The left condyle spins in the mandibular socket while the right condyle slides forward.

10. The thyroid cartilage

Functional Activity Questions

1. Mandibular depression

2. a. Mandibular elevation
   b. Side opposite the bread
   c. Same side as bread

3. Side-to-side motion—lateral deviation
Anterior-posterior motion—protraction/retraction

4. Motion: mandibular elevation
Muscle: temporalis, masseter, medial pterygoid

Clinical Exercise Questions

1. a. Mandibular lateral deviation
   b. Concentric
   c. Right temporalis and masseter, left medial and lateral pterygoid

2. a. Mandibular protraction
   b. Isometric
   c. Medial and lateral pterygoid

3. a. Mandibular depression
   b. Concentric
   c. Lateral pterygoid

Chapter 15 Neck And Trunk

General Anatomy Questions

1. a. Neck and trunk lateral bending
   b. Neck and trunk rotation
   c. Neck and trunk flexion, extension, and hyperextension

2. The cervical vertebra has a bifid spinous process, and there is a foramen in the transverse process. The thoracic vertebra has a long slender, downward-pointing spinous process with rib facets on the body and transverse processes; the superior articular processes face posteriorly. The lumbar vertebra has a large spinous process pointing straight back; the superior articular processes face medially.

3. The frontal plane position of the superior and inferior articular processes

4. The sagittal plane position of the superior and inferior articular processes

5. From the occiput to C7: nuchal ligament
From C7 to the sacrum: supraspinal ligament

6. Ligamentum flavum

7. Anterior and posterior longitudinal ligaments

8. The muscle's line of pull is through or close to the center of the frontal axis of trunk flexion and extension, thus making it ineffective in this motion. To be effective in rotation, the muscle's line of pull would have to be horizontal or diagonal. The quadratus lumborum has a vertical line of pull.

9. The erector spinae

10. A combination of trunk flexion and rotation to the right brought about by the rectus abdominis, left external oblique, and right internal oblique

Functional Activity Questions

1. Neck rotation and possibly some hyperextension
2. Neck lateral bending
3. Neck hyperextension
4. Neck flexion
5. Neck hyperextension
6. Trunk rotation to left
7. Trunk rotation to right
8. Trunk lateral bending
9. Trunk flexion
10. Trunk hyperextension

Clinical Exercise Questions
Head and Neck

1. a. Flexion of head on C1
   b. Neck extension
   c. Concentric
   d. Isometric
   e. Neck extensors (splenius capitis, splenius cervicis, erector spinae, interspinales and transversospinalis)
2. a. Lateral bending of head and neck
   b. Isometric
   c. Right sternocleidomastoid, right splenius capitis, right splenius cervicis, right scalenes, right erector spinae, and right intertransversarii
3. a. Neck lateral bending to the right
   b. Left neck lateral benders
   c. Right sternocleidomastoid, right scalenes, right splenius capitis and cervicis, right erector spinae, and right intertransversarii
   d. Right lateral benders
   e. Same as answer (c), except on right side
4. Left sternocleidomastoid
5. a. Flexion of head on C1
   b. Concentric
   c. Prevertebral muscles
   d. Neck flexion
   e. Concentric
   f. Sternocleidomastoid (bonus point if you included the longus colli of the prevertebral muscle group)
   g. Isometric

h. Sternocleidomastoid (another bonus point if you remembered the longus colli)
   i. Neck extension
   j. Eccentric contraction
   k. Sternocleidomastoid and longus colli

Trunk

1. a. Trunk flexion, especially lumbar region
   b. Trunk extensors
   c. Erector spinae, transversospinalis, interspinales
2. a. Trunk flexion
   b. Concentric
   c. Bilateral rectus abdominis, external and internal obliques
3. a. Yes
   b. Flexing
   c. Origin toward insertion
   d. Reversal of muscle action
   e. Iliopsoas
   f. Holding down the feet makes the distal segment more stable and the proximal segment more movable. This allows the hip flexors to flex the hip (and trunk) in a reversal of muscle action
4. a. Trunk flexion with rotation to the left
   b. Concentric
   c. Both rectus abdominis, right external oblique, and left internal oblique
5. a. Flexion of head on C1
   b. Concentric
   c. Isometric
   d. Prevertebral muscle group
   e. Neck extension
   f. Isometric
   g. Splenius capitis and cervicis, erector spinae
   h. Trunk hyperextension
   i. Concentric
   j. Erector spinae, transversospinalis, intertransversarii

Chapter 16 Respiratory System

General Anatomy Questions

1. The sternum, ribs, costal cartilages, and thoracic vertebrae
2. The bodies and transverse processes of the thoracic vertebrae articulate with the tubercle and neck of the ribs.
3. Elevation and depression bringing about inspiration and expiration

4. During inspiration, the ribs elevate and the diaphragm lowers, and during expiration, the ribs depress and the diaphragm muscle elevates.

5. The origin, or more stable attachment, is above the rib cage and in a position to pull the rib cage up.

6. The line of pull does not change from front to back, but the muscle moves 180 degrees around the rib cage, giving the appearance of changing direction from front to back.

7. The origin, or more stable attachment, has a bony attachment, but the insertion attaches to a central tendon. When the muscle is relaxed, it is dome-shaped. When it contracts, the muscle flattens out, allowing more room in the thoracic cavity.

8. You talk only during expiration when air is moving out through the airway.

9. The accessory muscles of inspiration pull up on the sternum and rib cage while the accessory muscles of expiration pull down.

10. Rib cage movement is compared to bucket handle movement; thoracic cavity movement is compared to movement of a bellows.

11. The person with a C3 injury will not have an innervated diaphragm; therefore, they will need the assistance of a ventilator to breathe. A person with a C5 injury will have a neurologically intact diaphragm and can breathe without mechanical assistance.

Functional Activity Questions

1. Forced inspiration followed by forced expiration
2. Deep inspiration
3. Forced expiration
4. Forced expiration
5. Quiet inspiration and expiration

Clinical Exercise Questions

1. a. Chest breathing
   b. Diaphragmatic breathing
2. Anterior trunk muscles—rectus abdominis, external and internal oblique, and transverse abdominis
3. a. Chest rose during sniffing
   b. Muscles contracted
   c. Sniffing requires deep inspiration. Accessory muscles of inspiration assisted by pulling up the rib cage in a reversal of muscle action. These muscles were the scalenes and sternocleidomastoid.

4. a. Ribcage moves up and out during inspiration.
   b. The pectoralis major is assisting in deep inspiration by pulling up on the ribs.
   c. This is a closed-chain activity.

Chapter 17 Pelvic Girdle

General Anatomy Questions

1. a. Anterior/posterior pelvic tilt
   b. Lateral tilt
   c. Pelvic rotation
2. To the left
3. The hip joints
4. a. Hip flexion
   b. Hip extension
   c. Hip abduction on the unsupported side and hip adduction on the weight-bearing side
5. a. Right hip medial rotation/left hip lateral rotation
   b. Right hip lateral rotation/left hip medial rotation
6. a. Hyperextension
   b. Flexion
   c. Lateral bending to opposite side
7. Back extensors, hip flexors

Functional Activity Questions

1. Posterior pelvic tilt
2. Anterior pelvic tilt
3. Posterior pelvic tilt
4. Left hip adducted and right hip abducted

Clinical Exercise Questions

1. Motions: posterior pelvic tilt, trunk flexion, hip extension
   Muscles: gluteus maximus and abdominals
2. Motions: left lateral pelvic tilt; left hip adduction and right hip abduction
   Muscles: right hip abductors (gluteus medius and minimus) and left quadratus lumborum

Chapter 18 Hip Joint

General Anatomy Question

1. a. Two hip bones, the sacrum, and the coccyx
   b. The fused bones of the ilium, ischium, and pubis
   c. Acetabulum of the hip bone and head of the femur

d. The ilium, ischium, and pubis

e. The ischium and pubis

f. The ilium and ischium

2. With the greater sciatic notch posterior and the body of pubis anterior, the acetabulum faces laterally. Therefore, if the acetabular opening is facing to the right in this position, it is a right hip bone.

3. With the femur in the vertical position, the linea aspera and lesser trochanter are posterior, and the head faces medially. Therefore, in this position the head of the right femur faces toward the left.

4. a. Number of axes: 3

b. Shape of joint: ball and socket

c. Type of motion allowed: flexion/extension, abduction/adduction, and rotation

5. a. Medial and lateral rotation

b. Flexion/extension

c. Abduction/adduction

6. The distal attachment of the iliofemoral ligament; because it splits into two parts, forming an upside-down Y

7. The acetabulum forms a deep socket holding most of the femoral head, and the joint is surrounded by three very strong ligaments.

8. The line of attachment of the ligaments is a spiral. This arrangement causes the ligaments to become taut as the joint moves into extension and to slacken with flexion, thus limiting hyperextension without impeding flexion.

9. The rectus femoris, sartorius, gracilis, semitendinosus, semimembranosus, biceps femoris (long head), and tensor fascia latae muscles

10. The sartorius muscle is involved in hip flexion, abduction, and lateral rotation; the tensor fascia latae muscle is involved in flexion and abduction.

11. When you lift your right foot off the floor, the left hip abductors and right trunk extensors contract to keep the right side of the pelvis from dropping. A force couple exists when the hip abductors are pulling down while the trunk extensors are pulling up.

12. Opposite

13. Hip flexion—soft tissue approximation; hip extension—soft tissue stretch

Functional Activity Questions

1. Hip extension and medial rotation, and maybe some adduction

2. a. Greater hip flexion is required with a low surface.

b. Medial rotation and adduction may accompany the increased flexion.

3. a. Adduction

b. Right hip adductors

c. Closed

4. a. Swing phase includes hip flexion, extension, and hyperextension.

b. Greater hip flexion than walking

c. Hip flexion and abduction

d. Combination of hip hyperextension, abduction, flexion, adduction as you swing your leg over the bike, and may also include some rotation

5. a. Posterior tilt

b. Anterior tilt with increased lumbar lordosis

6. a. It maintains the pelvis in a posterior tilt.

b. There is not sufficient length of the hip flexors to complete the range of motion.

c. Iliopsoas

d. The anterior hip muscles must be elongated more when the pelvis is in a posterior tilt position versus an anterior tilt position.

7. You may compensate by standing with the lumbar spine in lordosis and the pelvis in anterior tilt, or by leaning forward in a slightly flexed hip position.

8. a. The right hip is flexed, adducted, and medially rotated.

b. The left hip is extended, abducted, and laterally rotated.

9. Hip—closed chain; shoulder—open chain

Clinical Exercise Questions

1. a. Hip hyperextension

b. Strengthening

c. Gluteus maximus

2. a. Hip hyperextension

b. Stretching

c. Iliopsoas

3. a. Yes. The rectus femoris is being stretched over both joints at the same time.

4. a. Hip abduction

b. Strengthening

c. Hip abductors—gluteus medius and gluteus minimus

5. a. Combination of hip abduction and flexion

b. Strengthening

c. Tensor fascia latae

6. a. Concentric

b. Third class

7. a. No

b. By having the knee flexed, the hamstrings are already shortened. As the hip goes into more hyperextension, they will quickly become actively insufficient.

8. a. Hip abduction and flexion
   b. Stretching
   c. Adductors—pectineus, adductor longus, adductor brevis, adductor magnus
      Extensors (hamstrings)—semimembranosus, semitendinosus, biceps femoris

9. a. Exercise B is more difficult.
   b. With the knees in extension, the resistance arm is much longer than in exercise A. The force arm remains the same length in both.

10. a. Closed
    b. Hip extension
    c. Concentric
    d. Hip extensors—gluteus maximus and hamstrings
    e. Hip flexor—rectus femoris

Chapter 19 Knee Joint

General Anatomy Questions

1. a. *Number of axes:*
      Knee joint: 1
      Patellofemoral joint: 0
   b. *Shape of joint:*
      Knee joint: hinge
      Patellofemoral joint: irregular
   c. *Type of motion:*
      Knee joint: flexion/extension
      Patellofemoral joint: gliding

2. Knee flexion and extension occur in the sagittal plane around the frontal axis.

3. The Q angle is formed by the intersection of the line between the tibial tuberosity and middle of the patella and the line between the ASIS and the middle of the patella. The greater the angle, the higher the stress on the patellofemoral joint during knee flexion and extension.

4. Femur and tibia

5. Because it initiates knee flexion, moving the knee out of the "locked" position of extension

6. The distal attachments of the sartorius, gracilis, and semitendinosus muscles

7. Weakened knee extension (quadriceps = L2–L4) and no knee flexion (hamstrings = L5–S2)

8. a. Closed kinetic chain
   b. No. This could only happen as a closed-chain action.
   c. The gastrocnemius is pulling origin toward insertion—a reversal of muscle action.

9. Rotary

10. a. Bending
    b. Tensile stress on medial side
    c. Compressive stress on lateral side

Functional Activity Questions

1. a. Hamstring action: hip extension and knee flexion
   b. Hip position (see Fig. 19-25A): extension
   c. Hip position (see Fig. 19-25B): partly flexed
   d. Position of hamstring active insufficiency: hip extension and knee flexion
   e. See Figure 19-25B: hip partly flexed
   f. Keeping the hip in slight flexion keeps some elongation of the hamstrings while they are being shortened at the knee, thus avoiding active insufficiency. Keeping the hip in extension has the hamstrings shortened over the hip while they are shortening over the knee. Thus, active insufficiency will be reached more quickly.

2. a. Hip position in Figure 19-26A = partial hip flexion; the hip position in Figure 19-26B = greater hip flexion
   b. Vasti muscle
   c. Rectus femoris—hip flexion and knee extension
   d. The one-joint vasti muscles are elongated with knee flexion. Because they do not cross the hip, hip position has no effect on them. The two-joint rectus femoris is elongated in hip extension and knee flexion. Therefore, it is elongated more in position A. In position B, it is already shortened (on a slack) at the hip.
   e. If you want to strengthen the rectus femoris, use a more extended hip position (see Fig. 19-26A).
   f. If you want to isolate and strengthen only the vasti muscles, use a more flexed hip position (see Fig. 19-26B), where the rectus femoris is shortened and is not as strong.

3. a. Placing foot onto curb—knee flexion
   b. Moving up onto curb—knee extension

4. a. Preparing to kick—bringing knee into flexion and hip into hyperextension
   b. Rectus femoris is being stretched over both hip and knee.
   c. Point of ball contact—knee extension and hip extension
   d. Rectus femoris is shortening at the knee but is still elongated at the hip.
   e. Follow-through—knee remains in extension, hip going into flexion
   f. Rectus femoris is shortened over both joints and is becoming actively insufficient.

5. a. Left foot, not right foot, would lead
   b. Hip hiking (pelvic elevation on right side; also called *right trunk lateral bending* in a reversal of muscle action)

Clinical Exercise Questions

1. Slide down:
   a. Knee flexion
   b. Eccentric contraction
   c. Knee extensors (quadriceps)
   d. Closed chain
   Hold position:
   a. Isometric
   b. Knee extensors (quadriceps)
   Return to standing:
   a. Knee extension
   b. Concentric contraction
   c. Knee extensors (quadriceps)

2. a. Hip flexion and knee extension
   b. Stretching of hamstrings, which extend hip and flex knee
   c. Hamstrings consist of semimembranosus, semitendinosus, biceps femoris

3. a. Hip flexion and knee extension
   b. Strengthening
   c. Hip flexors (rectus femoris, iliopsoas, and pectineus) and knee extensors (quadriceps group)
   d. Open chain

4. a. Hip extension and knee flexion
   b. Stretching
   c. Rectus femoris (which does hip flexion and knee extension)

5. Flexion—soft tissue approximation; extension—soft tissue stretch

6. a. Position C is easier to hold.
   b. Force is the quadriceps muscle, resistance is the leg and foot, and axis is the knee joint. It is a third-class lever (AFR).
   c. Resistance arm shortens
   d. Force arm remains the same.

7. See Figure 19-28.
   Straighten knee:
   a. Knee extension
   b. Concentric contraction
   c. Knee extensors (quadriceps)
   d. Closed-chain activity
   Hold position:
   a. Knee extension
   b. Isometric contraction
   c. Knee extensors (quadriceps)

Bend knee:
   a. Knee flexion
   b. Eccentric contraction
   c. Knee extensors (quadriceps)

8. The clinician can apply greater force just above the ankle than just below the knee, because the force lever arm is longer. The axis is the knee joint. The resistance is being applied by the patient in this case. The resistance arm is the distance between the axis and the insertion of the quadriceps muscle, which does not change. The force arm is the distance between the axis and the place on the patient's leg where force is applied. Stated another way, the clinician does not need to apply as much force when using a longer force lever arm as she would with a shorter force lever arm to accomplish the same result.

Chapter 20 Ankle Joint and Foot

General Anatomy Questions

1. a. 1
   b. Hinge
   c. Dorsiflexion, plantar flexion
   d. Tibia and talus (primarily)

2. The subtalar joint involves the talus and calcaneus; the transverse tarsal joint involves the talus and calcaneus with the navicular and cuboid bone.

3. The function of the interosseous membrane, which is located between the tibia and fibula, is to hold the two bones together and to provide a large area for muscle attachment.

4. The deltoid ligament, made up of the tibionavicular, tibiocalcaneal, and posterior tibiotalar ligaments

5. The lateral ligament, made up of the posterior and anterior talofibular and calcaneofibular ligaments.

6. The medial and lateral longitudinal arches

7. The medial longitudinal arch is made up of the calcaneus and the navicular, cuneiform, and first three metatarsal bones. The lateral longitudinal arch is made up of the calcaneus, cuboid, and fourth and fifth metatarsals.

8. The transverse arch, made up of the cuboid and three cuneiform bones

9. The function of the arches is to provide some shock absorption, adjust to uneven terrain, and propel the body forward.

10. Tibialis posterior, flexor digitorum longus, and flexor hallucis longus muscles

11. Tibialis posterior, tibialis anterior, peroneus longus muscles

12. Peroneus longus and peroneus brevis muscles

13. Peroneus brevis and tertius muscles

14. Tibialis anterior and peroneus longus muscles; together, the peroneus longus and tibialis anterior muscles are sometimes referred to as the stirrup of the foot, because the peroneus longus muscle descends the leg laterally before crossing the foot medially to join the tibialis anterior muscle. The tibialis anterior muscle descends the leg medially to meet the peroneus longus muscle, forming a "U" or stirrup.

15. No, the strongest plantar flexors are the gastrocnemius and soleus, which are innervated at the S1–S2 levels. The posterior deep group is innervated at the L5–S1 level primarily.

Functional Activity Questions

1. Ankle plantar flexion

2. Ankle plantar flexion

3. Ankle dorsiflexion

4. Ankle plantar flexion

5. Ankle inversion/eversion

6. Ankle dorsiflexion

7. Ankle plantar flexion

Clinical Exercise Questions

1. Gastrocnemius:
   a. Number of joints crossed: 2
   b. Knee motion: knee flexion
   c. Ankle motion: ankle plantar flexion
   Soleus:
   a. Number of joints crossed: 1
   b. Knee motion: no knee motion
   c. Ankle motion: ankle plantar flexion

2. a. Left knee: extension
      Left ankle: dorsiflexion
   b. Left gastrocnemius is stretching
   c. Left soleus is stretching
   d. Gastrocnemius
   e. The gastrocnemius is stretched more because it has to stretch over the combined range of both knee and ankle joints, while the soleus is being stretched over only the ankle joint.

3. a. Left knee: flexion
      Left ankle: dorsiflexion
   b. The left gastrocnemius is slack at the knee.
   c. The left gastrocnemius is stretched at the ankle.
   d. The left soleus is not stretched at the knee, because it doesn't cross the knee.
   e. Yes. The left soleus is stretched at the ankle.
   f. Soleus
   g. The soleus is stretched more because there is more ankle ROM. With the gastrocnemius slack over the knee, more ankle motion is possible, which stretches the soleus more.

4. a. Left knee: extension
      Left ankle: plantar flexion
   b. The left gastrocnemius is elongating.
   c. The left gastrocnemius is shortening.
   d. The left soleus is not acting over the knee.
   e. The left soleus is shortening over the ankle.
   f. The two-joint gastrocnemius is able to elongate over the knee while shortening over the ankle, thus keeping more tension in the muscle through a greater range. The one-joint soleus is shortening over the ankle and will lose tension quickly.

5. a. Inversion
   b. Concentric, then isometric contraction to hold the feet in position
   c. Tibialis anterior and tibialis posterior

6. a. Ankle dorsiflexion, ankle dorsiflexion, ankle plantar flexion
   b. Concentric, isometric, eccentric
   c. Ankle dorsiflexion—tibialis anterior is the prime mover for all three phases.
   d. Open

Chapter 21 Posture

General Anatomy Questions

1. Cervical extensors

2. The side view

3. Hip flexors

4. The side

5. Level and not elevated or depressed

6. From the front or back

7. Slightly in front of the lateral malleolus

8. a. Knee—slightly posterior to the patella
   b. Hip—through the greater trochanter
   c. Shoulder—through the tip of the acromion process
   d. Head—through the earlobe

Functional Activity Questions

1. Shoulder girdle protraction
2. Shoulder girdle retraction, maybe some elevation
3. Cervical flexion and possibly some forward head
4. Right shoulder higher
5. The woman's COG shifts anteriorly
6. Anterior tilt
7. Increased lordosis
8. a. Posterior trunk—lumbar erector spinae and paraspinals become tight.
   b. Anterior trunk—abdominals become stretched.
9. Hip flexors

Clinical Exercise Questions

1. Cervical hyperextension
2. a. Cervical extensors—tighter
   b. Cervical flexors—stretched
3. Left side of pelvis is higher.
4. a. Left side muscles—tighter
   b. Right side muscles—stretched
5. a. Left side of disk more compressed
   b. Right side more distracted
   c. Intervertebral foramen—right side opened more
   d. Intervertebral foramen on left made smaller
6. a. Trunk extensors—posterior
   b. Anterior part
7. a. Trunk flexors—anterior
   b. Posterior part

Chapter 22 Gait

General Anatomy Questions

1. Both have the same components and sequence of events. Walking has a period of double support while running does not. Running has a period of nonsupport that walking does not have.
2. Traditional terminology refers to single points in a time frame, whereas RLA terminology refers to periods within a time frame.
3. Stance phase
4. Period of double support; between heel-off and toe-off of one foot and heel strike and foot flat on the opposite foot

5. During midstance of the stance phase
6. Swing phase
7. Step length lengthens and cadence increases
8. Walk with feet farther apart to widen the base of support.
9. Heel strike of stance phase and midswing of swing phase
10. Push-off stance phase

Functional Activity Questions

1. Shorter step length
   Flatter foot during stance
   Less arm swing
2. Narrower walking base
   Arms more out to side to help maintain balance
3. Wider walking base
   Greater horizontal displacement
4. Increased forward lean
5. Greater vertical displacement
   Greater arm swing
6. Circumducted gait during swing
   Greater horizontal displacement during stance
7. Curvilinear motion

Clinical Exercise Questions

1. a. Ankle—dorsiflexion
   b. Hip—flexion
   c. Pelvis—anterior pelvic tilt
   d. Lumbar spine—lordosis
2. a. Type of contraction: concentric contraction
      Muscle group involved: knee extensors
   b. Type of contraction: eccentric contraction
      Muscle group involved: ankle plantar flexors
   c. Type of contraction: concentric contraction
      Muscle group involved: hip extensors
   d. Type of contraction: isometric contraction
      Muscle group involved: contralateral hip abductors
   e. Type of contraction: eccentric contraction
      Muscle group involved: knee flexors
3. a. Increasing lateral pelvic tilt to involved side
   b. Leaning over the involved (shorter) leg during stance phase
   c. Walking in an equinus gait
   d. Flexing the knee of the uninvolved (longer) leg

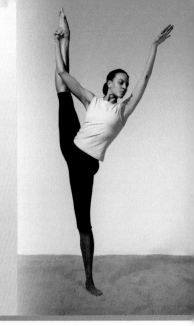

Index

Note: Page numbers followed by "f" and "t" indicate figures and tables, respectively.

Abdomen, 5
Abdominal muscles, 222–224
  external oblique, 223, 223f
  internal oblique, 223, 223f
  layers of, 223f
  rectus abdominis, 222f, 223
  transverse abdominis, 223f, 224
Abducted gait, 352
Abduction, 8–9, 8f, 132
  of ankle, 304
  of fingers, 173, 173f
  of hip joint, 262f
  horizontal, 8f, 9
  of shoulder, 8f
  of thumb, 172, 172f
Abductor digiti minimi muscle, 182f, 184–185
Abductor pollicis brevis muscle, 181, 181f
Abductor pollicis longus muscle, 177–178, 178f
Abnormal bony end feel, 32
Acceleration, 94, 346
Accessory expiratory muscles, 242, 243t
Accessory inspiratory muscles, 241, 243t
Accessory motion, 36, 171–172
  forces, 36, 37f
  terminology, 32
Acetabular labrum, 266
Acetabulum, 264
Achilles tendon, 292, 311
Achilles tendonitis, 323
Acquired bursae, 26
Acromioclavicular joint, 118, 118f
Acromioclavicular ligaments, 118, 118f
Acromioclavicular separation, 142
Acromion process, 133
Action-reaction, law of, 94
Active insufficiency, 43, 43f
Active tension, 42
Adam's apple, 238
Adduction, 8–9, 8f, 132, 172f
  of ankle, 304
  of fingers, 173, 173f

  of hip joint, 262f
  horizontal, 8f, 9
  of shoulder, 8f
  of thumb, 172
Adductor brevis muscle, 269–270, 269f
Adductor longus muscle, 268–269, 269f
Adductor magnus muscle, 270
Adductor pollicis muscle, 182, 182f
Adductor tubercle, 265, 286
Adhesive capsulitis, 143
Afferent impulses, 55
Afferent lymph vessels, 89
Agonist, 48
AIIS. *See* Anterior inferior iliac spine
Ala, of sacrum, 249
Alveolus, 238
Alzheimer's disease, 71
Amphiarthrodial joints, 22
Amyotrophic lateral sclerosis, 71
Anastomosis, 87, 87f
Anatomical position, 4, 4f
Anatomical snuffbox, 179, 179f
Anconeus muscle, 154, 154f
Aneurysm, 91
Angina, 91
Angion, 88, 88f
Angle of inclination, 275, 276f
Angle of pull, 121
Angle of torsion, 276, 277f
Angular force, 97, 98f
Angular motion, 6, 6f, 7f
Ankle. *See also* Foot
  joint capsule, 308
  joints of
    subtalar, 306–307
    talocrural (talotibial), 305–306, 305f
    tibiofibular, 305f
    transverse tarsal, 307, 307f
  ligaments of
    deltoid, 308
    lateral, 308, 308f

Ankle. *See also* Foot *(continued)*
    motions of, 304, 304f, 305f, 306-307, 306t
    muscles of
        anatomical relationships, 317-321
        anterior group, 314-315, 320f
        deep posterior group, 312-314
        extensor digitorum longus, 314-315
        extensor hallucis longus, 314, 315f
        extrinsic, 310-311, 311t
        flexor digitorum longus, 313-314, 313f
        flexor hallucis longus, 313, 313f
        gastrocnemius, 311-312, 311f
        innervation of, 321-322, 323t
        intrinsic, 317
        lateral group, 315-317, 320f
        peroneus brevis, 316, 317f
        peroneus longus, 315-316, 316f
        peroneus tertius, 316-317, 317f
        plantaris, 312
        soleus, 312, 312f
        superficial posterior group, 311-312
        tibialis anterior, 314, 315f
        tibialis posterior, 312-313, 312f
        triceps surae, 312
    pathologies of, 322-323
Ankle dorsiflexors, 350
Ankle fracture, 323
Ankle fusion, 352
Ankle sprains, 323
Ankylosing spondylitis, 230
Annular ligament, 151
Annulus fibrosus, 215
Antagonist, 48
Antalgic gait, 354
Anterior, 4, 4f
Anterior (ventral) ramus, 60, 62
Anterior cerebral arteries, 86
Anterior communicating artery, 86
Anterior cord syndrome, 71
Anterior cruciate ligament, 288, 288f
Anterior deltoid muscle, 135-136, 135f
Anterior horn, 58
Anterior inferior iliac spine (AIIS), 263, 285
Anterior longitudinal ligament, 218
Anterior position, 4, 333, 333f
Anterior root, 54
Anterior sacroiliac ligament, 251
Anterior scalene muscle, 220, 220f
Anterior shoulder dislocations, 143
Anterior superior iliac spine (ASIS), 254f, 255-256, 263, 285
Anterior tibial arteries, 83
Anterior tibial veins, 83
Anterior tilt, 253, 254f
Anteversion, 276, 277f
Antigravity muscles, 331, 331f
Aorta, 79, 82f
    ascending, 81, 82f
    descending, 82f
Aortic arch, 81t, 82f, 86f
Aortic valve, 77
Ape hand, 72
Aponeurosis, 26
Appendicular skeleton, 13, 14t, 15f

Approximation, 36
Arachnoid, 57
Arch
    of aorta, 81
    foot, 308-310, 309f
Arm, 5
Arteries, 79-80
    coronary, 81
    major, 81t, 84f, 85f, 86f
    pathways, 81-86
Arterioles, 79
Arteriosclerosis, 91
Arthokinematic motion (joint surface motion), 6, 32-37
    of knee, 284, 284f
    types of, 33-34
Arthrokinematics, 8, 31-38, 93-94
Articular cartilage, 22, 25, 25f
Articular disk, 164, 201-202
Articular fossa, 199
Articular process, 214
Articular system, 21-28
Articular tubercle, 199
Ascending aorta, 81, 81t, 82f
Assisting mover, 48
Asthma, 245
Ataxic gait, 353
Atherosclerosis, 91
Atlantoaxial joints, 213, 217, 217f
Atlanto-occipital joint, 213, 217
Atlas vertebra (C1), 215, 215f
Atria, 76-77
Atrioventricular (AV) valves, 77
Auditory meatus, 200
Auricular surface, 250
Autonomic dysreflexia, 71
Autonomic nervous system (ANS), 53, 53f
Axes, 27, 28f
    frontal, 27, 28f
    sagittal, 27, 28f
    vertical, 27, 28f
Axial extension, 213
Axial skeleton, 13, 14t, 15f
Axillary artery, 81t, 85
Axillary border, 133
Axillary nerve, 65, 66f
Axis (A), 102
Axis vertebra (C2), 215, 215f
Axons, 54, 54f
Axon terminal, 54

Back knees (genu recurvatum), 294
Baker's cyst, 295
Ball-and-socket joint, 24, 24f
Ballet dancers, 11f, 331-332, 332f
Basal ganglia, 56
Base of support (BOS), 99, 100f, 101, 101f, 102f
Basilar area, 213
Basilar artery, 86
Basilic vein, 85
Bell-clapper gait, 351-352, 351f
Bell's palsy, 72
Bending force, 36, 37f
Biaxial joint motion, 24

Biceps brachii muscle, 152–153, 152f, 156f
   supination action of, 153f
Biceps femoris muscle, 40, 271, 291, 292
Bicipital tendonitis, 144
Bicuspid valve, 77
Bilateral, 5
Bimalleolar fracture, 323
Biomechanics, 3, 93–94, 93f
   force, 95–97
   laws of motion, 94
   stability, 99–102, 102f
   torque, 97–99
Bipennate muscles, 41
Birth canal, 248
Blood, flow through heart, 77–78, 77f, 78f
Blood pressure, 80–81
Blood supply, 86–87
Blood vessels, 80f
   pathways, 81–86
   pulse and blood pressure, 80–81
   types of, 79–80
      arteries, 79–80
      capillaries, 79
      veins, 79–80
Body proportions, 99, 99f
Body segments, 5–6, 6f
Boggy end feel, 32
Bone markings, 18f
Bone(s). See also specific bones and body areas
   cancellous, 14
   compact, 14
   composition of, 13–14, 15f
   fractures, 17
   of human body, 14t
   irregular, 16, 16f
   joint structure and, 24–25
   longitudinal cross section of, 15f
   structure of, 14–16
   types of, 16–17, 16f, 17t
      flat, 16, 16f, 17t
      irregular, 17t
      long, 16, 16f, 17t
      sesamoid, 16–17
      short, 16, 16f, 17t
Bony end feel, 31–32
Boutonnière deformity, 187
Bow legs, 294
Brachial artery, 81t, 85
Brachialis muscle, 152, 152f
Brachial plexus, 64f, 65f
   terminal nerves of, 65–68, 66f
Brachial vein, 85
Brachiocephalic, 81t
Brachiocephalic trunk, 81
Brachioradialis muscle, 153, 153f
Brain, 55–58, 56f
   protection of, 57–58
Brainstem, 56, 60f
Breath-holding, 244–245
Breathing. See Respiration
Bronchial tree, 238
Bronchioles, 238
Bronchitis, 245

Brown-Séquard's syndrome, 71
Buccinator muscle, 207–208, 207f
Burner syndrome, 72
Bursae, 26, 26f, 288–289, 289f
   acquired, 26
   of knee, 289f, 290t
Bursitis, 29
   prepatellar, 295
   trochanteric, 277

C7 (vertebra prominens), 215
Cadence, 339–340
Calcaneal positions, 305f
Calcaneal tuberosity, 302
Calcaneus, 287, 302
Calcaneus foot, 322
Calcific tendonitis, 144
Cancellous bone, 14
Capillaries, 79
   lymph, 88
Capitate bone, 162, 163f
Capitulum, 149
Capsular ligaments, 25
Capsule, 25
Capsulitis, 29
Cardiac cycle, 78–79
Cardinal plane, 27
Cardiovascular system, 75–87
   blood vessels, 79–87
   common pathologies of, 90–91
   heart, 76–79
Carotid artery, 81, 85
Carpal tunnel syndrome, 72, 186
Carpometacarpal (CMC) joints, 24, 161–162, 171–173, 172f, 173f
   structure of, 24
Carrying angle, 148–149, 149f
Cartilage, 25
   articular, 25, 25f
   elastic, 26
   fibrocartilage, 25–26
   hyaline, 25
   types of, 22
Cartilaginous joint, 22, 22f
Cauda equina, 58, 58f
Caudal, 5
Cell body, 54
Center of gravity (COG), 27, 27f, 99–101, 99f, 100f, 101f, 102f, 218
Central cord syndrome, 71
Central nervous system (CNS), 53, 53f, 55–60
   brain, 55–58
   common pathologies of, 71
   spinal cord, 58–60
Cephalic vein, 85
Cerebellum, 56–57
Cerebral arteries, 86
Cerebral hemispheres, 55
Cerebral hemorrhage, 90
Cerebral palsy, 71
Cerebrospinal fluid, 57f, 58
Cerebrovascular accident, 91
Cerebrum, 55–56, 56f, 60f
Cervical nerves, 62f
Cervical orientation, 217f

Cervical plexus, 64, 64f
Cervical protraction, 213
Cervical spine, 213. *See also* Vertebral column
    functions of, 218–219
    joints of, 217
    motions of, 217–218
    muscles of, 219–222
        of mouth and hyoid bone, 220–221, 221t
        prevertebral, 220–221, 220f
        scalene, 220, 220f
        splenius capitis, 222, 222f, 222t
        splenius cervicis, 222, 222f, 222t
        sternocleidomastoid, 219–220, 219f
        suboccipital, 221, 221f, 221t
Cervical sprains, 229–230
Cervical vertebrae, 216f, 216t
Chambers, of heart, 76–77
Chest breathing, 244
Chrondromalacia patella, 295
Circle of Willis, 86, 87f
Circulatory system, 75–91
    cardiovascular system, 75–87
    common pathologies of, 90–91
    lymphatic system, 87–90
Circumducted gait, 352, 352f
Circumduction, 9, 9f, 161
Classical motion, 31
Clavicle, 116, 117, 117f
Clavicular fractures, 142
Clavicular portion, 136
Claw toe, 322
Closed kinetic chain, 49, 49f
Close-packed position, 35, 35t
Coccyx, 13
Cocontraction, 48
Collapsed lung, 245
Collateral ligaments
    of elbow, 151
    of knee, 288
Colles' fracture, 186
Common carotid, 81t, 85
Common iliac arteries, 81t, 82
Common iliac veins, 82
Common peroneal nerve, 68
Communicating arteries, 86
Compact bone, 14
Component movements, 32
Compression, 36, 36f
Compression fractures, 231
Concave-convex rule, 34–35
Concave joint surface, 34
Concentric contraction, 45, 45f, 46, 46f, 46t
Concurrent forces, 95–96, 95f
Condyle, 199
Condyloid joints, 24, 24f, 161
Congenital defects, 71
Congenital hip dislocation, 275
Congestive heart failure, 91
Congruent joints, 35
Contractility, 42
Contraction, muscle, 45–48, 45f
    concentric, 45
    eccentric, 45

isometric, 45
isotonic, 45
Contralateral, 5
Conus medullaris, 58, 58f
Convex joint surface, 34, 34f
Convex-concave rule, 34–35
Coracoacromial ligament, 118, 118f
Coracobrachialis muscle, 140, 140f
Coracoclavicular ligament, 118
Coracohumeral ligament, 134, 134f
Coracoid process, 149
Cords, 65
Coronal plane, 27
Coronary arteries, 81, 91
Coronoid process, 150, 199
Corpus callosum, 55
Cortex, 55
Corticospinal tract, 59, 60f
Costal facets, 215f
Costoclavicular ligament, 118
Costovertebral joints, 236, 236f
Counternutation, 249
Coxa plana, 275
Coxa valga, 275
Coxa vara, 275–276
Cranial, 5
Cranial nerves, 60, 61f, 62t
Cranium, bones of, 14t
Crouch gait, 353
Cubital fossa, 151–152
Cubital tunnel syndrome, 72
Cuboid, 302
Cuneiforms, 302
Curvilinear motion, 6, 6f
Cybex Orthotron, 47
Cylindrical grip, 190, 190f

Deceleration, 345t, 346, 347f
Deep, 5
Deep inspiration, 239, 243t
Deep palm muscles, 181, 182
Deep peroneal nerve, 321
Deep rotator muscles, 271, 271f, 272t
Degenerative diseases, 71
Degrees of freedom, 28
Deltoid ligament, 308
Deltoid muscle, 135–136, 135f
Demifacet, 215, 236
Demyelinating diseases, 71
Dendrites, 54, 54f
Dens, 215
Depression, 119, 119f, 120, 198
De Quervain's disease, 186
Dermatomes, 62–63, 63f
Descending aorta, 81t, 82f
Diaphragm, 238–240, 240f
Diaphragmatic breathing, 244
Diaphysis, 15, 15f
Diarthrodial joints, 23t
Digastric muscle, 205, 206, 206f
Disk pressure, 335f
Disks, 25–26
Dislocating force, 98

Dislocation, 29
Distal, 4f, 5
Distal carpal arch, 175, 175f
Distal interphalangeal (DIP) joint, 307
Distal radioulnar joint, 148
Distraction, 36
Dorsal, 4
Dorsal columns, 58
Dorsal interossei muscles, 182–183, 183f, 183t, 321f
Dorsalis pedis artery, 83
Dorsal radiocarpal ligament, 163f, 164
Dorsal scapular nerve, 65
Dorsiflexion, 7f, 8, 304
Double support, 340–341
Downward rotation, 119, 119f
Drop foot, 350
Dupuytren's contracture, 186
Dura matter, 57
Dynamics, 93
Dynamic systems, 3
Dysplasia, 275

Eccentric contraction, 45–47, 45f, 46t
Efferent impulses, 54
Efferent lymph vessels, 89
Elastic cartilage, 26
Elasticity, 42
Elastic tubing, 47
Elbow dislocation, 157
Elbow joint, 147, 147f
    bones and landmarks of, 149–151
        capitulum, 149
        coracoid process, 149
        coronoid process, 150
        humerus, 149–150
        infraglenoid tubercle, 149
        lateral epicondyle, 149
        lateral supracondylar ridge, 149
        medial epicondyle, 149
        olecranon fossa, 150
        olecranon process, 150
        radial notch, 150
        radial tuberosity, 150
        radius, 150, 151f
        scapula, 149
        styloid process, 150
        supraglenoid tubercle, 149
        trochlea, 149
        trochlear notch, 150
        ulna, 150
        ulnar tuberosity, 150
    interosseous membrane, of forearm, 151
    joint capsule, 151, 151f
    ligaments of
        annular, 151
        lateral collateral, 151
        medial collateral, 151
    motions of, 157f
    muscles of, 157f
        anatomical relationships, 155–156
        anconeus, 154, 154f
        biceps brachii, 152–153, 152f
        brachialis, 152, 152f
            brachioradialis, 153, 153f
            innervation of, 156, 158t
            pronator quadratus, 155, 155f
            pronator teres, 154–155, 155f
            supinator, 155
            triceps brachii, 154, 154f
        pathologies of, 156–158
        structure and motions of, 147–149
        structures of
            cubital fossa, 151–152
            interosseous membrane, 151, 151f
Elevation, 119, 119f, 120
Embolism, 91
Emphysema, 245
Empty end feel, 32
End feel, 31–32
    abnormal, 32
        boggy, 32
        empty, 32
        muscle spasm, 32
        springy block, 32
    firm, 32
    normal, 31
        bony, 31–32
        soft tissue approximation, 32
        soft tissue stretch, 32
Endosteum, 15, 15f
Epidural bleeds, 90
Epiphyseal lines, 15f
Epiphyseal plate, 14, 15f
Epiphysis, 14, 15f
    pressure, 15–16
    traction, 16, 18
    types of, in immature bone, 16f
Equilibrium
    neutral, 100, 100f
    stable, 100, 100f
    state of, 99, 100f
    unstable, 100, 100f
Equinus gait, 350, 350f, 354
Erb's palsy, 72
Erector spinae muscles, 221–222, 224, 225, 225f, 348f
Ethmoid, 237
Eversion, 10, 10f, 304, 307
Excursion, 42–43, 42f
Exercise
    isokinetic, 47–48
    kinetic chain, 49–50
    terminology, 50t
Expiration, 238–239, 238f
    forced, 239, 243t
    quiet, 239, 243t
Extensibility, 42
Extension, 7f, 8, 132
    of cervical spine, 213
    of elbow joint, 147, 148f
    of hip joint, 262f
    of knee, 284
    of thumb, 172, 172f
    of vertebral column, 212, 212f
    of wrist joint, 162
Extensor carpi radialis brevis muscle, 166, 166f

Extensor carpi radialis longus muscle, 165–166, 166f
Extensor carpi ulnaris muscle, 40, 166, 167f
Extensor digiti minimi muscle, 180, 180f
Extensor digitorum longus muscle, 314–315, 316f
Extensor digitorum muscle, 179–180, 179f
Extensor hallucis longus muscle, 314, 315f
Extensor hood, 175
Extensor indicis muscle, 180, 180f
Extensor pollicis brevis muscle, 178, 178f
Extensor pollicis longus muscle, 178–179, 179f
Extensor retinaculum, 167, 168f, 175, 175f
External carotid artery, 85
External iliac arteries, 81t, 82
External iliac veins, 82
External jugular vein, 86
External oblique muscle, 223
External rotation, 9

Face, bones of, 14t
Facet, 212, 215f, 236
Facet joints, 212, 217
False pelvis, 248
False ribs, 235
Femoral artery, 81t, 83, 84f, 266
Femoral nerve, 68, 68f, 69, 84f
Femoral triangle, 83, 84f
Femoral veins, 82, 83, 84, 84f, 266
Femur, 264–265, 264f, 286f
    landmarks of
        adductor tubercle, 265, 286
        body, 264, 286
        greater trochanter, 264, 286
        head, 264
        lateral condyle, 264
        lateral epicondyle, 264
        lesser trochanter, 264, 286
        linea aspera, 265, 286
        medial condyle, 264, 286
        medial epicondyle, 264
        neck, 264, 286
        patellar surface, 265, 286
        pectineal line, 265, 286
Festinating gait, 353
Fibrocartilage, 25–26
Fibrocartilaginous disk, 26
Fibrous joint, 21–22, 22f
Fibula, 286, 287f, 302f
    landmarks of
        head, 302
        lateral malleolus, 302
Fifth finger opposition, 173
Filum terminale, 58, 58f
Fingers
    joints of, 172f, 173–174
    motions of, 173–174
    muscles of, 176–186
Firm end feel, 32
First-class levers, 103–104, 103f, 104f
First-degree sprain, 142
Fixator, 48
Fixed pulley, 107, 108f
Flail chest, 245
Flat back, 230

Flat bones, 16, 16f, 17t
Flat foot, 322
Flexion, 6, 7f, 8, 132
    of cervical spine, 213
    dorsiflexion, 7f, 8
    of elbow joint, 147, 148f
    of hip joint, 262f
    of knee, 284
    lateral, 9
    palmar, 7f, 8
    plantar, 7f, 8
    of thumb, 172, 172f
    of vertebral column, 212, 212f
    of wrist joint, 162
Flexor carpi radialis muscle, 165, 165f
Flexor carpi ulnaris muscle, 164–165, 164f
Flexor digiti minimi muscle, 184
Flexor digitorum longus muscle, 313–314, 313f, 314f
Flexor digitorum profundus muscle, 176, 177f
Flexor digitorum superficialis, 176, 176f
Flexor hallucis longus muscle, 313, 313f
Flexor pollicis brevis muscle, 181, 181f
Flexor pollicis longus muscle, 176–177, 177f
Flexor retinaculum, 174, 174f
Floating ribs, 235
Foot, 5, 261f. *See also* Ankle
    arches, 308–310
        lateral longitudinal, 309, 309f
        medial longitudinal, 309, 309f
        transverse, 309, 309f
    bones of, 302–303, 303f
        metatarsals, 302–303
        phalanges, 303
        tarsal, 302
    eversion, 10f
    forefoot, 303
    functional aspects of, 303, 303f
    great toe, 303
    hindfoot, 303
    inversion, 10f
    joints of
        distal interphalangeal, 307
        interphalangeal, 307, 307f
        metatarsophalangeal, 307
        proximal interphalangeal, 307
    lesser toes, 303
    ligaments of
        long plantar, 310
        short plantar ligament, 310
        spring, 309–310
    midfoot, 303
    motions of, 304f, 306t
    muscles of
        anatomical relationships, 317–321
        anterior group, 314–315
        deep posterior group, 312–314
        extrinsic, 310–311, 311t
        innervation of, 318t, 321–322, 322t, 323t
        intrinsic, 317–319, 318t, 321f
        lateral group, 315–317
        plantar, 320f, 321f
        superficial posterior group, 311–312
    pathologies of, 322–323

plantar fascia, 310, 310f
    stirrup of the, 315
    support structures of, 309f, 310f
    toe motions, 308f
Foot drop, 72
Foot flat, 341t, 343, 343f, 344t
Foot slap, 350
Foramen magnum, 213
Foramina, 249
Force arm (FA), 103
Force couple, 97, 97f
    causing anterior pelvic tilt, 256f
    causing level pelvis, 257f
    causing posterior pelvic tilt, 257f
    of deltoid/rotator cuff muscles, 142f
    of scapula, 126f, 127f
    of shoulder girdle, 126
Forced expiration, 239, 243t
Forced inspiration, 239, 243t
Force(s), 94, 95–97, 102
    accessory motion, 36, 37f
    angular, 97, 98f
    approximation, 36
    bending, 36, 37f
    compression, 36f
    concurrent, 95–96, 95f
    dislocating, 98
    linear, 95, 95f
    moment of, 97–99
    parallel, 95, 96f
    resultant, 96, 96f, 97f
    shear, 36, 36f
    stabilizing, 97, 98
    traction, 36
Forearm, 5
    interosseous membrane, 151
    motions of, 147–149
    muscles of, 152–156. See also Elbow joint
    pronation and supination, 6, 9–10, 9f
Forefoot, 303, 303f
Fracture, 17
Fractures with dislocation, 231
Freedom, degrees of, 28
Friction, 94
Frontal axis, 27, 28f
Frontal lobe, 56, 56f
Frontal plane, 27, 27f, 217, 217f
Frozen shoulder, 143
Fundamental position, 4, 4f
Fused hip, 351
Fusiform muscle, 41

Gait
    abnormal (atypical), 349–354
        due to muscular weakness/paralysis, 349–351, 349f, 350f
        leg length discrepancy and, 354
        neurological involvement in, 352–353
        pain and, 353–354
    age-related patterns, 348–349
    definitions of, 339–342
    determinants of, 347–348
    due to joint/muscle range-of-motion limitation, 351–352
    terminology, 341t, 342t

Gait cycle (stride), 339
    key events of, 344–345t
    phases of, 340f
    stance phase, 340, 340f, 342–346, 342f, 343f
    swing phase, 340, 340f, 346–347, 346f, 347f
    terminology, 340f
Gamekeeper's thumb, 186
Ganglion cyst, 186
Gastrocnemius muscle, 292–293, 292f, 311–312, 311f
Geniohyoid muscle, 205
Genu recurvatum (back knees), 294
Genu recurvatum gait, 350f
Genu valgum (knock-knees), 294
Genu varum (bowlegs), 294
Glenohumeral joint. See Shoulder joint
Glenohumeral ligaments, 134
Glenohumeral subluxation, 143
Glenoid fossa, 132
Glenoid labrum, 133, 134, 134f
Glide, 33, 33f
Glottis, 238
Gluteus maximus gait, 349, 349f
Gluteus maximus muscle, 270–271, 270f
Gluteus medius gait, 349–350, 349f
Gluteus medius muscle, 272, 272f
Gluteus minimus muscle, 272–273, 273f
Golfer's elbow, 157
Gomphosis, 21–22, 22f
Gracilis muscle, 270, 270f, 293
Gravitational force, 99
Gravity, 99
Gravity-eliminated position, 47
Gray matter, 54, 58, 59f
Greater sciatic notch, 264
Greater trochanter, 264, 286
Great saphenous vein, 84
Great toe, 303
Greenstick fracture, 186

Hallux rigidus, 322
Hallux valgus, 322
Hamate bone, 162, 163f
Hammer toe, 322
Hamstring muscles, 271, 272f, 275, 291–293, 291f, 350
    active insufficiency of, 43f
    optimal length-tension relationship, 43f
    passive insufficiency of, 44f
Hamstring strain, 277
Hand, 5, 171
    anatomical relationships, 185–186
    bones and landmarks of, 174
    extrinsic muscles of
        abductor pollicis longus, 178f, 177–178
        extensor digiti minimi, 180, 180f
        extensor digitorum, 179–180, 179f
        extensor indicis, 180, 180f
        extensor pollicis brevis, 178, 178f
        extensor pollicis longus, 178–179, 179f
        flexor digitorum profundus, 176, 177f
        flexor digitorum superficialis, 176, 176f
        flexor pollicis longus, 176–177, 177f
    fingers, 173–174
    functional position of the, 189, 189f

Hand (continued)
  function of, 189–192
  grasps, 189–192
  intrinsic muscles of, 181t
    abductor digiti minimi, 184, 184f
    abductor pollicis brevis, 181, 181f
    adductor pollicis, 182, 182f
    deep palm, 181
    dorsal interossei, 182–183, 183f, 183t
    flexor digiti minimi, 184
    flexor pollicis brevis, 181, 181f
    hypothenar, 181
    lumbricales, 184, 184f, 185f
    opponens digiti minimi, 185
    opponens pollicis, 181–182, 182
    palmar interossei, 182, 183f, 184t
    thenar, 181
  ligaments of
    distal carpal arch, 175, 175f
    extensor retinaculum, 175, 175f
    flexor retinaculum, 174, 174f
    palmar carpal, 174
    proximal carpal arch, 175, 175f
    transverse carpal, 174, 174f
  muscle innervation, 187–189, 187f, 188t
  pathologies of, 186–187
  power grips, 189–191, 189f
    cylindrical, 190, 190f
    hook, 190–191, 191f
    spherical, 190, 190f
  precision grips, 189, 190f
    lumbrical, 191, 192f
    pad-to-pad, 191
    pad-to-side, 191, 191f
    pincer, 191
    pinch, 191, 191f
    side-to-side, 191–192, 192f
    three-jaw chuck, 191, 191f
    tip-to-tip, 191
  prime movers of, 187t
  sensation, 189
  thumb, 171–173
Hand of benediction, 72
Hangman's fracture, 231
Hard end feel, 32
Head, 5
Heart, 76
  blood flow through, 77–78, 77f, 78f
  cardiac cycle, 78–79
  chambers, 76–77, 77f
  location of, 76, 76f, 77f
  valves, 77, 77f
Heart attack, 91
Heart murmur, 91
Heart sounds, 78
Heel cord, 292, 311
Heel-off, 341t, 343, 343f, 344t
Heel strike, 341t, 342–343, 343f, 344t
Heimlich maneuver, 239
Hemiplegic gait, 352–353, 353f
Hemorrhage, 90
Herniated disks, 230
Hiccups, 245
Hindfoot, 303, 303f

Hinge joint, 23, 23f
Hip, 262
Hip bone (os coxae), 13, 251f, 262, 263f. See also
  Pelvic girdle (pelvis)
  landmarks of
    acetabulum, 264
      greater sciatic notch, 264
      obturator foramen, 264
Hip flexion contracture, 351, 351f
Hip fractures, 277
Hip hiking, 226–227, 255
Hip joint, 261, 262f
  bones and landmarks of, 262–265
    femur, 264–265, 264f
    ilium, 263
    ischium, 263
    pubis, 264
    tibia, 265, 265f
  joint capsule, 265, 265f, 266f
  ligaments of
    acetabular labrum, 266
    iliofemoral, 265
    iliotibial, 266–267
    inguinal, 266, 267f
    ischiofemoral, 265
    ligamentum teres, 266, 266f
    pubofemoral, 265
    spiral attachment of, 266f
  muscles of
    action of, 278t
    adductor brevis, 269–270, 269f
    adductor longus, 268–269, 269f
    adductor magnus, 270
    anatomical relationships, 274–275
    anterior deep, 274f
    anterior superficial, 274f
    biceps femoris, 271
    deep rotator, 271, 271f, 272t
    gluteus maximus, 270–271, 270f
    gluteus medius, 272, 272f
    gluteus minimus, 272–273, 273f
    gracilis, 270f
    hamstring, 271
    iliopsoas, 267, 267f
    innervation of, 277–278, 278–279t
    lateral, 276f
    medial, 275f
    pectineus, 268, 268f
    posterior deep, 276f
    rectus femoris, 268, 268f
    reversal of muscle function, 272–273, 273f
    sartorius, 268, 268f
    semimebranous, 271
    semitendinosus, 271
    tensor fascia latae, 273–274, 273f
  pathologies of, 275–277
  structure and motions of, 262, 262f
Hip pointer, 277
Hook grip, 190–191, 191f
Horizontal abduction, 8f, 9, 132
Horizontal adduction, 9, 85, 132
Horizontal displacement, 347
Horizontal plane, 27
Humeral neck fracture, 142–143

Humerus, 133–134, 133f, 150f
    bony landmarks of, 149–150
    fractures of, 143–144
Hyaline, 22
Hyaline cartilage, 25
Hydrocephalus, 71
Hyoid bone, 201, 201f, 220, 221t
Hyperextension, 7f, 8, 132
    of hip joint, 262f
    of vertebral column, 212, 212f
Hyperreflexia, 71
Hyperventilation, 245
Hypothalamus, 56, 56f
Hypothenar muscles, 181

Iliac crest, 263
Iliac fossa, 263
Iliocostalis muscles, 225
Iliofemoral ligament, 265
Iliolumbar ligament, 252
Iliopsoas muscle, 267, 267f
Iliotibial band syndrome, 277
Iliotibial band/tract, 266–267, 273
Ilium, 13, 250, 263
    landmarks of
        anterior inferior iliac spine, 263
        anterior superior iliac spine, 263
        iliac crest, 263
        iliac fossa, 263
        posterior inferior iliac spine, 263
        posterior superior iliac spine, 263
Impingement syndrome, 143
Inchworm effect, 135–136
Inclined plane, 109–110, 110f
Inertia, 94
Inferior, 4f, 5
Inferior gluteal nerve, 68
Inferior pubic ligament, 252
Inferior radioulnar joint, 148
Inferior ramus, 252, 264
Inferior tibiofibular joint, 304
Inferior vena cava, 82
Infraglenoid tubercle, 149
Infrahyoid muscles, 206, 208
Infraspinatus muscle, 138, 139f
Infraspinous fossa, 133
Inguinal ligament, 266, 267f
Insertion, 39–40, 39f, 40f
Inspiration, 238, 238f
    deep, 239, 243t
    forced, 239, 243t
    quiet, 239, 243t
Intercarpal joints, 161
Intercellular fluid, 88
Interclavicular ligament, 118
Intercondylar eminence, 286
Intercostal muscles, 240–241
    external, 240f
    internal, 240f, 241f
Intercostal nerves, 63, 64f
Internal carotid artery, 85
Internal iliac arteries, 82
Internal jugular vein, 86

Internal oblique muscle, 223
Internal rotation, 9
Interneurons, 55
Interosseous membrane, 151, 151f, 301, 301f
Interosseous sacroiliac ligament, 251
Interphalangeal (IP) joints, 171
    of fingers, 173–174
    of great toe, 307, 307f
Interspinales muscles, 226
Interspinal ligament, 218
Interstitial fluid, 88
Interstitial spaces, 88
Intertransversarii muscles, 226, 226f
Intervertebral disks, 25, 214–215, 214f
    landmarks of
        annulus fibrosus, 215
        nucleus pulposus, 215
Intervertebral foramen, 58, 59f, 214
Intracapsular ligaments, 287–288
Inversion, 10, 10f, 304, 307
Ipsilateral, 5
Irregular bones, 16, 16f, 17t
Irritability, 42
Ischemia, 91
Ischial tuberosity, 263
Ischiofemoral ligament, 265
Ischium, 13, 250, 263
    landmarks of
        body, 263
        ischial tuberosity, 263
        ramuss, 263
        spine, 263
Isokinetic contraction, 47–48, 48t
Isometric contraction, 45, 45f, 48t
Isotonic contraction, 45, 46, 48t

Jaw, 198
Joint capsule, 25, 25f
    of ankle joint, 308
    of elbow, 151, 151f
    of hip, 265, 265f
    of radiocarpal joint, 164
    of shoulder, 134, 134f
    of temporomandibular joint, 201, 202f
Joint congruency, 35, 35–36, 35t
Joint mobilization, 32
Joint movements (osteokinematics), 6–10, 31–32
    of abduction and adduction, 8–9, 8f
    around axes, 27–28
    convex-concave rule, 34–35
    degrees of freedom, 28, 28f
    of flexion and extension, 7f
    protraction, 10, 10f
    retraction, 10, 10f
    rotation, 9–10, 9f
    of shoulder joint, 131–132, 132f
    of shoulder girdle, 119–121
    types of
        biaxial, 24
Joint play, 32, 36
Joint(s). See also specific joints
    classification, 23t
    close-packed (closed-pack) position, 35, 35t

Joint(s). *See also specific joints (continued)*
  degrees of freedom, 28
  loose-packed position, 35t, 36
  motion, by plane and axis, 28t
  open-packed position, 35t, 36
  pathologies of, 29
  pivot, 23–24
  sellar, 33, 33f
  structure of, 24–26
  surface shape, 32–33
    ovoid, 32, 33f
    sellar (saddle-shaped), 33, 33f
  types of, 21–24
    amphiarthrodial, 22
    ball-and-socket, 24, 24f
    cartilaginous, 22, 22f
    condyloid, 24, 24f
    diarthrodial, 23t
    fibrous, 21–22, 22f
    gomphosis, 21–22, 22f
    hinge, 23, 23f
    nonaxial, 22
    ovoid, 32, 33f
    pivot, 24f
    plane, 22, 23f
    saddle, 24, 24f
    synarthrosis, 21
    syndesmosis, 21, 22f
    synovial, 7–8, 22, 22f, 25f
    triaxial, 24
    uniaxial, 23
Joint surface movement, 8, 32–37
Joint surface positions, 35–36, 35t
Jugular veins, 86
Jumper's knee (patellar tendonitis), 294

Kienböck's disease, 187
Kinematics, 3, 93
Kinesiology, 3
Kinetic chains, 49–50
  closed, 49, 49f
  open, 49, 50f
Kinetics, 3, 93, 94
Knee flexion contracture, 352
Knee fusion, 352, 352f
Knee/knee joint, 283f
  arthrokinematic motion of, 33–34
  bones and landmarks of
    calcaneus, 287
    femur, 286
    fibula, 286–287, 287f
    intercondylar eminence, 286
    lateral condyle, 286
    medial condyle, 286
    patella, 287, 287f
    plateau, 286
    tibia, 286, 287f
  bursae, 289f, 290t
  extension of, 284f, 288
  flexion of, 284f, 287f, 288
  lateral meniscus, 288
  ligaments of
    anterior cruciate, 288, 288f
    intracapsular, 287–288
    lateral collateral, 288

    medial collateral, 288
    posterior cruciate, 288, 288f
  medial meniscus, 288
  muscles of, 290t
    anatomical relationships, 293–294, 293f, 294f
    anterior, 290–291
    biceps femoris, 291, 292
    gastrocnemius, 292–293, 292f
    gracilis, 293
    innervation of, 294, 295t
    pes anserine, 289, 289f
    popliteus, 292, 292f
    posterior, 291–293
    rectus femoris, 290–291, 291f
    sartorius, 293
    semimebranous, 291, 291f
    semitendinosus, 291–292
    tensor fascia latae, 293
    vastus intermedialis, 291
    vastus lateralis, 291
    vastus medialis, 291
  pathologies of, 294–296
  pes anserine muscle group, 289, 289f
  popliteal space, 289, 289f
  Q angle of, 285, 285f
  right, anterior view, 287f
  right, superior view, 288f
  screw-home motion of, 284f
  structure and motions of, 283–285, 284f
Knock knees (genu valgum), 294
Kyphosis, 230

Labrum, 26, 26f
Lamina, 214
Laryngopharynx, 238
Larynx, 201, 238, 245
Lateral, 4, 4f
Lateral atlantoaxial joints, 217
Lateral bending, 8f, 9, 212, 212f
Lateral collateral ligament, 151, 288
Lateral condyle, 264, 286
Lateral deviation, 198
Lateral epicondyle, 149, 264, 286
Lateral epicondylitis, 156–157
Lateral flexion, 9
Lateral head, 154
Lateral ligament, 201, 308, 308f
Lateral longitudinal arch, 309, 309f
Lateral malleolus, 108f
Lateral menisci, 288
Lateral muscles, 276f
Lateral pelvic tilt, 330, 348, 348f
Lateral position, 332–333
Lateral pterygoid muscle, 204–205, 204f
Lateral pterygoid plate, 200
Lateral rotation, 9, 9f, 132, 262f
Lateral supracondylar ridge, 149
Lateral tilt, 253–254, 255f
Latissimus dorsi muscle, 137, 137f
Law of acceleration, 94
Law of action-reaction, 94
Law of inertia, 94
Leg, 5, 261f. *See also* Ankle; Foot; Hip joint
  anterior deep muscles of, 274f
  anterior superficial muscles of, 274f

bones of, 301, 301f, 302
  interosseous membrane, 301, 301f
  lateral muscles of, 276f
  medial muscles of, 275f
  muscle innervation, 322t
  posterior deep muscles of, 276f
  posterior superficial muscles of, 275f, 319f
Leg advancement, 340
Legg-Calvé-Perthes disease, 17, 275
Leg length discrepancy, 354
Lengthening contractions, 45–46
Lesser toes, 303
Lesser trochanter, 264, 286
Levator costarum muscles, 242f
Levator scapula muscle, 123, 123f
Levers, 102–107
  classes of, 103–107
    factors that change, 107
  components of, 103f
  first-class, 103–104, 103f, 104f
  second-class, 104f, 105f, 106f, 107f
  third-class, 105–107, 105f, 106f, 107f, 108f
Ligaments, 25, 25f. See also specific ligaments
Ligamentum flavum, 218
Ligamentum teres, 266, 266f
Linea alba, 26, 222
Linea aspera, 265, 286
Linear forces, 95, 95f
Linear motion, 6, 7, 7f
Line of gravity (LOG), 99, 100f, 101
Little League elbow, 157
Lobar bronchi, 238
Lobes, brain, 55–56, 56f
Long bones, 16, 16f, 17t
Long head
  of biceps brachii muscle, 152
  of biceps femoris muscle, 271
  of triceps brachii muscle, 154
Longissimus muscle group, 225
Longitudinal arch
  of foot, 309, 309f
  of hand, 175, 175f
Longitudinal axis, 27
Long plantar ligament, 310
Long posterior sacroiliac ligament, 252
Loose-packed position, 35t, 36
Lordosis, 230, 330
Lower extremity, 5, 261–262
  bones of, 14t, 261f, 262t
Lower motor neurons, 60
Lower respiratory infection (LRIS), 245
Lower respiratory tract, 237
Lower trapezius muscle, 121–123, 121f, 122f
Lumbar orientation, 217f
Lumbar plexus, 64f
Lumbar spine, 218
Lumbar vertebrae, 216f, 216t
Lumbosacral angle, 249, 253, 253f
Lumbosacral joint, 247, 247f
  ligaments of, 252–253
  structure of, 252
Lumbosacral ligament, 252–253
Lumbosacral plexus, 68, 68f
  terminal nerves of, 69–70, 69f, 70f

Lumbricales, 184, 184f, 185f
Lumbrical grip, 192, 192f
Lunate bone, 162, 163f
Lungs, 238
Lymph, 87–89
Lymph capillaries, 88
Lymph glands, 89
Lymph nodes, 88, 89f, 90f
Lymph vessels, 88, 88f, 89, 89f
Lymphatic ducts, 89, 90f
Lymphatic system, 75, 87–90
  drainage patterns, 89–90, 90f
  functions of, 87–89
Lymphatic trunks, 89
Lymphedema, 91

Main stem bronchi, 238
Mallet finger, 187
Mallet toe, 322
Mandible, 198–199
  joint motion during depression of, 203f
  landmarks of, 199f
    angle, 198
    body, 198
    condyle, 199
    coronoid process, 199
    mental spine, 199
    neck, 199
    notch, 199
    ramus, 199
  motion during lateral deviation of, 203f
Mandibular bone, 198
Mandibular elevation, 198
Mandibular motion, 203f
Manipulation, 32
Manubrium, 117, 117f, 236, 236f
Mass, 94
Masseter muscle, 204, 204f, 207f
Mastoid process, 200
Maxilla (maxillary bone), 201
Mechanical advantage, 107–108, 109f
Mechanics, 93, 93f
Medial, 4, 4f
Medial collateral ligament, 151, 288
Medial condyle, 264, 286
Medial epicondyle, 149, 264, 286
Medial epicondylitis, 157
Medial head, 154
Medial longitudinal arch, 309, 309f
Medial meniscus, 288
Medial muscles, 275f
Medial pterygoid muscle, 204, 204f
Medial rotation, 9, 9f, 132, 262f
Medial tibial stress syndrome, 322
Median atlantoaxial joint, 217
Median cubital vein, 85
Median nerve, 65, 67, 67f
Mediastinum, 76, 76f, 238
Medulla oblongata, 56
Medullary canal, 15, 15f
Meninges, 57–58, 59f
Meningocele, 71
Menisci, 25
Mental spine, 199

Metacarpophalangeal (MCP) joint, 171, 173, 173f
Metaphysis, 15, 15f, 16
Metatarsalgia, 322
Metatarsals, 302–303
Metatarsophalangeal (MTP) joints, 307
Midbrain, 56
Midcarpal joints, 161
Middle cerebral artery, 86
Middle deltoid muscle, 135–136, 135f
Middle scalene muscle, 220, 220f
Middle trapezius muscle, 121–123, 121f, 122f
Midfoot, 303, 303f
Midhumeral fractures, 143
Midstance, 341t, 343, 343f, 344t
Midswing, 345t, 346, 346f
Miserable malalignment syndrome, 296
Mitral valve, 77
Moment arm, 97, 97f, 98f
Moment of force, 97–99, 97f
Morton's neuroma, 72, 322–323
Motion
    angular, 6, 6f, 7f
    arthrokinematic, 6, 32–37
    attachment of, 40f
    circumduction, 9, 9f
    curvilinear, 6, 6f
    joint, 7–10
    laws of, 94
    linear, 6, 7, 7f
    osteokinematic, 31–32
    rectilinear, 5f, 6
    types of, 6–7
Motor (efferent) neurons, 54, 54f, 59–60, 61t
Motor endplate, 54
Motor impulses, 54, 55
Mouth
    bones of, 237
    muscles of, 220–221, 221t
Moveable pulley, 107, 109f
Multiaxial joint, 24
Multipennate muscles, 42
Multiple sclerosis, 71
Muscle(s). See also specific muscles
    angle of pull, 48–49, 49f
    attachment of, 39–40, 39f
    contraction, types of, 45–48, 45f, 46f, 46t, 48t
    fiber arrangement, 41–42
    innervation levels of, 63–64, 64f
    kinetic chains, 49–50, 49f, 50f
    names, 40–41
    role of, 48
    tissue
        functional characteristics of, 42
        length-tension relationship, 42–44, 43f
Muscle spasm, 32
Muscular dystrophy, 71
Musculocutaneous nerve, 65, 65–66, 66f
Myasthenia gravis, 71
Myelin, 54
Myelomeningocele, 71
Mylohyoid muscle, 205
Myocardial infarction, 91

Nasal cavity, 237
Nasal nares, 237
Nasal pharynx, 237
Nasal septum, 237
Navicular, 302
Neck, 5
    anatomical relationships, 227–229
    motions of, 212f
    muscle innervation, 229
    muscles of, 219–222, 227–228, 227f, 228f, 230t
        erector spinae group, 221–222
        prevertebral, 220–221, 220f, 221t
        scalene, 220, 220f
        splenius capitis, 222, 222f
        splenius cervicis, 222, 222f
        suboccipital, 221, 221f, 221t
    rotation, 9, 9f
Nerve fibers, 54
Nervous system, 53–73, 53f
    autonomic, 53, 53f
    central, 53, 53f, 55–60
        brain, 55–58
        common pathologies of, 71
        spinal cord, 58–60
    peripheral, 53, 53f, 60–70
        common pathologies of, 71–72
        cranial nerves, 60, 61f, 62t
        spinal nerves, 60, 62–63
Neural arch, 58, 213
Neurons (nervous tissue), 54–55, 54f
    interneurons, 55
    motor, 54, 54f, 59–60
    sensory, 54f, 55, 55f
Neuropathy, 71–72
Neutral equilibrium, 100, 100f
Neutralizer, 48
Neutral position, 162
Node of Ranvier, 54
Nonaxial joint, 22
Nonsupport, 341
Normal resting strength, 42
Nose, 237
Nostrils, 237
Nuchal ligament, 219f
Nuchal line, 213
Nucleus pulposus, 215
Nursemaid's elbow, 157
Nutation, 249

Oblique line, 174
Oblique muscle fibers, 41
Obturator foramen, 264
Obturator nerve, 68, 69, 69f
Occipital bone, 213
Occipital condyles, 213
Occipital lobe, 56, 56f
Occipital protuberance, 213
Occlusion, 91
Odontoid process, 215
Olecranon fossa, 150
Olecranon process, 150
Omohyoid muscle, 207

Open kinetic chain, 49–50, 50f
Open-packed (loose-packed) position, 35t, 36
Opponens digiti minimi muscle, 185
Opponens pollicis muscle, 181–182, 182f
Opposition, 172, 172f
Oral cavity, 237
Oral pharynx, 237–238
Origin, 39–40, 39f, 40f
Osgood-Schlatter disease, 18, 295
Osteoarthritis, 29, 277
Osteoclasts, 15
Osteokinematic motion, 31–32
Osteokinematics (joint movements), 7–10. *See also* Joint movements
Osteomyelitis, 17
Osteoporosis, 17, 231
Ovoid joint, 32, 33f

Pad-to-side grip, 191, 191f
Pain, abnormal gait and, 353–354
Palmar carpal ligament, 174
Palmar fascia, 164, 164f
Palmar flexion, 7f, 8
Palmar interossei muscles, 183, 183f, 184t
Palmar radiocarpal ligament, 163–164, 163f
Palmaris longus muscle, 165, 165f
Parallel forces, 95, 96f
Parallel muscle fibers, 41
Parallelogram method, 96, 96f
Paraplegia, 71
Parasympathetic nervous system, 53
Parietal lobe, 56, 56f
Parkinsonian gait, 353, 353f
Passive insufficiency, 43
  of hamstring, 43–44, 44f
Passive tension, 42
Patella, 287, 287f
Patellar surface, 265, 286
Patellar tendon, 290
Patellar tendonitis, 294
Patellofemoral angle, 285, 285f
Patellofemoral joint, 285, 285f
Patellofemoral pain syndrome, 295
Pathological fractures, 143
Pectineal line, 265, 286
Pectineus muscle, 268, 268f
Pectoralis major muscle, 41, 136–137, 136f, 242f
Pectoralis minor muscle, 41, 124–125, 125f
Pedicle, 214
Pelvic cavity, 248
Pelvic girdle (pelvis), 261f
  bones of, 247, 263f
  false pelvis, 248
  joints of, 247, 247f
    lumbrosacral, 252–253
    pubic symphysis, 252, 252f
    sacroiliac, 247–252, 249f
  ligaments of, 251–252, 251f
  male versus female, 248f
  motions of, 253–257, 256t
    anterior tilt, 253, 254f
    in frontal plane, 254f
    lateral tilt, 253–254, 255f

  pelvic rotation, 255–256, 255f
  posterior tilt, 253, 254f
  in sagittal plane, 254f
  muscle control, 256–257, 256f, 257f
  structure and function of, 247
  true pelvis, 248
Pelvic inlet, 248, 248f
Pelvic outlet, 248, 248f
Pelvic rotation, 255–256, 255f
Pelvic surface, 250
Periosteum, 15, 15f
Peripheral nerves, 65
Peripheral nervous system (PNS), 53, 53f, 60–70
  common pathologies of, 71–72
  cranial nerves, 60, 61f, 62t
  plexus, 64–69
  spinal nerves, 60, 62–63
Peroneal nerves, 70, 70f, 321
Peroneus brevis muscle, 316, 317f
Peroneus longus muscle, 315–316, 316f
Peroneus tertius muscle, 316–317, 317f
Pes anserine muscle group, 289, 289f
Pes cavus, 322
Pes planus (flat foot), 322
Phalanges
  of foot, 303, 303f
  of hand, 172f, 173–174
Pharynx, 237–238
Phlebitis, 91
Phrenic nerve, 64
Physiological motion, 31
Pia mater, 57
Pincer grip, 191
Pinch grip, 191, 191f
Pisiform bone, 162, 163f
Pivot joint, 23–24, 24f
Plane joint, 22, 23f
Plane joints, 161
Plane(s)
  cardinal, 27
  frontal, 27, 27f
  sagittal, 27, 27f
  transverse, 27, 27f
Plantar fascia, 310, 310f
Plantar fasciitis, 323
Plantar flexion, 7f, 8, 304
Plantar interossei, 321f
Plantar ligaments, 310
Plantaris muscle, 312
Plantigrade, 322
Plate grip, 192
Platysma muscle, 227f
Pleura, 238
Pleurisy, 245
Plexus
  brachial, 65–68, 65f
  cervical, 64
  formation, 64–69
  lumbosacral, 68–70, 68f, 69f
  sacral, 68
Pneumonia, 245
Pneumothorax, 245

Pope's blessing, 72
Popliteal artery, 81t, 83
Popliteal cyst, 295
Popliteal space, 289, 289f
Popliteal vein, 83
Popliteus muscle, 292, 292f
Positions
    anatomical, 4, 4f
    descriptive, 4f
    fundamental, 4, 4f
    intervertebral disk pressure and, 335f
Posterior, 4, 4f
Posterior (dorsal) ramus, 60
Posterior cerebral arteries, 86
Posterior columns, 58
Posterior communicating artery, 86
Posterior cruciate ligament, 288, 288f
Posterior deltoid muscle, 135-136, 135f
Posterior horn, 58
Posterior inferior iliac spine, 263
Posterior longitudinal ligament, 218
Posterior position, 4, 333, 333f
Posterior scalene muscle, 220, 220f
Posterior superior iliac spine, 263
Posterior tibial arteries, 83
Posterior tibial veins, 83
Posterior tilt, 253, 254f
Posterior trunk muscles, 224-227, 224t
Postglenoid tubercle, 199
Postural sway, 331, 331f
Posture
    deviations, 334t, 336
    intervertebral disk pressure and, 335f
    kneeling stool, 335f
    lying, 336f
    postural curves, 330-332
        primary, 330
        secondary, 330
    sitting, 334-336, 335f, 336f
    slouched, 335f
    standing, 332-334, 332f, 333f
    supine, 336, 336f
    vertebral alignment, 329-332
Power grips, 189-191, 189f
Precision grips, 189, 190f, 191-192, 191f, 192f
Prehension, 189
Prepatellar bursitis, 295
Pressure epiphysis, 15-16
Preswing period, 345, 346f
Prevertebral muscles, 220-221, 220f
Primary curve, 330, 330f
Prime mover, 48
Pronation, 9-10, 9f, 148, 304
Pronator quadratus muscle, 155, 155f
Pronator teres muscle, 154-155, 155f
Prone, 5
Propulsion phase, 345
Protraction, 10, 10f, 119, 119f, 120
Protrusion, 198
Proximal, 4f, 5
Proximal carpal arch, 175
Proximal interphalangeal (PIP) joint, 307
Proximal radioulnar joint, 148
Pterygoid muscle, 207f

Pubic symphysis, 252, 252f
Pubic tubercle, 264
Pubis, 13, 252, 264
Pubofemoral ligament, 265
Pulled elbow, 157
Pulled hamstring, 277
Pulleys, 107-108
    fixed, 107, 108f
    moveable, 107, 109f
Pulmonary circuit, 75, 76f
Pulmonary valve, 77
Pulmonic valve, 77
Pulse, 80-81, 80f
Pump-handle effect, 236, 237f
Push-off, 342, 343, 345

Q angle, 285, 285f
Quadratus lumborum muscle, 226-227, 226f
Quadriceps muscles, 290f, 350
    gait due to weakness/paralysis of, 350f
    moment arm of, 285f
    paralysis of, 293f
Quadriplegia, 71
Quiet expiration, 239, 243t
Quiet inspiration, 239, 243t

Radial artery, 85
Radial collateral ligament, 163
Radial deviation, 8f, 9, 162
Radial nerve, 65, 66, 66f
Radial nerve injury, 143
Radial notch, 150
Radial tuberosity, 150
Radial vein, 85
Radiocarpal joint, 161
Radiocarpal ligament
    dorsal, 163f, 164
    palmar, 163, 163f
Radioulnar joint, 147-148, 148f
Radius, 147-148, 148f, 150, 151f
Ramus
    of ischium, 263
    of pubis, 264
    of skull, 199
Range of motion (ROM), 31
Rectilinear motion, 5f, 6
Rectus abdominis muscle, 40, 222-223, 222f,
    241f, 242
Rectus femoris muscle, 268, 268f, 290-291, 290f
Reposition, 172-173, 172f
Resistance, 47, 102-103
Resistance arm (RA), 103
Respiration
    diaphragmatic versus chest breathing, 244
    mechanics of, 238-239
    muscles of, 243f
        accessory expiratory, 242, 243t
        accessory inspiratory, 241, 243t
        anatomical relationships, 242-244
        diaphragm, 239-240, 240f
        innervation of, 244
        intercostal, 240-241, 240f, 241f
    phases of, 239, 243t
    structures of, 237-239, 237f

Respiratory system, 235–245
  pathologies of, 245
  structures of, 237–239, 237f
Resting position, 36
Resultant force, 96, 96f, 97f
Retraction, 10, 10f, 119, 119f, 120
Retroversion, 276, 277f
Retrusion, 198
Reversal of muscle action, 40, 126–127
Reversal of muscle function, 272–273, 273f
Rhomboidal muscle, 41
Rhomboids, 123–124, 124f
Rib cage, 235–237, 236, 236f
Rib dislocation, 245
Rib separation, 245
Right lymphatic duct, 89
Roll, 33
Rotary motion, 6
Rotation, 9–10, 9f
  of cervical spine, 213
  downward, 119
  of hip, 262
  lateral, 9, 9f, 132
  medial, 9, 9f, 132
  of shoulder girdle, 116
  of shoulder joint, 132
  of thoracic spine, 217
  upward, 119
  of vertebral column, 212, 212f
Rotator cuff, 134–135, 139, 139f
  torn, 143–144
Ruptured Achilles tendon, 323

Sacral plexus, 64f, 68
Sacroiliac joint (SI joint), 247–249, 247f
  bones and landmarks of, 249–251
    ala, 249
    auricular surface, 250
    base, 249
    foramina, 249
    greater sciatic foramen, 250
    greater sciatic notch, 250
    iliac crest, 250
    ilium, 250
    ischium, 250
    lesser sciatic notch, 250
    pelvic surface, 250
    posterior inferior iliac spine, 250
    posterior superior iliac spine, 250
    promontory, 249
    sacrum, 249–250, 250f
    spine, 250
    superior articular process, 249
    tuberosity, 250
  cross section of, 251f
  ligaments of, 251f
    anterior sacroiliac, 251
    iliolumbar, 252
    interosseous sacroiliac, 251
    long posterior sacroiliac, 252
    sacrospinous, 252
    sacrotuberous, 252
    short posterior sacroiliac, 251–252
  motion of, 249, 249f

Sacrospinous ligament, 252
Sacrotuberous ligament, 252
Sacrum, 13, 249–250, 250f
Saddle joint, 24, 24f
Saddle-shaped joint, 33
Sagittal axis, 27, 28f
Sagittal plane, 27, 27f, 217, 217f
Sartorius muscle, 268, 268f, 293
Saturday night palsy, 72
Scalar, 94
Scalene muscles, 220, 220f, 241
Scaphoid bone, 162, 163f
Scaption, 132
Scapula, 115–117, 116f, 133f
  bony landmarks of, 116, 116f, 132–133, 149
  resting position of, 116f
Scapular plane, 132
Scapular tilt, 119, 119f
Scapular winging, 72
Scapulohumeral rhythm, 120
Scapulothoracic articulation, 115–116
Sciatica, 72, 230
Sciatic nerve, 68, 69, 69f
Scissors gait, 353, 353f
Scoliosis, 230, 330, 336
Screw-home mechanism, 284, 284f
Secondary curves, 330
Second-class levers, 104–105, 104f, 105f, 106f, 107f
Second-degree sprain, 142
Sellar joint, 33, 33f
Semilunar (SL) valves, 77
Semilunar notch, 150
Semimembranosus muscle, 271, 291, 291f
Semispinalis muscles, 226
Semitendinosus muscle, 271, 291–292
Sensation, 189
Sensory (afferent) neurons, 55, 55f
Sensory fibers, 62
Sensory impulses, 55
Sensory neurons, 54f
Sentinel node, 89
Serratus anterior muscle, 40f, 124, 124f
Serratus posterior inferior muscle, 242f
Serratus posterior superior muscle, 242f
Sesamoid bones, 16–17
Shear forces, 36, 36f
Shin splints, 322
Short bones, 16, 16f, 17t
Short head, 152
Short plantar ligament, 310
Short posterior sacroiliac ligament, 251–252
Shoulder
  abduction of, 8f
  adduction of, 8f
  dislocations, 143
Shoulder complex, 115, 115f
Shoulder girdle, 115–129
  bones and landmarks of, 116–117
    clavicle, 117, 117f
    scapula, 116–117, 116f
  joint motions of, 119–121, 119f, 120f
  joints of
    acromioclavicular, 118, 118f
    sternoclavicular, 117–118, 117f

Shoulder girdle *(continued)*
  ligaments of
    acromioclavicular, 118, 118f
    coracoacromial, 118, 118f
    coracoclavicular, 118
    costoclavicular, 118
    interclavicular, 118
    sternoclavicular, 118
  muscles of, 121–127
    anatomical relationships, 125–126, 125f, 140
    force couples, 126, 127f
    innervation of, 127, 127t
    levator scapula, 123, 123f
    pectoralis minor, 124–125, 125f
    reversal of muscle action, 126–127
    rhomboids, 123–124, 124f
    trapezius, 121–123, 121f, 122f
  serratus anterior muscle, 124, 124f
  sternum, 117, 117f
Shoulder joint (glenohumeral joint), 116, 131, 131f
  bones and landmarks of, 132–134
    glenoid labrum, 134
    humerus, 133–134, 133f
    rotator cuff, 134–135
    scapula, 132–133, 133f
    thoracolumbar fascia, 135
  joint motions of, 131–132, 132f
  ligaments of
    coracohumeral, 134, 134f
    glenohumeral, 134
  motions of, 120
  muscles of, 141f
    anatomical relationships, 140–141
    coracobrachialis, 140, 140f
    deltoid, 135f, 135036
    glenohumeral movement, 141–142
    infraspinatus, 138, 139f
    innervation of, 142, 143t
    latissimus dorsi muscle, 137, 137f
    muscle action, 142
    pectoralis major, 136–137, 136f
    subscapularis, 139, 140f
    supraspinatus, 138, 138f
    teres major, 137–138, 138f
    teres minor, 138–139, 139f
  pathologies of, 142–144
Side-to-side grip, 191–192, 192f
SI joint. *See* Sacroiliac joint
Simple machines, 102–110
  inclined plane, 109–110, 110f
  levers, 102–107
  pulleys, 107–108
  wheel and axle, 108–109, 109f, 110f
Single leg support, 340
Single support, 341
SIT muscles, 139
SITS muscles, 139
Sitting posture, 334–336, 335f, 336f
Sit-ups, 222–223
Skeleton
  appendicular, 13, 14t, 15f
  axial, 13, 14t, 15f
  bones of, 201

functions of, 13
  pathologies of, 17–18
Skier's thumb, 186
Skull, 57–58, 57f, 198, 211
  bones of, 198–201, 199f, 213, 213f
    hyoid, 201, 201f
    mandible, 198–199, 199f
    occipital bone, 213
    sphenoid, 200, 200f
    temporal, 199–200, 200f, 213
    zygomatic, 200–201
Slide, 33
Slipped femoral capital epiphysis, 17, 275
Small saphenous vein, 84
Smith's fracture, 186
Soft end feel, 32
Soft tissue approximation, 32
Soft tissue stretch, 32, 132
Soleus muscle, 312, 312f
Sphenoid bone, 200, 200f, 237
  landmarks of
    greater wing, 200
    lateral pterygoid plate, 200
    spine, 200
Sphenomandibular ligament, 201, 202f
Spherical grip, 190, 190f
Spin, 33, 34f
Spina bifida, 71
Spina bifida occulta, 71
Spinal column, 211
Spinal cord, 58–60, 58f, 59f, 211–212
  cross section of, 55f
  level, functional significance of, 63–64
  sensory and motor pathways, 60f
Spinal cord injury (SCI), 71
Spinalis muscle group, 224
Spinal nerves, 60, 62–63
  branches of, 60, 62
  dermatomes, 62–63, 63f
  formation of, 62f
  plexuses and, 64f
  thoracic nerves, 63
Spinal stenosis, 230
Spine, 211–212, 263
Spinous process, 214
Splenius capitis muscle, 222, 222f, 222t
Splenius cervicis muscles, 222, 222f, 222t
Spondylolisthesis, 230
Spondylolysis, 230
Spondylosis, 230
Sprain(s), 29
  ankle, 323
  cervical, 229
  shoulder, 142
Spring ligament, 309–310
Springy block, 32
Stability, 99–102, 102f
Stabilizer, 48
Stabilizing force, 97, 98
Stable equilibrium, 100, 100f
Stance phase, 340, 340f, 342–346, 342f, 343f
Standing posture, 332–334, 332f, 333f
State of equilibrium, 99, 100f

Static systems, 3
Statics, 93
Stenosing tenosynovitis, 186
Step, 339
Step length, 339
Steppage gait, 350, 350f
Sternal portion, 136
Sternoclavicular joint, 117–118, 117f
Sternoclavicular ligament, 118
Sternocleidomastoid muscle, 40, 41f, 219–220, 219f, 241f
Sternohyoid muscle, 206, 207
Sternothyroid muscle, 206–207
Sternum, 117, 117f, 235
Stinger syndrome, 72
Stirrup of the foot, 315
Stitch, 245
Strains, 29
Strap muscles, 41
Stretching, 44
Stride, 339
Stride length, 339
Stroke, 90, 91
Stylohyoid ligament, 201
Stylohyoid muscle, 206
Styloid process, 150, 200
Stylomandibular ligament, 201
Subarachnoid space, 58
Subclavian, 81t
Subclavian artery, 84–85
Subdural bleeds, 90
Subluxation, 29
Subluxing of the biceps tendon, 144
Suboccipital muscles, 221, 221f, 221t
Subscapular fossa, 133
Subscapularis muscle, 139, 140f
Subtalar joint, 306–307
Superficial, 5
Superficial peroneal nerve, 321
Superficial posterior group, 311–312
Superior, 4f, 5
Superior gluteal nerve, 68
Superior pubic ligament, 252
Superior radioulnar joint, 148
Superior ramus, 252, 264
Superior tibiofibular joint, 304
Supination, 9–10, 9f, 148, 304
Supinator muscle, 155, 155f, 156f, 157f
Supine, 5
Supine posture, 336, 336f
Supracondylar fractures, 157–158
Supraglenoid tubercle, 149
Suprahyoid muscles, 205, 208
Suprascapular nerve, 65
Supraspinal ligament, 218
Supraspinatus muscle, 138, 138f
Supraspinous fossa, 133
Sustentaculum tali, 302
Swan neck deformity, 186–187
Swayback, 230
Swimmer's shoulder, 143
Swing phase, 247f, 340, 340f, 345t, 346–347, 346f
Sympathetic nervous system, 53
Symphysis pubis, 247, 247f, 264

Synapse, 54
Synarthrosis, 21
Syndesmosis, 21, 22f
Synergist, 48
Synovial fluid, 25, 25f
Synovial joints, 7–8, 22, 22f, 25f
Synovial membrane, 25, 25f
Synovitis, 29
Systemic circuit, 75–76, 76f

Talocrural (talotibial) joint, 305–306, 305f
Talus, 302
Tarsal bones, 302
    calcaneal tuberosity, 302
    calcaneus, 302
    cuboid, 302
    cuneiforms, 302
    navicular, 302
    sustentaculum tali, 302
    talus, 302
    tuberosity of navicular, 302
Temporal bone, 199, 213
    landmarks of
        articular fossa, 199
        articular tubercle, 199
        external auditory meatus, 200
        mastoid process, 200
        postglenoid tubercle, 199
        styloid process, 200
        zygomatic process, 200
Temporal fossa, 200, 201f
Temporalis muscle, 203–204, 203f, 207f
Temporal lobe, 56, 56f
Temporal process, 200
Temporomandibular joint (TMJ), 197, 197f
    articular disk, 201–202
    bones and landmarks of, 198–201, 200f
        hyoid, 201, 201f
        mandible, 198–199
        maxilla, 201
        sphenoid, 200
        temporal, 199–200
        zygomatic bone, 200
    joint capsule, 201
    ligaments of, 202f
        lateral, 201
        sphenomandibular, 201
        stylohyoid, 201
        stylomandibular, 201
        temporomandibular, 201
    mechanics of movement of, 202–203, 203f
    muscles of
        anatomical relationships, 207–208
        digastric, 205, 206, 206f
        geniohyoid, 205
        infrahyoid, 206
        innervation of, 208, 208t
        lateral pterygoid, 204–205, 204f
        masseter, 204, 204f
        medial pterygoid, 204, 204f
        mylohyoid, 205
        omohyoid, 207
        sternohyoid, 206

Temporomandibular joint (TMJ) *(continued)*
    sternothyroid, 206–207
    stylohyoid, 206
    summary of muscle action, 208
    suprahyoid, 205
    temporalis, 203–204, 203f
    thyrohyoid, 207
  structure and motions of, 197–198, 198f
Temporomandibular ligament, 201
Tendon action of a muscle, 44, 44f
Tendonitis, 29
Tendons, 26
Tendon sheaths, 26
Tennis elbow, 156–157
Tenodesis, 44, 44f
Tenon and mortise joint, 305
Tenosynovitis, 29, 186
Tension, 36, 42–43
  active, 42
  passive, 42
Tensor fascia latae muscle, 273–274, 273f, 293
Teres major muscle, 137–138, 138f
Teres minor muscle, 138–139, 139f
Terminal stance, 343f, 345
Terminal swing, 346, 347f
Terminology
  accessory motion, 32
  of common pathologies, 28
  descriptive, 4–5, 4f
    for quadruped, 5f
  exercise, 50t
  of gait cycle, 339–342, 341t
Terrible triad, 295–296
Thalamus, 56, 56f
Thenar muscles, 181
Thigh, 5, 261f
Third-class levers, 105–107, 105f, 106f, 107f, 108f
Third-degree sprain, 142
Thoracic cage, 235–237, 236f
Thoracic duct, 90
Thoracic nerves, 63
Thoracic orientation, 217f
Thoracic outlet syndrome, 72, 91, 229
Thoracic spine, 218
Thoracic vertebrae, 216f, 216t, 236, 236f
Thoracolumbar fascia, 135
Thorax, 5, 115–116
  bones of, 14t
  movements of, 236–237, 237f
  resting position of, 116f
Three-jaw chuck grip, 191, 191f
Thrombophlebitis, 91
Thrombosis, 91
Thumb
  joints of, 171–173, 172f
  motions of, 171–173
  muscles of, 176–186
Thyrohyoid muscle, 207
Thyroid cartilage, 201
Tibia, 265, 265f, 287f, 302
  landmarks of
    crest, 302
    intercondylar eminence, 286

lateral condyle, 286, 302
medial condyle, 286, 302
medial malleolus, 302
plateau, 286
tibial tuberosity, 265, 286
Tibialis anterior, 40
Tibialis anterior muscle, 314, 315f
Tibialis posterior muscle, 312–313, 312f
Tibial nerve, 68, 70, 70f, 321
Tibial tuberosity, 265, 286
Tibiofibular joints, 305f
Tip-to-tip grip, 191
TMJ. *See* Temporomandibular joint (TMJ)
Toe motions, 308f
Toe-off, 341t, 345, 345t, 346f
Tone, 42
Torn rotator cuff, 143–144
Torque, 94, 97–99, 97f, 98f
Torque arm, 97, 97f, 98f
Torticollis, 229
Trabeculae, 14
Trachea, 238
Tract, 54
Traction epiphysis, 16, 18
Traction force, 36, 36f
Translatory motion, 6
Transverse abdominis muscle, 224
Transverse arch, 309, 309f
Transverse carpal ligament, 174, 174f
Transverse foramen, 215f
Transverse plane, 27, 27f
Transverse process, 214
Transverse tarsal joint, 307, 307f
Transversospinalis (transverse spinal) muscle group, 225–226, 225f
Trapezium bone, 162, 163f
Trapezius muscle, 40, 121–123, 121f, 122f
Trendelenburg gait, 349–350
Trendelenburg sign, 348
Triangular muscle, 41
Triaxial joint, 24
Triceps, 139f, 154
Triceps brachii muscle, 40, 154, 154f
Triceps surae contracture, 352
Triceps surae muscle, 312, 351
Tricuspid valve, 77
Trigger finger, 186
Trimalleolar fracture, 323
Triplanar, 217f, 305–306
Triple arthrodesis, 323, 352
Triquetrum bone, 162, 163f
Trochanteric bursitis, 277
Trochlea, 149
Trochlear notch, 150
True pelvis, 248
True ribs, 235
Trunk, 5, 65
  anatomical relationships, 227–229
  lateral bending, 8f
  motions of, 212f
  muscle innervation, 229
  muscles of, 222–229, 228f, 229f, 230t
    erector spinae, 224, 225f
    external oblique, 223

iliocostalis, 225
internal oblique, 223
interspinales, 226
intertransversarii, 226, 226f
longissimus, 225
posterior, 224–227, 224t
quadratus lumborum, 226–227, 226f
rectus abdominis, 222–223, 222f
spinalis, 224
transverse abdominis, 224
transversospinalis, 225–226, 225f
Tubercle, 252
Tuberosity
calcaneal, 302
of ischium, 250
of navicular, 302
radial, 150
of sacroiliac joint, 250
ulnar, 150
Turf toe, 323

Ulna, 147–148, 148f, 150, 150f
Ulnar artery, 85
Ulnar collateral ligament, 163
Ulnar deviation, 8f, 9, 162
Ulnar nerve, 65, 67–68
Ulnar tuberosity, 150
Ulnar vein, 85
Uniaxial joint, 23
Unipennate muscles, 41
Unstable equilibrium, 100, 100f
Upper extremity, 5, 14t
Upper motor neurons, 59–60
Upper respiratory infection (URI), 245
Upper respiratory tract, 237
Upper trapezius muscle, 121, 121f, 122, 122f
Upward rotation, 119, 119f

Valgus, 304
Valsalva's maneuver, 244–245
Valves, heart, 77
Varicose veins, 91
Varus, 304
Vastus intermedialis muscle, 291
Vastus lateralis muscle, 291
Vastus medialis muscle, 291
Vaulting gait, 352
Vector, 94
Vector quantities, 95
Veins, 79–80
major, 83f, 84f, 85f, 86f
pathways, 81–86
Velocity, 94
Vena cavae, 79, 82f
Ventral, 4
Ventricles, 58, 76–77
Venules, 79
Vertebra, 59f
Vertebrae, 213–214
anterior arch, 215
atlas (C1), 215, 215f
axis (C2), 215, 215f
C7 (vertebra prominens), 215
cervical, 216f, 216t

dens, 215
lumbar, 216f, 216t
parts of, 214f
articular process, 214
body, 213
intervertebral foramen, 214
lamina, 214
neural arch, 213
pedicle, 214
spinous process, 214
transverse process, 214
vertebral foramen, 214
vertebral notches, 214
thoracic, 216f, 216t, 236, 236f
Vertebral alignment, 329–332
Vertebral artery, 86
Vertebral column, 211, 212f
bones of, 14t
curves, 329–330, 330f
joint motions of, 212–213
joints of
atlantoaxial, 217, 217f
atlanto-occipital, 217
facet, 217
ligaments of, 218f
anterior longitudinal, 218
interspinal, 218
posterior longitudinal, 218
supraspinal, 218
muscles of, 219t
cervical spine, 219–222
erector spinae group, 221–222
trunk, 222–227
pathologies of, 229–231
Vertebral curves, 211
Vertebral foramen, 58, 58f, 59f, 214
Vertebral notches, 214
Vertebral segments, 212
Vertebral vein, 86
Vertical axis, 27, 28f
Vertical displacement, 347, 347f
Volkmann's ischemic contracture, 158

Waddling gait, 351, 351f
Walking base width, 347f
Walking speed, 339–340
Watersheds, 90
Weight acceptance, 340
Wheel and axle, 108–109, 109f, 110f
White matter, 54, 58–59, 59f
Width of walking base, 347, 347f
Willis, Thomas, 86
Windpipe, 238
Wrist
radial deviation, 8f
ulnar deviation, 8f
Wrist drop, 72
Wrist joint, 162f
bones and landmarks of
capitate, 162, 163f
carpal bones, 162
hamate, 162, 163f
hook of the hamate, 162
lateral epicondyle, 163

Wrist joint *(continued)*
  lunate, 162, 163f
  medial epicondyle, 162
  pisiform, 162, 163f
  scaphoid, 162, 163f
  styloid process, 162
  supracondylar ridge, 163
  trapezium, 162, 163f
  triquetrum, 162, 163f
  ligaments of
    dorsal radiocarpal, 163f, 164
    palmar radiocarpal, 163, 163f
    radial collateral, 163
    ulnar collateral, 163
  motions of, 162, 163f
  muscle action of, 167, 168t
  muscles of
    anatomical relationships, 166–167, 168f
    extensor carpi radialis brevis, 166, 166f
    extensor carpi radialis longus, 165–166, 166f
    extensor carpi ulnaris, 166, 167f
    flexor carpi radialis, 165, 165f
    flexor carpi ulnaris, 164–165, 164f
    innervation of, 167–168, 168t
    palmaris longus, 165, 165f
  pathologies of, 186–187
  structures of, 161–162
    articular disk, 164
    joint capsule, 164
    palmar fascia, 164, 164f
  terminology, 162t
Wry (twisted) neck, 229

Xiphoid process, 5, 117

Zygomatic arch, 200
Zygomatic bone, 200
Zygomatic process, 200